Symmetry in Vision

Special Issue Editors

Marco Bertamini

Lewis Griffin

MDPI • Basel • Beijing • Wuhan • Barcelona • Belgrade

MDPI

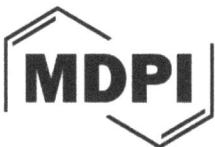

Special Issue Editors

Marco Bertamini
University of Liverpool
UK

Lewis Griffin
University College London
UK

Editorial Office
MDPI AG
St. Alban-Anlage 66
Basel, Switzerland

This edition is a reprint of the Special Issue published online in the open access journal *Symmetry* (ISSN 2073-8994) from 2016–2017 (available at: http://www.mdpi.com/journal/symmetry/special_issues/symmetry_vision).

For citation purposes, cite each article independently as indicated on the article page online and as indicated below:

Author 1, Author 2. Article title. *Journal Name*. **Year**. Article number/page range.

First Edition 2017

ISBN 978-3-03842-496-3 (Pbk)
ISBN 978-3-03842-497-0 (PDF)

Table of Contents

Part 1

Part 2

About the Special Issue Editors

Marco Bertamini studied Psychology at the University of Padova, Italy, and then at the University of Virginia, USA. He moved to Liverpool, UK, in 1999 where he established the Visual Perception Lab. His interests are broad across visual perception and cognition; in particular, he has a long-standing interest in perception of shape, including symmetry, contour curvature and part structure. To study shape, he has made use of a special case of figure-ground, which is that of a visual hole (Bertamini, 2006). Starting from work on symmetry (Bertamini, Friedenberg and Kubovy, 1997), he has worked on neural responses to regularity (Bertamini and Makin, 2014) and he has explored the link between perception and emotion, or more specifically what visual properties drive visual preference (Bertamini, Makin and Pecchinenda, 2013). Work on preference, however, has not been confined to symmetry; he has studied other aspects, such as composition (Bertamini Bode and Bruno, 2011). For more information: www.bertamini.org/lab/.

Lewis Griffin received a BA in Mathematics and Philosophy from Oxford University, UK, in 1988, and a PhD from the University of London in 1995 for a thesis "Descriptions of Image Structure" in the area of computational vision. Following positions at Aston University (Vision Sciences) and Kings College London (Imaging Sciences), he has been at University College London (Computer Science) since 2005, where is now a Reader. His research interests include image structure, colour vision, machine learning and biomedical modelling, with applications in security science, biomedicine and geoscience. He has developed theory on how V1 simple cells are sensitive to symmetries (Griffin and Lliholm 2010), and used that to define a system of Basic Image Features (Crosier and Griffin 2010) with applications to handwriting authorship recognition (Newell and Griffin 2010) and other problems.

Preface to "Symmetry in Vision"

It is not uncommon to dismiss symmetry as a mere curiosity for vision, something often mentioned by scientists, mathematicians and artists, but not an important part of the normal content for which vision evolved. This unfortunate stance misses the central role of symmetry in relation to the content of images, and in particular how symmetry is relevant for both biological and artificial visual systems.

At its essence, symmetry is a concept closely related to structure and regularity. In particular, symmetrical structures can be described as containing self-similarities. Although the concept of symmetry has ancient origins, in modern times, abstracted and formalized into Group Theory, symmetry has found spectacular applications, far beyond the field of perception or visual art.

The concept of symmetry is broader than its application to spatial content of images but if we take 2D images, then self-similarity can exist when there are rigid transformations that map one part of an image onto another. The four types of symmetric patterns in common understanding take their names from these transformations: reflections, rotations, translations and glide reflections. Examples of all of these can be found in visual art, in different cultures and across the centuries. Mathematical and artistic analysis (especially by Escher) extended and refined the catalogue of possible image symmetries. For instance, for periodically repeating patterns that cover the plane, known as wallpaper patterns, there are 17 possible distinct groups. The proof was provided by Evgraf Fedorov in 1891.

In terms of empirical studies, the history is relatively more recent, but is rich and has contributions from a number of fields. An early reference in visual psychology is the discussion in Ernst Mach's classic book on sensations (1886). Mach showed that regularities in the image are useful when compared and contrasted with perceived regularities. In particular, he claimed that vertical reflectional symmetry was the only type of symmetry that human observers could perceive without effort. This observation has later been confirmed empirically. Another classic book that outlines the preponderance of symmetry in nature is that by Hermann Weyl (1955).

Short reviews focused on symmetry within neuroscience are available in Wagemans (1997), Bertamini and Makin (2014) and Cattaneo (2017). With respect to applications, symmetry contributes to the attention and selection of some salient regions of an image. Therefore, computer and machine vision applications have used symmetry in relation to image segmentation, target detection, image compression, and human–robot interaction (e.g., Brady and Asada, 1984; Li, Pizlo, and Steinman, 2009; Zabrodsky, Peleg, and Avnir, 1995). A mathematical treatment of the classes of symmetries relevant to images can be found in Griffin (2008; 2009).

Symmetry also has a key role in psychological literature. For instance, Gestalt psychologists recognized it as a factor in perceptual organization (Koffka, 1935). Empirical work on the role of symmetry in figure-ground organization was started by Bahnsen (1928), a student of Edgar Rubin, and continues to this day (Bertamini, Friedenberg and Kubovy 1997; Kanizsa and Gerbino, 1976; Makin et al., 2016; Mojica and Peterson, 2014).

The wide range of areas in which symmetry has been used as a tool is reflected in the diversity of the papers published in the journal *Symmetry*.

This book collects papers that have appeared in two recent Special Issues. The first was titled "Symmetry in Vision" (Editors: Bertamini and Griffin). The original idea for a Special Issue came from a symposium at the European Conference on Visual Perception, August 2015 in Liverpool (www.ecvp.org/2015/). The topic of the symposium was brain responses to visual symmetry, but the Special Issue extended the scope. This Special Issue provided a shared place for cutting edge studies on how and why symmetry is processed and exploited by biological and artificial visual systems.

In June 2017, there was a one-day event on Neuroscience of Symmetry held in Liverpool. The meeting, supported by the Experimental Psychology Society (EPS), brought together many of the leading scientists working on symmetry perception and neuroscience. From this workshop, and from other work in the field, we organized a second Special Issue, as a follow-up to the one on "Symmetry in Vision". The title was more specific: "Symmetry-Related Activity in Mid-Level Vision", and there were three Editors: Bertamini, Makin and Cattaneo.

We are very pleased to collect within this book all published contributions to both Special Issues. We have organized them in two groups. The first deals with more formal uses of symmetry for image processing. The second deals with symmetry in human vision. The papers are a testament to the reach of symmetry within vision. Within image analysis, their coverage includes natural image statistics (Hu, and Victor, 2016), computational aesthetics (Brachmann and Redies, 2016), camera modeling (Turski, 2016), fractals (Bies et al. 2016) and salience maps (Sharma, 2016); within human vision, the coverage includes 3D vision (Michaux et al. 2017), cross-modal matching (Bianchi et al., 2017a), perceptual structures (Gillam, 2017, and Bianchi et al., 2017b), aesthetics (Dresp-Langley, 2016), reading (Erlikhman et al. 2017) and illusion (Sugihara, 2016).

Marco Bertamini and Lewis Griffin

Special Issue Editors

Part 1:
Symmetry in Images

Article

Two-Dimensional Hermite Filters Simplify the Description of High-Order Statistics of Natural Images

Qin Hu [1] and Jonathan D. Victor [2],*

[1]   Microsoft Research, One Microsoft Way, Redmond, WA 98052, USA; huqinpku@hotmail.com
[2]   Feil Family Brain and Mind Research Institute, Weill Cornell Medical College, 1300 York Ave, New York, NY 10065, USA
*   Correspondence: jdvicto@med.cornell.edu; Tel.: +1-212-746-2343

Academic Editor: Marco Bertamini
Received: 27 June 2016; Accepted: 18 September 2016; Published: 21 September 2016

Abstract: Natural image statistics play a crucial role in shaping biological visual systems, understanding their function and design principles, and designing effective computer-vision algorithms. High-order statistics are critical for conveying local features but they are challenging to study, largely because their number and variety is large. Here, via the use of two-dimensional Hermite (TDH) functions, we identify a covert symmetry in high-order statistics of natural images that simplifies this task. This emerges from the structure of TDH functions, which are an orthogonal set of functions that are organized into a hierarchy of ranks. Specifically, we find that the shape (skewness and kurtosis) of the distribution of filter coefficients depends only on the projection of the function onto a one-dimensional subspace specific to each rank. The characterization of natural image statistics provided by TDH filter coefficients reflects both their phase and amplitude structure, and we suggest an intuitive interpretation for the special subspace within each rank.

Keywords: image statistics; skewness; kurtosis; orthogonal functions; steerable filters

1. Introduction

Achieving a thorough understanding of the statistics of our visual environment is important from both a biological point of view and an engineering point of view. The biological relevance is that the statistics of the natural environment are a strong constraint under which visual systems evolve, develop and function [1]. The engineering relevance is that a knowledge of image statistics is important for many problems in computer vision [2], including image de-noising, image classification [3–6], image compression and texture synthesis [7]. However, understanding image statistics is hampered by the simple fact that the space of image statistics is so large. Here, we describe some progress in this direction: a specific filter-based approach that identifies a hidden symmetry, providing a simplified description of high-order natural image statistics, specifically those of order three and four.

The reason for our focus on high-order statistics is that they carry local visual features, such as lines, corners and edges [8,9], but, because of the curse of dimensionality, they are challenging to analyze. In contrast, second-order statistics are concisely captured by the power spectrum, because it is the Fourier transform of the autocorrelation function. As is well known, the power spectrum of natural images is approximately k^{-2} (where k is spatial frequency) [10,11]. However, while the power spectrum captures important spatial regularities of natural images, such as distance-independent scaling [12], it is far from a complete statistical description of natural images. For example, a synthetic image consisting of Gaussian noise with a k^{-2} power spectrum looks drastically different from a real natural image, even though the spectra are similar. Conversely, modifying a natural image by flattening its power spectrum but preserving its phases leaves its salient spatial features readily recognizable. Thus, most of the features that make an image look "natural", such as edges and contours, are coded in its phases, as well as its Fourier amplitudes [8,9,13]. Translated into the spatial domain, these phase correlations correspond to image statistics that are ignored by the power spectrum: joint distributions of image intensities at three or more points and aspects of the pairwise intensity distributions beyond their variances and covariances.

Since a direct tabulation of the joint distribution of multiple pixel values is impractical, a natural strategy is to focus on specific univariate distributions, namely the distribution of outputs of filters ("filter coefficients") placed on images. Typically, this approach is implemented with filter profiles that have a prominent orientation and dominant spatial frequency, either Gabor functions or Gabor-like wavelets, a choice motivated by concepts of visual processing and independent components analysis of natural images [14,15]. For natural images, the distributions of wavelet coefficients are highly kurtotic, having sharp peaks and much longer tails compared to a Gaussian distribution with the same variance [16]. Interestingly, [3] showed that this could be used to distinguish natural images from synthetic ones (including realistic computer-generated scenes), by applying linear classifiers to a feature space of wavelet coefficients. Other investigators have also used wavelet coefficients as a starting point, but focused on the extent to which wavelet coefficients are independent [17,18]. Thus, the filter approach provides a useful characterization of natural image statistics, but even with a filter-based approach, the number of parameters required to describe high-order image statistics is still large: a two-dimensional basis set is a two-parameter family.

Here, we show that the description of these filter coefficient distributions is simplified when, instead of Gabor-like filters, we use the two-dimensional Hermite functions (TDH) as filters. TDH functions [19–25] form an orthonormal basis that is halfway between the pixel basis and the Fourier basis, and their shapes are quite different from that of Gabor-like filters or one-dimensional wavelets.

We note that symmetry plays two distinct roles in this study: the purely mathematical symmetry properties of the TDH functions and the empirical finding that they reveal a hidden symmetry in the statistics of natural images. Specifically, the TDH functions at each rank form a representation of the surfaces of spheres of progressively ascending dimensions: the functions of rank two correspond to the points on the surface of an ordinary sphere; the functions of rank three correspond to the points on the surface of a hypersphere, etc. The statistics of their filter coefficients, in particular, their skewnesses and kurtoses, may therefore be regarded as functions on these spheres. A priori, these functions could have any behavior, but we find that their behavior is surprisingly simple: they are either constant or depend only on the projection onto a single axis. This simplification depends on both the phase and amplitude characteristics of natural scenes and, critically, encompasses the distribution of filter coefficients of nonstandard combinations of TDH functions (see Section 3.2 below) that do not have Cartesian or polar symmetry.

2. Materials and Methods

2.1. Two-Dimensional Hermite Functions: Definition and Properties

We analyze image statistics via the distribution of values that result from filtering them with two-dimensional Hermite (TDH) functions. Symmetry thus plays two roles in this work: first, the intrinsic symmetries of the TDH functions themselves and, second, an empirical symmetry of natural image statistics that emerges from this analysis.

We first describe the mathematical properties of TDH functions, with a focus on their symmetries. TDHs (Figure 1) are a set of two-dimensional functions consisting of a product of Hermite polynomials multiplied by a Gaussian envelope. Like wavelets, they are filter functions that are limited in space and spatial frequency. However, they have several other mathematical properties, including additional symmetries. First, the TDHs are symmetrical with respect to space and spatial frequency: other than a multiplicative constant, each TDH is its own Fourier transform. Second, they are orthonormal functions and, as a set, form a complete basis set for functions of two variables. Third, the TDHs are grouped into "ranks": the sole member of the zeroth rank is an ordinary Gaussian; higher ranks contain functions of increasing spatial complexity. Finally, within each rank, the TDHs have an extended steerability property. This includes ordinary steerability (the filters can be rotated by forming simple linear combinations), but also, linear combinations within rank provide equivalent basis sets that are separable in Cartesian coordinates (see the rows of Figure 1).

Below, we define these functions in abstract terms and then give an explicit expression for their polynomial portions; the former makes their key properties transparent, while the latter is necessary for computation. For further details on this approach, see [25]; other descriptions of the properties of these functions in the context of image processing may be found in [19–24].

Taking inspiration from [26,27], we define the TDHs as the eigenvectors of the operator $D^{1/2}BD^{1/2}$, where D consists of spatial windowing by a two-dimensional Gaussian function (i.e., pointwise multiplication) and B consists of filtering by a two-dimensional Gaussian spatial frequency window (i.e., pointwise multiplication in the spatial frequency domain). Note that D is diagonal in the natural (pointwise spatial) basis, since it consists of pointwise multiplication by the Gaussian; similarly, B is diagonal in the Fourier basis, since it consists of pointwise multiplication by a Gaussian function of spatial frequency. Since the multiplying factors in both cases are positive real numbers, both operators have a naturally-defined principal square root, which we denote as $D^{1/2}$ and $B^{1/2}$. Based on these and other considerations, it can be shown that the operator $D^{1/2}BD^{1/2}$ is self-adjoint and has a discrete set of eigenvalues [25]. The approach of [28] shows that the eigenvalues are of the form $\lambda = \eta^{1+r}$, for a positive constant $\eta < 1$, where the rank, r, ranges over the non-negative integers [25]. It also shows that the r-th rank contains $r + 1$ linearly-independent functions [25]. Note that this setup is symmetric under the interchange of space and spatial frequency, i.e., under the interchange of D and B, so the above properties (and those mentioned below) also hold for $B^{1/2}DB^{1/2}$.

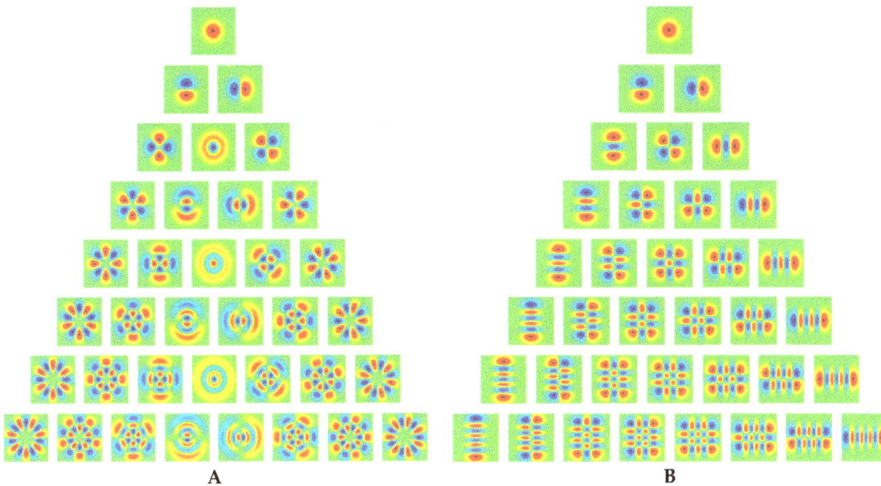

Figure 1. Two-dimensional Hermite (TDH) functions of rank 0–7 in (**A**) polar form and (**B**) Cartesian form. The pseudocolor scale (red positive, blue negative) is chosen separately for each function to cover the entire range. Modified with permission from Figure 1 in [29], Victor et al., J. Neurophysiol. 95, 375-400. American Physiological Society. 2006.

Since D corresponds to confinement in space and B corresponds to confinement in spatial frequency, a TDH function f has the property that successive windowing in space and spatial frequency results in multiplication by a constant (the eigenvalue λ): $D^{1/2}BD^{1/2}f = \lambda f$. That is, for functions f corresponding to eigenvalues λ close to 1, these windowing operations have a small effect, which formalizes the notion that f is confined in both space and spatial frequency.

The eigenfunction of the largest eigenvalue (i.e., the TDH function of rank $r = 0$) is a Gaussian, and its eigenvalue is given by $\eta = \left(\frac{2c}{1+\sqrt{1+4c^2}}\right)^2$, where c is the product of the standard deviation of the Gaussians that define the projections of D or B on either coordinate axis.

Since the eigenvalues are all of the form $\lambda = \eta^{1+r}$, the TDH function of rank $r = 0$ has the eigenvalue that is closest to 1 and is therefore the most confined. Successive ranks have exponentially-declining eigenvalues and are therefore progressively less confined (i.e., more extensive spatially and containing a progressively broader range of spatial frequencies). TDH functions at different ranks are orthogonal, since they correspond to different eigenvalues of the self-adjoint operator $D^{1/2}BD^{1/2}$.

The extended steerability of the TDH functions is a consequence of combining this setup with the fact that a circularly-symmetric Gaussian is separable both in Cartesian and polar coordinates. As a consequence, both D and B have polar symmetry and separability in Cartesian coordinates, These symmetries are inherited by $D^{1/2}BD^{1/2}$ as well, and must be retained by the eigenspaces, so the existence of Cartesian and polar-symmetric eigenvectors is guaranteed. Since any set of $r + 1$ linearly-independent eigenvectors forms a basis for each rank, it follows that we can express the Cartesian and polar basis sets as linear combinations of each other.

The second role played by symmetry, the empirical symmetry identified in natural images, is distinct from the spatial symmetries of the Cartesian or polar TDH functions themselves. Rather, this emerges from an analysis that is motivated by the eigenstructure of the operator $D^{1/2}BD^{1/2}$ (or $B^{1/2}DB^{1/2}$). Since the eigenspace of rank r has dimension $r + 1$, the complete set of unit-norm eigenvectors for each eigenvalue can be considered as points on an r-sphere (i.e., the surface of an ordinary sphere for $r = 2$ or of a hypersphere for $r = 3$, etc.) This spherical surface includes not only the Cartesian and polar basis sets, but other eigenfunctions (see Section 3.2 below) that are mixtures of the two and have no intrinsic symmetry. Descriptors of filter functions' distributions (such as the skewness and kurtosis) for the complete set of eigenvectors can thus be viewed as functions on these spheres. While these functions could have any behavior, we will show that they depend primarily only on the projection onto a single axis, even for filter shapes that are highly irregular.

2.2. Two-Dimensional Hermite Functions: Explicit Expressions

As described in Section 2.1, there are two natural basis sets for the TDH functions of rank r: polar and Cartesian. The polar basis functions are specified by their rotational symmetry (an integer μ, for which a rotation by $2\pi/\mu$ leaves the function unchanged) and the number of zero-crossings along each radius (an integer ν). These indices are related to the rank r by $r = \mu + 2\nu$. For $\mu > 0$, the basis functions form "cosine" and "sine" pairs:

$$A^{\cos}_{\mu,\nu,\sigma}(R,\theta) = \frac{K}{\sigma}\cos(\mu\theta)\left(\frac{R}{\sigma}\right)^{\mu} P_{\mu,\nu}\left(\frac{R^2}{\sigma^2}\right)\exp\left(-\frac{R^2}{4\sigma^2}\right) \tag{1}$$

and

$$A^{\sin}_{\mu,\nu,\sigma}(R,\theta) = \frac{K}{\sigma}\sin(\mu\theta)\left(\frac{R}{\sigma}\right)^{\mu} P_{\mu,\nu}\left(\frac{R^2}{\sigma^2}\right)\exp\left(-\frac{R^2}{4\sigma^2}\right), \tag{2}$$

where σ sets the overall size of the filter set, K is a normalization constant and $P_{\mu,\nu}(u)$ is a radial polynomial defined by:

$$P_{\mu,\nu}(u) = \sum_{p=0}^{\nu}(-2)^{\nu-p}\frac{(\mu+\nu)!\nu!}{(\mu+p)!p!(\nu-p)!}u^p. \tag{3}$$

For each even rank, there is also an unpaired basis function, corresponding to $\mu = 0$ and $\nu = r/2$. These basis functions have no angular dependence (central column of Figure 1A) and are given by $A^{\cos}_{0,r/2,\sigma}(R,\theta)$.

A typical Cartesian basis function has the appearance of a vignetted $(j+1) \times (k+1)$ checkerboard, where there are j vertical zero-crossings and k horizontal crossings, and these indices are related to the rank by $r = j + k$. It is given by:

$$C_{j,k,\sigma}(x,y) = \frac{K}{\sigma} h_j(\frac{x}{\sigma}) h_k(\frac{y}{\sigma}) \exp(-\frac{x^2 + y^2}{4\sigma^2}),$$

where $h_j(u)$ and $h_k(u)$ are Hermite polynomials, normalized so that they have the generating function:

$$\sum_{n=0}^{\infty} \frac{z^n}{n!} h_n(u) = \exp(uz - \frac{z^2}{2}).$$

As detailed in Section 2.4, we calculate image statistics of natural images filtered by the polar TDHs and then use steerability to calculate the statistics of images filtered by other TDHs of a given rank, including the Cartesian TDH filters (as indicated in Figure 2) and intermediate ones. Note that this "steerability" is much more than geometric rotation, as it allows for filters of different shapes, including asymmetric ones (see Sections 3.1 and 3.2 below), to be represented in terms of a small basis set.

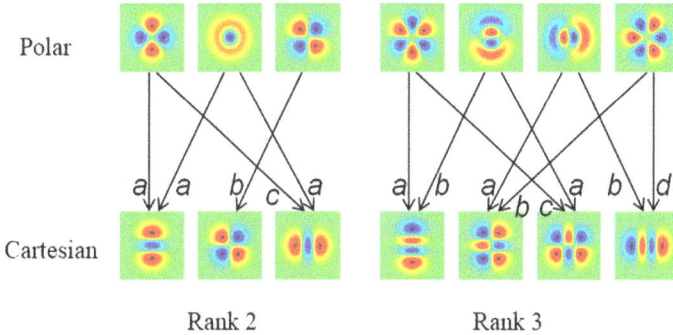

Figure 2. Cartesian TDH functions are a linear combination of polar TDH functions. Examples are shown for rank 2 (**left**) and rank 3 (**right**). For rank 2, the coefficients are $a = \sqrt{2}/2$, $b = 1$, $c = -\sqrt{2}/2$. For rank 3, the coefficients are $a = 1/2$, $b = \sqrt{3}/2$, $c = -\sqrt{3}/2$, $d = -1/2$.

2.3. Natural Images

All 4167 images from the van Hateren natural image database [15] (van Hateren and van der Schaaf, 1998) were chosen for analysis. Each image is 1536 by 1024 pixels, with each pixel's intensity represented by a 16-bit unsigned integer, reflecting an effective bit depth of 12. The images mainly contain landscapes and plants, but occasionally, manmade objects such as houses, appear.

2.4. Analysis

To characterize high-order statistics of natural images, we calculated the skewness and kurtosis (as "excess kurtosis") of the distribution of filter coefficients, i.e., the distribution of values that result from convolving the images with TDH functions. To focus on the structure of the individual scenes (rather than the overall differences across scenes), skewness and kurtosis were calculated individually for each image, and values were then averaged across the image database.

As shown in Figure 3, this calculation was carried out across 7 spatial scales, spaced in approximately octave steps. The smallest scale used was $\sigma = 7/12$ (0.58) pixels and the largest, $\sigma = 511/12$ (42.6) pixels. At each scale, the image was convolved with polar TDH functions of ranks 0–7 (36 filters in all), and the convolution was sampled at points placed in a rectangular grid on the filtered image. Filters' centers were separated by 10 pixels for scales 1–5 and 50 pixels for scales 6 and 7. We then calculated the pure and mixed moments of these distributions up to order 4 and used the extended steerability property (detailed below) to go from the moments for the polar TDH functions to the moments for arbitrary TDH functions. From these moments, skewness and kurtosis were then calculated in the standard fashion.

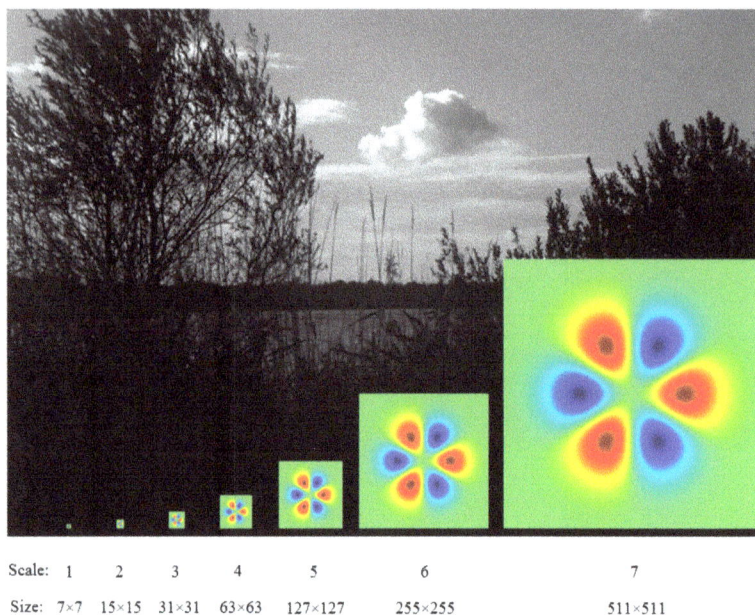

Scale:	1	2	3	4	5	6	7
Size:	7×7	15×15	31×31	63×63	127×127	255×255	511×511

Figure 3. The seven filter sizes used to calculate image statistics, compared to the size of natural images used in this study (1536 × 1024).

In detail, the computation of the skewness and kurtosis for all TDH functions F of rank r was carried out in parallel, as follows. For each image I, we calculated the pure moments for each polar basis function f, given by

$$M_m(f) = \left\langle ((f * I)(x,y))^m \right\rangle_{x,y}, \qquad (4)$$

up to $m = 4$, along with the mixed moments for each pair of functions f and f', given by

$$M_{m,m'}(f,f') = \left\langle ((f * I)(x,y))^m ((f' * I)(x,y))^{m'} \right\rangle_{x,y}, \qquad (5)$$

up to $m + m' = 4$ and, analogously, the mixed moments $M_{1,1,1}(f,f',f'')$, $M_{2,1,1}(f,f',f'')$ and $M_{1,1,1,1}(f,f',f'',f''')$.

To use the extended steerability property, we wrote the filter function F as a linear combination of the polar basis functions of that rank:

$$F(x,y) = \sum_{n=1}^{r+1} b_n f_n(x,y).$$

Therefore, the convolution of F with an image I can be calculated as a linear combination of the convolutions of the basis functions with the image,

$$(F * I)(x,y) = \sum_{n=1}^{r+1} b_n (f_n * I)(x,y). \tag{6}$$

Expressions relating the moments of the distribution of the filter coefficients for F to the moments for the basis functions f_n follow via multinomial expansion of (6), using (4) and (5):

$$M_1(F) = \langle (F * I)(x,y)\rangle_{x,y} = \sum_n b_n M_1(f_n), \tag{7}$$

$$M_2(F) = \left\langle ((F * I)(x,y))^2 \right\rangle_{x,y} = \sum_n b_n{}^2 M_2(f_n) + 2\sum_{n_1 < n_2} b_{n_1} b_{n_2} M_{1,1}(f_{n_1}, f_{n_2}), \tag{8}$$

$$M_3(F) = \left\langle ((F * I)(x,y))^3 \right\rangle_{x,y} = \sum_n b_n{}^3 M_3(f_n) + 3\sum_{n_1 \neq n_2} b_{n_1}{}^2 b_{n_2} M_{2,1}(f_{n_1}, f_{n_2})$$
$$+ 6\sum_{n_1 < n_2 < n_3} b_{n_1} b_{n_2} b_{n_3} M_{1,1,1}(f_{n_1}, f_{n_2}, f_{n_3}) \tag{9}$$

and

$$M_4(F) = \left\langle ((F * I)(x,y))^4 \right\rangle_{x,y} = \sum_n b_n{}^4 M_4(f_n) + 4\sum_{n_1 \neq n_2} b_{n_1}{}^3 b_{n_2} M_{3,1}(f_{n_1}, f_{n_2})$$
$$+ 6\sum_{n_1 < n_2} b_{n_1}{}^2 b_{n_2}{}^2 M_{2,2}(f_{n_1}, f_{n_2}) + 12\sum_{n_1 \neq n_2, n_1 \neq n_3, n_2 < n_3} b_{n_1}{}^2 b_{n_2} b_{n_3} M_{2,1,1}(f_{n_1}, f_{n_2}, f_{n_3}) \ . \tag{10}$$
$$+ 24\sum_{n_1 < n_2 < n_3 < n_4} b_{n_1} b_{n_2} b_{n_3} b_{n_4} M_{1,1,1,1}(f_{n_1}, f_{n_2}, f_{n_3}, f_{n_4})$$

As is standard, the cumulants of the distribution of the filter outputs of F are determined from its moments by:

$$\kappa_2 = M_2(F) - (M_1(F))^2, \tag{11}$$

$$\kappa_3 = 2(M_1(F))^3 - 3M_1(F)M_2(F) + M_3(F), \tag{12}$$

and

$$\kappa_4 = -6(M_1(F))^4 + 12(M_1(F))^2 M_2(F) - 3(M_2(F))^2 - 4M_1(F)M_3(F) + M_4(F). \tag{13}$$

Skewness and (excess) kurtosis are ratios of the cumulants:

$$\gamma_3 = \kappa_3 / \kappa_2{}^{3/2} \tag{14}$$

and

$$\gamma_4 = \kappa_4 / \kappa_2{}^2. \tag{15}$$

3. Results

We characterized the high-order statistics of natural images via the distribution of filter coefficients for two-dimensional Hermite (TDH) functions. We present the findings for rank two first because this low rank allows for a detailed visualization and then turn to higher ranks.

3.1. Statistics of Rank Two TDH Filter Coefficients for Natural Images

To visualize the results for rank two, we note that the full set of rank two filters can be regarded as points on the surface of an ordinary sphere (Figure 4). This follows from the general observation that the r-th rank of TDH functions is spanned by $r + 1$ orthonormal filters, so the full set of unit-magnitude filters of rank r (i.e., the full set of unit-magnitude linear combinations of these $r + 1$ basis elements) may be regarded as the surface of a sphere in $(r + 1)$-space. In this spherical representation of rank two TDH functions shown in Figure 4, the polar filters correspond to one set of orthogonal directions, the Cartesian filters to a second orthogonal set of directions, and intermediate directions correspond to mixtures of polar or Cartesian filters. The latitude (altitude) indicates the size of the projection onto the target-like TDH function. For TDH functions at the same latitude, the azimuth on the sphere corresponds to the orientation (i.e., the in-plane rotation angle) of the filter function.

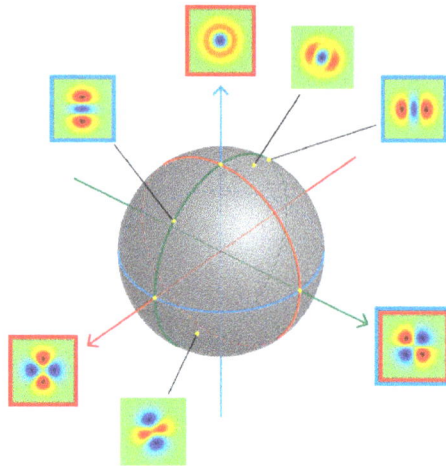

Figure 4. Generalized steerability of the rank two TDH filters. Each unit-magnitude filter corresponds to a point on the surface of a sphere. The polar and Cartesian basis functions form two sets of orthogonal coordinate axes. Filters with a red frame are polar TDH filters; filters with a blue frame are Cartesian TDH filters; one filter is in both sets as indicated by its two frames. Filters without a frame are intermediate filters; they can be constructed from a linear combination of either polar or Cartesian filters.

Figure 5 shows the skewness and kurtosis of the distributions for all TDH filters of rank two, plotted on the filter space shown in Figure 4. Skewness and kurtosis depend strongly on latitude, but are largely independent of orientation, although there is a small dependence of kurtosis at the orientation at the two largest scales. Skewness is maximal for the circularly-symmetric (target-like) filters at the poles and is zero for filters on the equator, while kurtosis is minimal for the target-like filters and is maximal for filters on the equator.

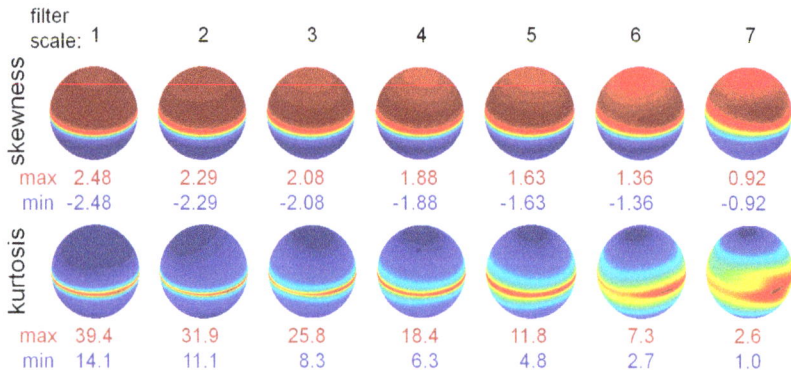

Figure 5. Skewness and kurtosis for natural images filtered by rank two TDH filters across seven spatial scales. Each sphere represents the filter space of unit-length rank two TDH filters (oriented as shown in Figure 4). Skewness and kurtosis are averaged across all filtered images and plotted as a function of direction in the filter space. The pseudocolor scales for each skewness and kurtosis map are set to range from blue (minimum) to red (maximum). The minimum and maximum skewness and kurtosis values are shown under each sphere.

3.2. Statistics of Higher-Rank TDH Filter Coefficients for Natural Images

For higher ranks, a similar visualization strategy is not possible, so we begin with the skewness and kurtosis for each of the filters in the polar basis set (Figure 6). We focus on filter scale four, the middle of the range studied; other filter scales gave a similar pattern of results.

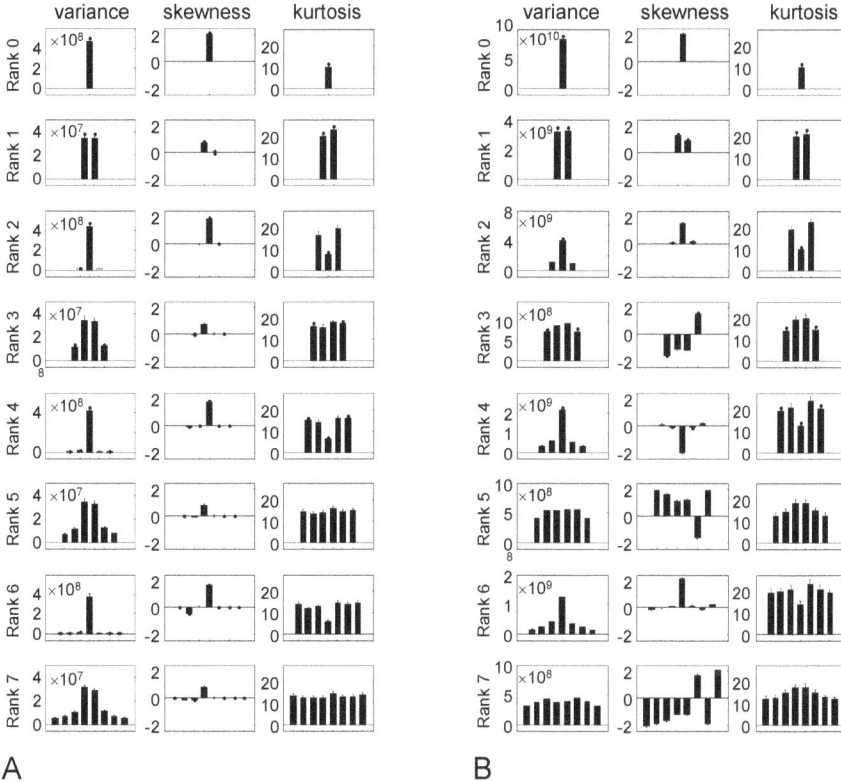

Figure 6. Variance, skewness and kurtosis for (**A**) natural images filtered by polar TDH filters of rank 0–7 (spatial scale four) and (**B**) modified TDH filters in which the polynomial component is replaced by its sign. Error bars are three standard errors of measurement (SEM).

With regard to skewness (Figure 6A, second column), there is a single polar filter within each rank for which skewness is large; for the others, it is close to zero. For even ranks (consistent with the rank two results shown in Figure 5), the single polar filter that has a large skewness is the target-like filter $A^{\cos}_{0,r/2}$; this is the only polar filter with a nonzero mean. For odd ranks, the filter with the largest skewness is the filter with a single horizontal inversion axis, $A^{\sin}_{1,(r-1)/2}$; this filter is specifically sensitive to vertical gradients.

With regard to kurtosis (Figure 6A, third column), the pattern is also a simple one. For even ranks (also consistent with Figure 2), kurtosis is uniform for all filters except the target-like one $A^{\cos}_{0,r/2}$, shown as the middle bar of each histogram in the right column; for the target-like filter, kurtosis is approximately half the size of the others. For odd ranks, the kurtosis is large, but uniform across all filters. Thus, we find that for each rank, skewness and kurtosis are either uniform across all polar basis functions or uniform for all basis functions, except for one special filter, the odd-rank filter with a single horizontal inversion axis, or the even-rank filter that is target-like.

For completeness, the first column of Figure 6A shows the variance of each filter's outputs. This is large for target-like filters (center filter in even ranks) and small for all other filters, with sine and cosine pairs resulting in similar variances. As variance is a second-order statistic, this behavior is a consequence of the k^{-2} power spectrum of the images.

The simple behavior of skewness and kurtosis for the TDH functions is not merely a consequence of their polar symmetry. To see this, we repeated the analysis of Figure 6A, but with the polar TDH functions replaced by binarized variants, in which positive values of the polynomial component (all terms except for the exponentials in Equations (1) and (2)) are replaced by +1 and negative values by −1. The binarized variants have the same polar symmetry and sine/cosine pairing as the original TDH functions and, within ranks, are mutually orthogonal, as well. However, when the polynomial portions of the TDH functions are replaced by ±1, neither skewness nor kurtosis have the same simple behavior seen in Figure 6A. Specifically, while the skewness and kurtosis vary over a wide range (approximately 0–2 for skewness, 10–20 for kurtosis) and this substantial variation is captured in a single basis function at each rank for the original TDH functions, it is spread across many basis functions for the modified ones (Figure 6B).

While Figure 6A suggests that the skewness and kurtosis of a general TDH filter depends only on its projection onto the special axis, it only examines filters that are orthogonal to the special axis. For oblique directions, it is possible that this result will not hold. The reason that more complex behavior may arise in oblique directions is that for moments of order three and higher, the steering equations (Equations (9) and (10) in Section 2.4) include contributions from mixed moments of the polar TDHs.

Figure 7 shows that despite this potential complication, the skewness and kurtosis of a TDH filter's output depends chiefly on the projection of the filter onto the single special axis identified in Figure 6A. It is noteworthy that this holds not only for the Cartesian TDHs, but also for generic TDHs, which typically lack rotational symmetry. Moreover, for ranks $r \geq 3$, TDH functions that share the same projection onto this axis are intrinsically different in shape and are not merely physical rotations of one another.

In sum, within each rank, skewness and kurtosis of the filter coefficient distribution is either uniform or uniform in all but one direction in filter space. This axis has a simple interpretation: it is either the target-like TDH function or the single TDH function that is sensitive to a top-to-bottom gradient. In other words, although the TDH filter space has a high dimensionality (equal to the rank + 1), the behavior of skewness and kurtosis is always low-dimensional, either uniform or rotationally symmetric. This simplification constitutes a symmetry of natural image statistics and goes beyond the overt spatial symmetries of the TDHs themselves: on the one hand, it applies to filter functions that lack either Cartesian or polar symmetry (Figure 7); on the other hand, this simplification fails when the polynomial portion of a TDH filter is replaced by ±1 (Figure 6B), even though this replacement retains all of the spatial symmetries of the filters.

Figure 8 uses this finding to describe the distribution of TDH filter coefficients across all spatial scales in a concise manner. Skewness is characterized by its value for the target-like filter at even ranks ($\gamma_{3,target}$; Figure 8A) and for the filter with a single horizontal inversion axis at odd ranks ($\gamma_{3,horiz}$; Figure 8B). $\gamma_{3,target}$ is a decreasing function of scale and rank, and $\gamma_{3,horiz}$ is an increasing function of scale and (except for rank one) nearly independent of rank. Kurtosis is characterized by its value for the target-like filter at even ranks ($\gamma_{4,target}$; Figure 8C) and by its value for the remaining filters, at both even and odd ranks ($\gamma_{4,non-target}$; Figure 8D). Both kurtosis quantities are decreasing functions of scale and rank. It would be of interest to characterize the scaling behaviors of the skewness and kurtosis parameters more precisely, but this is beyond the scope of the present study.

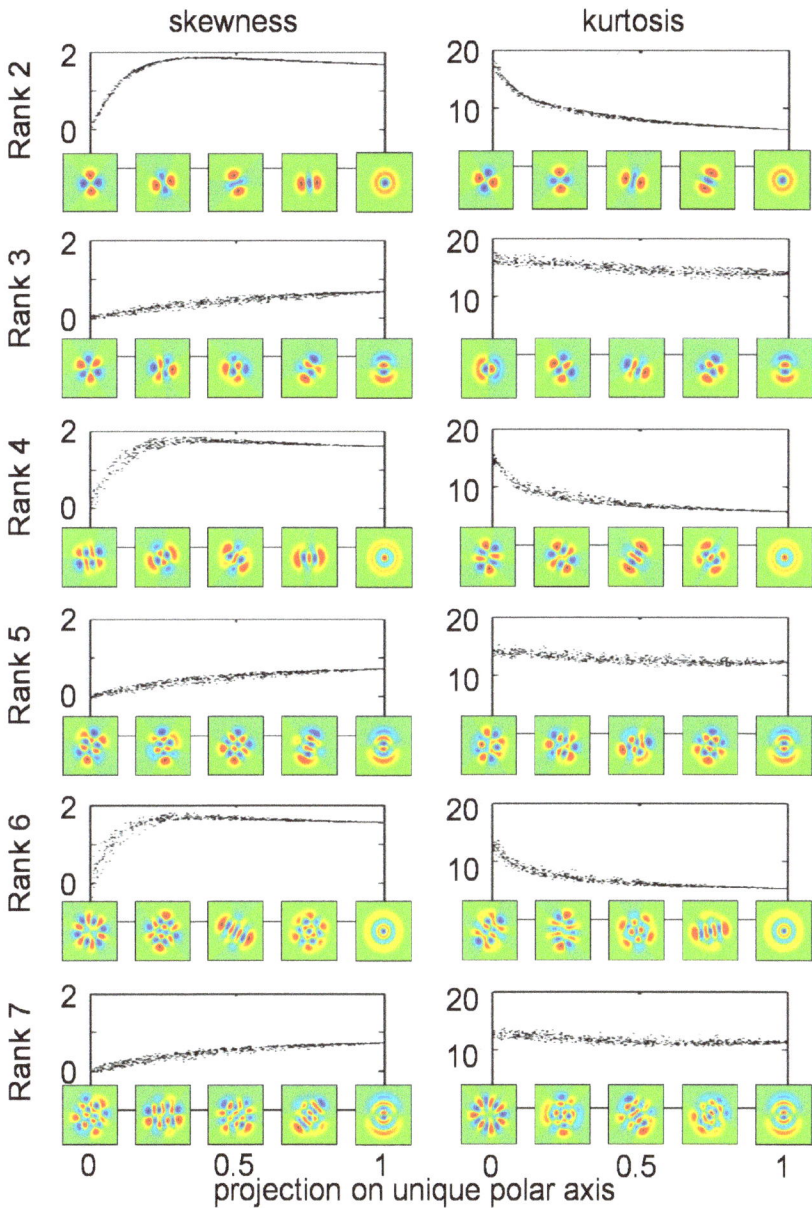

Figure 7. Skewness and kurtosis of natural images filtered by 1000 random TDH filters of rank 2–7, at scale four. The abscissa is the projection of each random TDH filter onto the polar TDH filter shown at the lower right of each plot, which is the target-like filter for even ranks and the filter with a single, horizontal inversion axis for odd ranks. The filters placed along the abscissa are examples of filters whose projections onto the rightmost polar filter are 0, 0.25, 0.5 and 0.75. They illustrate the diversity of filters with a given value of the projection; the examples shown for the skewness and kurtosis columns at corresponding points along the abscissa are interchangeable.

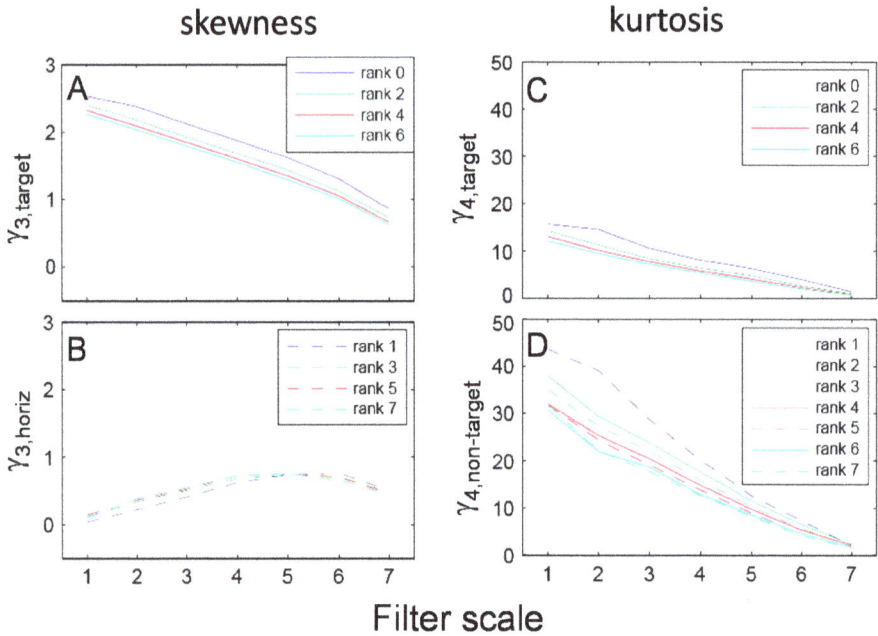

Figure 8. At each spatial scale, the skewness of TDH-filtered images is characterized by two values: $\gamma_{3,target}$ (**A**) for even ranks and $\gamma_{3,horiz}$ for odd ranks (**B**); and kurtosis is characterized by $\gamma_{4,target}$ (**C**) for even ranks and $\gamma_{4,non-target}$ for all ranks (**D**).

3.3. Statistics TDH Filter Coefficients for Altered Images

To understand the attributes of natural images that underlie the above findings, we carried out parallel analyses for natural images that were manipulated in several ways prior to the determination of filter coefficients.

First, we examined the role of local mean luminance. To do this, we repeated the analysis of Figure 6, but with subtraction of the local mean luminance over a disk of radius 6σ prior to computing TDH filter outputs (Figure 9A). This manipulation eliminated the difference between the kurtosis for the target-like filter and the others, so that kurtosis was uniform within each rank. Subtraction of the local mean reduced, but did not eliminate, the value of the skewness for the target-like filter. As expected, subtraction of the local mean did not change the distributions for the polar TDH filters that were not target-like, since for $\mu \neq 0$, the trigonometric terms in Equations (1) and (2) necessarily integrate to zero.

To distinguish the roles of spatial frequency content and phase correlations, we analyzed the distribution of filter coefficients for phase-scrambled images and for images that are spectrally flattened. To isolate the role of spatial frequency content, we created phase-scrambled images by randomizing the phases of the Fourier components in the original images. This effectively results in samples of a spatial Gaussian noise whose power spectrum matches that of the original image. As expected, analysis of these images yielded distributions of TDH filter outputs whose variances matched those of the original images, but for which skewness and kurtosis were zero (data not shown). This confirms that spatial frequency content alone does not carry the high-order statistics observed in natural images [8].

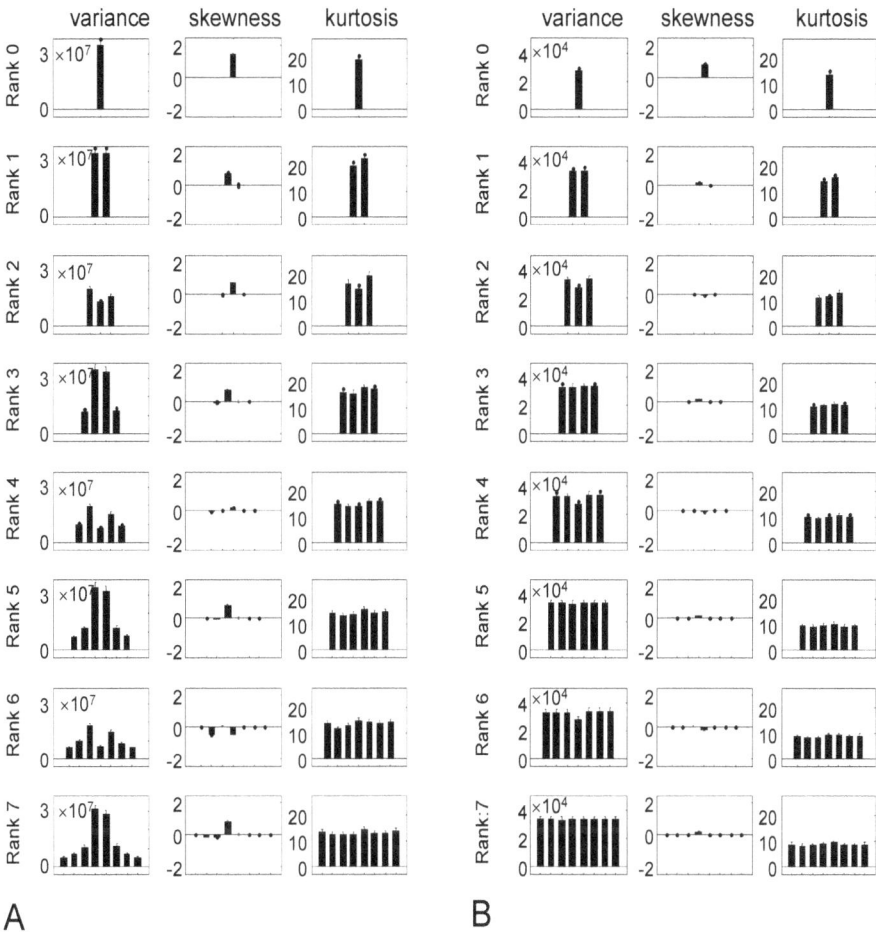

Figure 9. Variance, skewness and kurtosis for (**A**) natural images filtered by polar TDH filters of rank 0–7 (spatial scale four) after local mean subtraction; (**B**) as in (**A**), but natural images are whitened prior to analysis. Error bars are three SEM.

To isolate the role of phase correlations, we set the Fourier component amplitudes in the original images to unity, but retained their phases. As in Figure 9A, calculation of filter outputs was carried out with subtraction of the local mean, to retain the isotropy of the kurtosis. Other than for the rank zero filter, this eliminated the skewness (Figure 9B). The kurtosis remains isotropic. Thus, the heavy-tailed nature of the coefficient distributions depends not only on phase, but also on amplitude.

Finally, to determine the role of the luminance distribution, we calculated the filter coefficient distributions for images subjected to the manipulation of the pixel histogram: logarithmic transformation, histogram equalization and transformation of the intensity histogram to a Gaussian, truncated to 2.56 standard deviations (Figure 10). All of these reduced both skewness (by approximately a factor of 10) and kurtosis (by approximately a factor of five), with near-complete elimination of skewness following the logarithmic transformation. Skewness was concentrated in the filter with a single horizontal inversion axis at odd ranks, and kurtosis was approximately constant within rank.

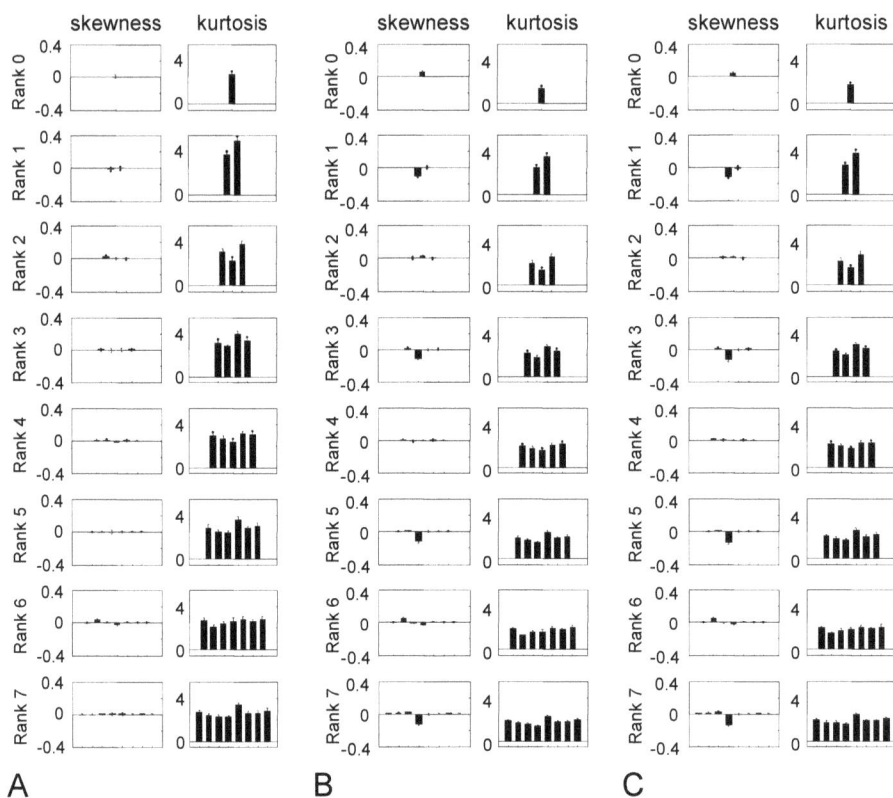

Figure 10. Skewness and kurtosis TDH filters of rank 0–7 (spatial scale four) processed by pointwise nonlinearities prior to analysis. (**A**) Logarithmic transformation; (**B**) histogram equalization; (**C**) Gaussian luminance distribution. Error bars are three SEM.

4. Discussion

Here, we show that two-dimensional Hermite (TDH) filters, an orthogonal basis set with a high degree of symmetry, simplify the description of high-order statistics of natural images, both locally and over wide areas. The significance of this result is that high-order statistics carry the local features that distinguish natural images from Gaussian processes [3,8,17,18,30], but they are challenging to analyze because of their high dimensionality. By identifying a hidden symmetry in high-order statistics, TDH functions provide a kind of dimensional reduction, and therefore, a needed simplification. We emphasize that our goal is focused on understanding natural images, not neural computations per se. Specifically, we do not intend to suggest that the visual system uses TDH filters; rather, our point is that they simplify the description of the stimulus set with which the visual system must grapple. This application of TDH functions to characterize natural image statistics is distinct from two other applications of them to vision: a body of work in image processing [19,21,23,24] that uses them to extract local features and neurophysiologic studies that use them as visual stimuli to analyze the properties of neuronal receptive fields [29,31].

It is worth noting that the TDH filters constitute a set of functions with an unusually high degree of symmetry. They can be written as a product of functions in either Cartesian or polar coordinates and, thus, have both rotational symmetry and steerability. The steerability includes not only the ordinary rotational transformations of the plane, but also rotations in the hyperspheres that correspond to each rank of TDH filters. Moreover, other than a constant factor, each TDH filter is its own Fourier transform, an explicit symmetry relating space and spatial frequency.

Our findings can be viewed as building on [17,32], which also focus on the high-order image statistics of natural images. Specifically, these authors examined the distributions of outputs of filters acting on whitened natural images and the joint distributions of outputs of pairs of filters identified by independent components analysis. The work in [17] showed that the joint distribution is approximately circular, and [32] showed that an improved characterization of the joint distribution could be obtained using an L^p-norm, rather than the Euclidean norm. This near-circularity implies that for any filter, the distribution of outputs has a qualitatively similar heavy-tailed shape. The observation that bandpass filter outputs have similar kurtoses has also been made in other studies [33,34]. However, this similarity is only a loose approximation: when analyzed quantitatively (e.g., Figure 5 of [17]), the kurtoses of these distributions varied by at least a factor of two. Here, we show that analysis in terms of TDH filters concisely summarizes this variation: at each rank, the kurtosis of a filter's output is determined by its projection onto a specific direction in filter space.

Examination of the polar TDH filters (Figure 1) suggests the reasons that specific axes are singled out. For the even-rank filters, the special axis is the only filter whose mean is nonzero; all other filters necessarily have a mean of zero because of their sinusoidal dependence on angle. Thus, these filters are the ones that are sensitive to the distribution of local luminance, which is well known to be heavy-tailed in natural images, both in terms of skewness [35,36] and kurtosis [37]. For the odd-rank filters, the identified axis has a horizontal mirror-inversion, with large lobes above and below the horizon. These filters are likely to be highly sensitive to vertical gradients, and thus, the distributions of their outputs will be skewed by the tendency of illumination to come from above. Consistent with these hypotheses, removal of the local mean (Figure 9A) eliminated the distinctive behavior of the target-like filter for kurtosis and reduced its skewness. When the low spatial frequencies were reduced by spectral flattening, the skewness was eliminated for the odd-rank filters, as well. Figure 10 provides further evidence that the distinctive kurtosis for the target-like filters is primarily a consequence of luminance distributions, as it is reduced by attenuating the tails of the luminance distribution via log transformation, histogram-equalization or Gaussianization.

The simplification we observe is not simply a consequence of the arrangement of the positive and negative lobes of the TDH filters and, thus, has deeper roots than the overt spatial symmetries of the TDH filters. The evidence for this is that replacing the Hermite polynomial values by ± 1, which preserves the arrangement of their lobes, does not result in a similar simplification of the skewness and kurtosis (Figure 6B). Thus, the crucial factor in our findings is the interaction between the polynomial gradations of the TDHs and the properties of natural images.

5. Conclusions

Two-dimensional Hermite filters provide a simple description of third- and fourth-order statistics of natural images across a range of scales. This simplification is a consequence of the high degree of symmetry of this orthogonal basis set and the phase, amplitude and luminance characteristics of natural images.

Acknowledgments: We thank Eyal Nitzany and Matthias Bethge for comments on an earlier version of this manuscript. Supported in part by NIH EY07977 and NIH EY09314 to J.D.V.

Author Contributions: J.D.V. and Q.H. designed the experiments. Q.H. carried out the analysis. J.D.V. and Q.H. wrote the paper.

Conflicts of Interest: The authors declare no conflict of interest.

Abbreviations

TDH   Two-dimensional Hermite

References

1. Elder, J.H.; Victor, J.; Zucker, S.W. Understanding the statistics of the natural environment and their implications for vision. *Vis. Res.* **2016**, *120*, 1–4. [CrossRef] [PubMed]
2. Pouli, T.; Cunningham, D.W.; Reinhard, E. Image statistics and their applications in computer graphics. Proceedings of Eurographics. *State Art Rep.* **2010**, *72*, 83–112.
3. Farid, H.; Lyu, S. Higher-order wavelet statistics and their application to digital forensics. In Proceedings of the IEEE Computer Society Conference on Computer Vision and Pattern Recognition, Madison, WI, USA, 16–22 June 2003; pp. 94–101.
4. Lyu, S.W.; Farid, H. Steganalysis using higher-order image statistics. *IEEE Trans. Inf. Forensics Secur.* **2006**, *1*, 111–119. [CrossRef]
5. Lyu, S.; Farid, H. Detecting hidden messages using higher-order statistics and support vector machines. *Inf. Hiding* **2003**, *2578*, 340–354.
6. Lyu, S.; Rockmore, D.; Farid, H. A digital technique for art authentication. *Proc. Natl. Acad. Sci. USA* **2004**, *101*, 17006–17010. [CrossRef] [PubMed]
7. Chainais, P. Infinitely divisible cascades to model the statistics of natural images. *IEEE Trans. Pattern Anal. Mach. Intell.* **2007**, *29*, 2105–2419. [CrossRef] [PubMed]
8. Oppenheim, A.V.; Lim, J.S. The importance of phase in signals. *Proc. IEEE* **1981**, *69*, 529–541. [CrossRef]
9. Morrone, M.C.; Burr, D.C. Feature detection in human vision: a phase-dependent energy model. *Proc. R. Soc. Lond. B Biol. Sci.* **1988**, *235*, 221–245. [CrossRef] [PubMed]
10. Field, D.J. Relations between the statistics of natural images and the response properties of cortical cells. *J. Opt. Soc. Am. A* **1987**, *4*, 2379–2394. [CrossRef] [PubMed]
11. Tolhurst, D.J.; Tadmor, Y.; Chao, T. Amplitude spectra of natural images. *Ophthalmic Physiol. Opt.* **1992**, *12*, 229–232. [CrossRef] [PubMed]
12. Ruderman, D.L. Origins of scaling in natural images. *Vis. Res.* **1997**, *37*, 3385–3398. [CrossRef]
13. Tadmor, Y.; Tolhurst, D.J. Both the phase and the amplitude spectrum may determine the appearance of natural images. *Vis. Res.* **1993**, *33*, 141–145. [CrossRef]
14. Van Hateren, J.H.; Ruderman, D.L. Independent component analysis of natural image sequences yields spatio-temporal filters similar to simple cells in primary visual cortex. *Proc. R. Soc. Lond. B Biol. Sci.* **1998**, *265*, 2315–2320. [CrossRef] [PubMed]
15. Van Hateren, J.H.; van der Schaaf, A. Independent component filters of natural images compared with simple cells in primary visual cortex. *Proc. Biol. Sci.* **1998**, *265*, 359–366. [CrossRef] [PubMed]
16. Simoncelli, E.P. Statistical modeling of photographic images. In *Handbook of Image and Video Processing*; Bovic, A.C., Ed.; Academic Press: Burlington, MA, USA, 2005; pp. 431–441.
17. Lyu, S.; Simoncelli, E.P. Nonlinear extraction of independent components of natural images using radial gaussianization. *Neural Comput.* **2009**, *21*, 1485–1519. [CrossRef] [PubMed]
18. Zetzsche, C.; Nuding, U. Nonlinear and higher-order approaches to the encoding of natural scenes. *Network* **2005**, *16*, 191–221. [CrossRef] [PubMed]
19. Martens, J.B. The Hermite Transform—Applications. *IEEE Trans. Acoust. Speech Signal Process.* **1990**, *38*, 1607–1618. [CrossRef]
20. Martens, J.B. The Hermite Transform—Theory. *IEEE Trans. Acoust. Speech Signal Process.* **1990**, *38*, 1595–1606. [CrossRef]
21. Martens, J.B. Local orientation analysis in images by means of the Hermite transform. *IEEE Trans. Image Process.* **1997**, *6*, 1103–1116. [CrossRef] [PubMed]
22. VanDijk, A.M.; Martens, J.B. Representation and compression with steered Hermite transforms. *Signal Process.* **1997**, *56*, 1–16. [CrossRef]
23. Refregier, A.; Shapelets, I. A method for image analysis. *Mon. Not. R. Astron. Soc.* **2003**, *338*, 35–47. [CrossRef]
24. Silvan-Cardenas, J.L.; Escalante-Ramirez, B. The multiscale hermite transform for local orientation analysis. *IEEE Trans. Image Process.* **2006**, *15*, 1236–1253. [CrossRef] [PubMed]
25. Victor, J.D.; Knight, B.W. Simultaneously band and space limited functions in two dimensions, and receptive fields of visual neurons. In *Springer Applied Mathematical Sciences Series*; Kaplan, E., Marsden, J., Sreenivasan, K.R., Eds.; Springer: New York, NY, USA, 2003; pp. 375–420.

26. Slepian, D.; Pollack, H. Prolate spheroidal wave functions, Fourier analysis and uncertainty—I. *Bell Syst. Tech. J.* **1961**, *40*, 43–64. [CrossRef]
27. Slepian, D. Prolate spheroidal wave functions, Fourier analysis and uncertainty—IV: Extensions to many dimensions; generalized prolate spheroidal functions. *Bell Syst. Tech.* **1964**, *43*, 3009–3057. [CrossRef]
28. Knight, B.; Sirovich, L. The Wigner transform and some exact properties of linear operators. *SIAM J. Appl. Math.* **1982**, *42*, 378–389. [CrossRef]
29. Victor, J.D.; Mechler, F.; Repucci, M.A.; Purpura, K.P.; Sharpee, T. Responses of V1 neurons to two-dimensional Hermite functions. *J. Neurophysiol.* **2006**, *95*, 379–400. [CrossRef] [PubMed]
30. Ruderman, D.L. The statistics of natural images. *Netw. Comput. Neural Syst.* **1994**, *5*, 517–548. [CrossRef]
31. Sharpee, T.O.; Victor, J.D. Contextual modulation of V1 receptive fields depends on their spatial symmetry. *J. Comput. Neurosci.* **2009**, *26*, 203–218. [CrossRef] [PubMed]
32. Sinz, F.H.; Simoncelli, E.; Bethge, M. Hierarchical modeling of local image features through L_p-nested symmetric distributions. *Adv. Neural Inf. Process. Syst.* **2010**, *22*, 1696–1704.
33. Bethge, M. Factorial coding of natural images: how effective are linear models in removing higher-order dependencies? *J. Opt. Soc. Am. A Opt. Image Sci. Vis.* **2006**, *23*, 1253–1268. [CrossRef] [PubMed]
34. Zhang, X.; Lyu, S. Using projection kurtosis concentration of natural images for blind noise covariance matrix estimation. In Proceedings of the IEEE Conference on Computer Vision and Pattern Recognition, Columbus, OH, USA, 23–28 June 2014.
35. Motoyoshi, I.; Nishida, S.Y.; Sharan, L.; Adelson, E.H. Image statistics and the perception of surface qualities. *Nature* **2007**, *447*, 206–209. [CrossRef] [PubMed]
36. Graham, D.; Schwarz, B.; Chatterjee, A.; Leder, H. Preference for luminance histogram regularities in natural scenes. *Vis. Res.* **2016**, *120*, 11–21. [CrossRef] [PubMed]
37. Portilla, J.; Simoncelli, E.P. A parametric texture model based on joint statistics of complex wavelet coefficients. *Int. J. Comput. Vis.* **2000**, *40*, 49–71. [CrossRef]

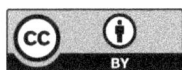

symmetry

MDPI

Article

Using Convolutional Neural Network Filters to Measure Left-Right Mirror Symmetry in Images

Anselm Brachmann and Christoph Redies *

Experimental Aesthetics Group, Institute of Anatomy, University of Jena School of Medicine,
Jena University Hospital, 07743 Jena, Germany; anselm.brachmann@med.uni-jena.de
* Correspondence: christoph.redies@med.uni-jena.de; Tel.: +49-3641-938-511

Academic Editor: Marco Bertamini
Received: 03 August 2016; Accepted: 28 November 2016; Published: 1 December 2016

Abstract: We propose a method for measuring symmetry in images by using filter responses from Convolutional Neural Networks (CNNs). The aim of the method is to model human perception of left/right symmetry as closely as possible. Using the Convolutional Neural Network (CNN) approach has two main advantages: First, CNN filter responses closely match the responses of neurons in the human visual system; they take information on color, edges and texture into account simultaneously. Second, we can measure higher-order symmetry, which relies not only on color, edges and texture, but also on the shapes and objects that are depicted in images. We validated our algorithm on a dataset of 300 music album covers, which were rated according to their symmetry by 20 human observers, and compared results with those from a previously proposed method. With our method, human perception of symmetry can be predicted with high accuracy. Moreover, we demonstrate that the inclusion of features from higher CNN layers, which encode more abstract image content, increases the performance further. In conclusion, we introduce a model of left/right symmetry that closely models human perception of symmetry in CD album covers.

Keywords: symmetry perception; continuous symmetry; convolutional neural networks; aesthetics

---

1. Introduction

Symmetry is ubiquitous. It can be found in formations that have emerged in evolution, such as bird wings and bugs, and in physical structures like crystals, as well as in man-made objects like cars, buildings, or art. Symmetry as a concept refers to any manner, in which part of a pattern can be mapped onto another part of itself [1]. While this can be done by translation (translational symmetry) or rotation (rotational symmetry), reflectional symmetry, in which a part of a pattern is mirrored along an axis, is special because it is highly salient for human observers [2]. Reflectional symmetry has been linked to attractiveness in faces [3] and it is thought to serve as an indicator of normal development, general health or the ability to withstand stress [4–6]. Symmetry was linked to beauty not only in natural stimuli, but also in abstract patterns [7]. Together, these findings suggest that the perception of symmetry is a general mechanism that plays an important role in our aesthetic judgment.

In mathematics, symmetry is a clean, formal concept of group theory. In contrast, symmetry detection in computer vision is faced with real world data, which can be noisy, ambiguous and even distorted. Nevertheless, several algorithms to detect symmetry in real world data have been proposed [8–10]. Much work has been done regarding the detection of axes of symmetry in an image. Continuous symmetry, as described by [11], measures the degree to which symmetry is present in a given shape (defined by a set of points). In the present article, we introduce a novel measure of continuous symmetry, which approximates the perception of natural images by human observers. The aim of this measure is to indicate to which degree reflectional symmetry is present in an arbitrary image. While this task is easily accomplished by humans, it is much harder for computers.

One possibility to assign a measure of continuous symmetry to images is to compare luminance values along an axis of the image, as proposed in [12]. However, this approach differs substantially from how humans perceive real-world scenes. Instead of comparing pixels, humans detect edges and group them into shapes, textures and, finally, into objects. Such grouping contributes to symmetry perception by humans. Shaker and Monadjemi [13] proposed a symmetry measure that uses edge information in gray-scale images. Although this approach goes beyond the restricted usage of luminance intensity information, it does not take into account color and shapes. In the present article, we propose a novel algorithm that detects symmetry in a manner that is closer to how humans perceive symmetry. To this aim, we use filter responses from Convolutional Neural Networks (CNNs), which have gained huge popularity among computer vision researchers in recent years. The novelty of our measure is twofold: First, by using CNN filter responses, we take color and spatial frequency information into account, as done by the human visual system, namely by encoding color-opponent edges as well as color blobs and spatial frequency information [14,15]. Second, we show that features from higher CNN layers, where more abstract image content is represented [16], can improve the prediction of symmetry judgements of human observers even further.

Although CNNs were first proposed more than two decades ago [17,18], they have become state-of-the-art technology for many computer vision tasks only recently, due to progress in computing technology, such as the introduction of graphic cards for calculations, and the availability of huge amounts of data for training. Currently, CNNs are being applied to object recognition tasks [19,20], image description [21], and texture synthesis [22], and they have conquered other areas like speech recognition [23]. CNNs learn a hierarchy of different filters that are applied to an input image, enabling them to extract useful information. The training algorithm works in a supervised manner, which means that, given an input image, the output is compared to the target output so that an error gradient can be computed. Using backpropagation, parameters of the model are changed so that the error is minimized and the network gets better at solving the task at hand.

In our study, we use filter responses from CNNs that were trained on millions of images of objects [24] for measuring continuous symmetry in images. To validate our results, we collected a dataset of 300 different CD album covers and asked human observers to rate them according to their left/right symmetry. CD album covers are especially suited for this task because they offer a wide variety and different degrees of symmetry. For each of the 300 images, the subjective symmetry ratings were compared to the symmetry measure obtained by our algorithm.

2. Materials and Methods

2.1. Measuring Continuous Symmetry Using Filter Responses from Convolutional Neural Networks

As mentioned above, CNNs learn a hierarchy of different filters that are applied to an input image. Filters reside on layers, where higher layers tend to extract more and more abstract features from an image, compared to the previous ones. Different layer types have been proposed and are investigated in ongoing research. The model we use in our experiments, referred to as *CaffeNet*, was proposed by [19] and is provided as a part of the Caffe Library [24]. It consists of a total of 8 building blocks, each consisting of one or more different layer types: *Convolutional layers*, in which the output of a previous layer is convolved with a set of different filters, *pooling layers*, in which a subsampling of the previous layer is performed by taking the maximum over equally sized subregions, and *normalization layers*, which perform a local brightness normalization. Several fully-connected layers that are stacked on top of a network learn to map extracted features onto class labels. Interestingly, the filters on the first layer tend do develop oriented Gabor-like edge detectors, akin to those found in human vision, when trained on huge datasets containing millions of natural images [25] (see Figure 1). In our experiments, we drop the fully connected layers on top, which allows us to resize the input to have a dimension of 512×512 pixels. Using this modification of the *CaffeNet* model [24], we propose an algorithm that measures continuous left/right mirror symmetry of natural images, as follows.

First, every image is fed to the network, which yields 96 filter response maps after the first convolutional layer, 256 after the second, 384 after the third and fourth, and 256 after the last convolutional layer. Using these filter responses, we then build a histogram of the maximum responses of equally sized, non-overlapping subregions of these maps, i.e., we perform a max-pooling operation over a grid of equally sized areas (*patches*). In the remainder of this article, a *patch level* of *n* refers to a tiling of the filter response maps into $n \times n$ subregions.

Using convolutional layer $l \in \{1, 2, ..., 5\}$, this procedures provides us with a max-pooling map I_l, which has three dimensions: two positional parameters of the subimage, on which the max-pooling was performed, and one dimension that holds the maximum responses in that subimage for each filter. We then flip the image along the middle vertical axis and repeat the same procedure for the flipped version, which provides us with another five max-pooling maps F_l.

In order to measure the reflectional symmetry of an image, we measure the asymmetry of the max-pooling maps I_l and F_l by calculating how different the right and the left side of any given image are, using the following equation:

$$A(I_l, F_l) = \frac{\sum_{x,y,f} |I_l(x, y, f) - F_l(x, y, f)|}{\sum_{x,y,f} \max(I_l(x, y, f), F_l(x, y, f))} \tag{1}$$

where x and y iterate over all subimages and f iterates over all filters on layer l. Subtracting $A(I_l, F_l)$ from one yields our final measure of symmetry:

$$S(I_l, F_l) = 1 - A(I_l, F_l) \tag{2}$$

This measure is bounded between zero and one (for asymmetric images and for highly symmetric ones, respectively).

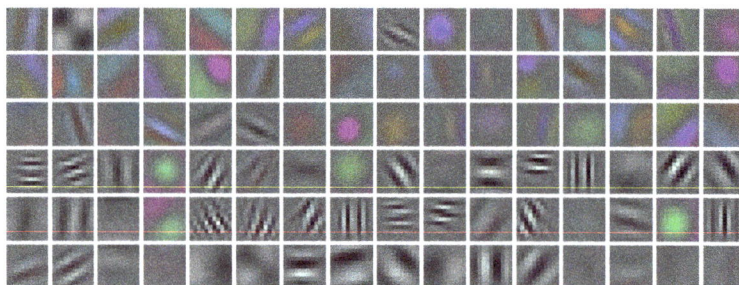

Figure 1. Filters of the first convolutional layer (conv1) of the Convolutional Neural Networks (CNN) architecture used in our experiment (*CaffeNet*; [24]). The filters detect oriented luminance edges and different spatial frequencies. Color is detected in form of oriented color-opponent edges and color blobs.

2.2. Image Dataset

In order to evaluate the algorithm proposed in Section 2.1, we used a dataset of 300 CD album covers that were collected from the internet in 2015 (kindly provided by Ms. Maria Grebenkina, University of Jena School of Medicine). Images were equally distributed between three different music genres (classic music, pop music and metal music). All cover images had a resolution of 500×500 pixels, or were down-sampled to this size by bicubic interpolation if the original image had a higher resolution. A complete list of the 300 CD covers used in this study is provided in Supplementary Table S1. The dataset is made available on request for scientific purposes (please contact author C.R.).

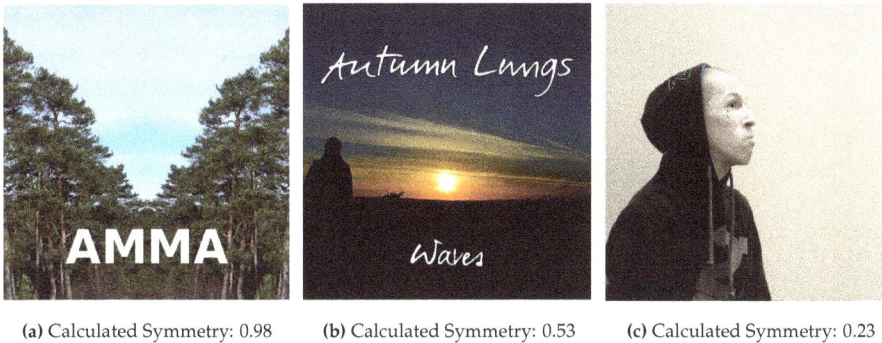

(a) Calculated Symmetry: 0.98   (b) Calculated Symmetry: 0.53   (c) Calculated Symmetry: 0.23

Figure 2. Representative covers and their respective calculated left/right symmetry values, which were obtained with first-layer filters at patch level 17. The images are of high symmetry (**a**); intermediate symmetry (**b**); and low symmetry (**c**); respectively. Due to copyright issues, we cannot reproduce covers used in our study here. Copyright: (**a**) author A.B.; (**b**) Graham James Worthington, CC BY-SA 4.0; and (**c**) Musiclive55, CC BY-SA 4.0.

2.3. Rating Experiment

Images of the 300 CD album covers (see above) were rated for their symmetry. Twenty participants (21–62 years old; Mean = 36 years; 6 male), mostly medical students or employees of the basic medical science department, participated in the experiment. All participants reported to have corrected-to-normal vision. Images were presented on a calibrated screen (EIZO ColorEdge CG241W, 1920×1200 pixels resolution) on a black background. A chin rest ensured a constant viewing distance of 70 cm. The images extended 500×500 pixels on the screen (135 mm $\times$ 135 mm, corresponding to 11×11 degrees of visual angle).

The study design was conducted in line with the ethical guidelines of the Declaration of Helsinki on human participants in experiments. The Ethics Committee of Jena University Hospital approved the procedure. Prior to participating in the study, all participants provided informed written consent on the procedure of the study. The participants were tested individually in front of the screen in a shaded room with the windows covered by blinds. First, the experimenter gave the instructions for the experiment. The participant was asked to rate the presented image according its left/right symmetry. The participants started the experiment with a mouse click. Then, for the first trial, a fixation cross appeared on the screen for between 300 and 800 ms followed by the first image. The question displayed on the screen below the image was "How symmetric is this image?" The participant rated the presented images on a continuous scale that was visualized as a white scoring bar on the bottom of the screen. The extremes of the scale were labeled as "not symmetric" and "very symmetric", respectively. Immediately after the response, the second trial with the next image was initiated, and so on. Images were presented in random order. After each of 100 trials, participants were allowed to take a rest for as long as they wished. The final symmetry rating value for each cover was defined as the median of the ratings of all 20 participants. To test for normality of the resulting data, D'Agostino and Pearson's normality test [26] was used.

3. Results

In order to validate the computer algorithm proposed in the present work, 20 participants rated the left/right symmetry of 300 covers from CD albums featuring pop music, metal music or classic music. For 97 covers, the distribution of ratings was not normally distributed ($p < 0.05$). As a representative value for a cover, we thus decided to use the median of all ratings for this cover. Figure 3 shows box-plot diagrams of the resulting subjective ratings for the three music genres. Median symmetry is highest for covers of metal music, intermediate for pop music, and lowest for covers of the classic genre. The symmetry ratings for all three music genres span a wide range of values, including extreme values. Consequently, the cover images seem sufficiently diverse with respect to their symmetry to serve as the ground truth in the validation of our model of left/right symmetry perception by human observers.

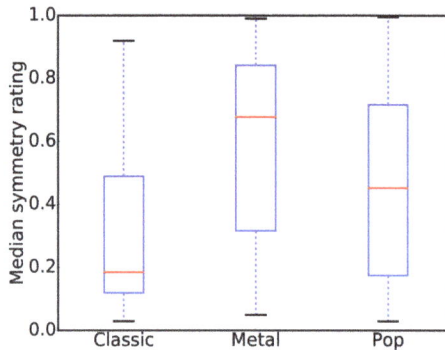

Figure 3. Subjective ratings for left/right symmetry in CD album covers of three music genres.

In order to maximize the correlation between the subjective ratings and the symmetry values calculated with our algorithm (see Section 2.1), we modified the following two parameters: First, we are free to chose which of the five convolutional layers of the CaffeNet model serves as a basis for the calculations. Second, we can decide how many subregions to use in the max-pooling operation. We therefore tested all five layers of the model. In addition, for layers conv1 and conv2, we obtained results for patch levels 2–32 and, for the upper layers, for patch levels 2–31 (note that the number of patches is restricted by the size of the response maps, which is 31×31 pixels for layers above conv2). We calculated our measure of symmetry for each of these parameter configurations (see Figure 2 for examples) and compared results with the human ratings. Because the distribution of ratings for many covers was not normally distributed ($p < 0.05$, D'Agostino and Pearson's normality test), Spearman's rank coefficients were calculated. Figure 4a plots the coefficients for the different model configurations. The correlation coefficients obtained for our model ranged from 0.64 (for convolutional layer 1 using patch level with 2 patches squared) to 0.90 (for convolutional layer 5 with 6 patches squared). Additionally, we provide the RMSE of a linear fit (Figure 4b), a quadratic fit (Figure 4c) and a cubic fit of the distributions (Figure 4d) to better understand the relation between our measure and the subjective ratings. Resulting trends are similar to those of the correlation analysis (Figure 4a); the quadratic and cubic models have a lower RMSE than the linear model, which indicates they provide a better fit of the relation between ratings and our measure.

For comparison, we implemented the symmetry measure recently proposed by [12] and measured a correlation of 0.34 for their model. Thus, all configurations tested in our model outperformed the previously proposed method. We also tried to compare our results with the approach described in [13]. However, due to missing details regarding the filtering process used in [13], we were not able to reproduce their results.

In our model, convolutional layer 1 performed worst with 2 patches squared, but results for this layer improved when more patches were used, i.e., when we use more, but smaller max-pooling regions. A plateau is reached at around 10 patches squared with a maximum correlation of 0.80 peak at 17 patches (Figure 4a).

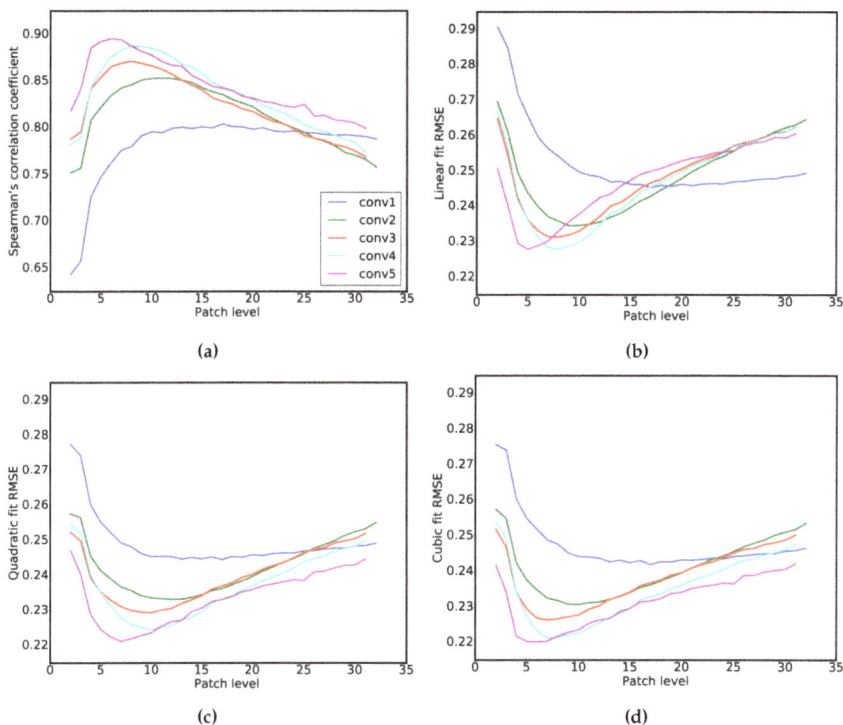

Figure 4. (**a**) Spearman's rank coefficients for the correlation between the subjective ratings and calculated values of left/right symmetry. Subjective ratings are plotted as a function of the number of subimages in the model for different layers of the CaffeNet model. The model parameters were systematically varied. The patch level squared corresponds to the number of subimages. The RMSE values of (**b**) a linear fit; (**c**) a quadratic fit and (**d**) a cubic fit show similar trends for all configurations. With quadratic and cubic polynomials, lower errors were obtained compared to the linear fit, which indicates that the relation between our measure and the subjective ratings is not linear.

Interestingly, the correlations between human ratings and our measure increase when higher layers of the network are used. For the second convolutional layer, the correlation peaks at 0.85 with 11 patches and then drops steadily as more patches are used, performing even worse than convolutional layer 1 at around 24 patches and above. The same can be observed for layers above layer 2 where the correlations peak at smaller number of patches and then drop rapidly. Specifically, the peak is reached at around 8 patches squared for layer 3 and 4, and at 6 patches squared for the highest (fifth) layer (see Figure 4).

In Figure 5, median symmetry ratings for each image are plotted as a function of the values calculated for two model configurations with high correlations. For both configurations, the rated and calculated values seem to correspond better at the extremes of the spectrum, i.e., for symmetry values closer to 0 or 1. In the mid-part of the spectrum, the two values correlated less well for the individual images. To visualize whether similar difference can also be observed at the level of individual observers, Figure 6 plots the standard deviation of all ratings for each cover over its median rating. The resulting plot shows an inverse u-curve shape, which means that the standard deviation of ratings is lower for highly symmetric covers and highly asymmetric covers, i.e., at the extremes, compared to symmetry values at the mid-part of the rating spectrum. In conclusion, while people tended to agree whether an image is highly symmetric or highly asymmetric, judgments show a higher deviation for images not falling into one of the extremes.

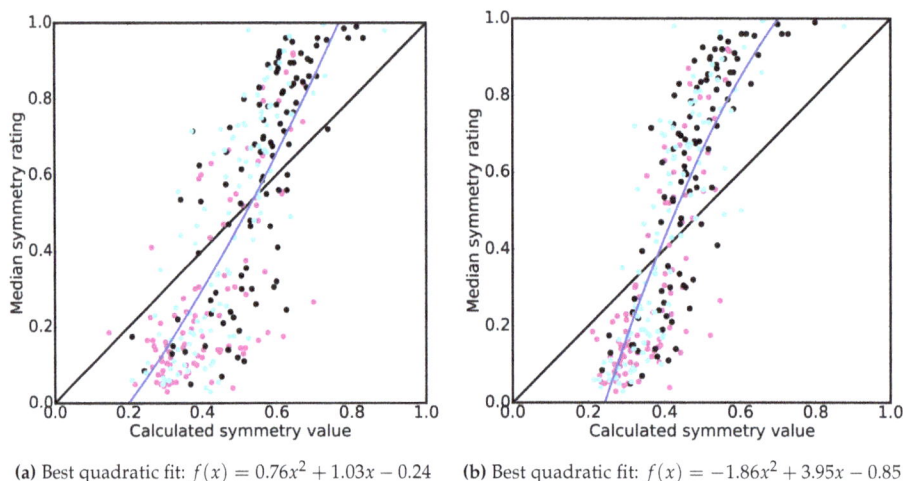

(a) Best quadratic fit: $f(x) = 0.76x^2 + 1.03x - 0.24$ **(b)** Best quadratic fit: $f(x) = -1.86x^2 + 3.95x - 0.85$

Figure 5. Scatter plot of rated symmetry values versus calculated symmetry values for two different configurations of the model (**a**, layer 1 with 17 patches squared, correlation of 0.80; **b**, layer 2 with 11 patches squared, correlation of 0.85). Each dot represents one cover image. Metal music covers are shown in black, pop music covers in cyan and classic music covers in magenta. The blue curve represents the best quadratic fit, as determined from the plots shown in Figure 4c.

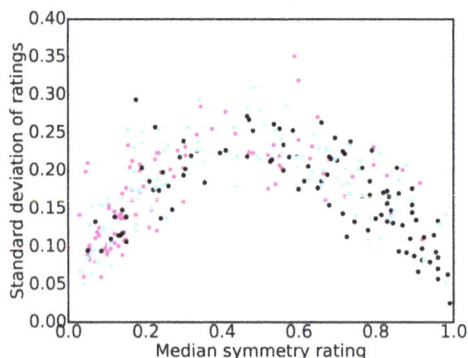

Figure 6. Standard deviation of the ratings of 20 participants for 300 CD album cover images, plotted as a function of the median rating for the covers. Each dot represents one cover image. Metal music covers are shown in black, pop music covers in cyan and classic music covers in magenta.

4. Discussion

In the present study, we introduce a novel computational measure of left/right symmetry that closely matches human perception, as exemplified for symmetry ratings of 300 CD album covers by human participants. Using CNN filter responses in our measure has two main advantages. First, CNN filters of the first layer are thought to resemble edge detectors akin to those found in the human visual system (Gabor-like filters [27]), as well as color detectors in form of color blobs and opponent color edges [19,25] (see Figure 1 for an illustration of filters used on conv1, the first layer). Similar to human vision, we can take luminance, color and spatial frequencies in an image into account simultaneously by using features from lower layers of the CNN. Second, because features are becoming increasingly abstract when using higher layers for the max-pooling maps, our symmetry measure is more likely to reflect human perception of symmetry because it takes into account the grouping of visual elements in the images as well as more abstract image features.

The first advantage may explain why our method outperforms the symmetry measure based on intensity values [12], which ignores color completely and does not deal with structural features like oriented edges. Furthermore, we group image regions over subimages (called *patches* in the present work), which makes our measure more robust with regard to image features that are somewhat symmetric but not exactly mirrored. Comparing intensity values of pixels alone does not address this issue. However, although we demonstrated that our approach works well for music cover art, it remains to be investigated whether it can also be applied to other types of images.

The emergence of increasingly abstract features at higher layers of the CNN can explain some of the trends that we observed in our experiment at different layers and for different patch sizes. On the one hand, when the patches become too big, our measure does not perform well because there is not much local detail taken into account. On the other hand, when regions become exceedingly small, grouping of luminance values is no longer possible over larger areas and, consequently, our measure does not correlate well with the ground truth data (i.e., the subjective symmetry ratings). Higher-layer features seem to resemble human symmetry perception more closely, if patch size is optimal at higher layers (Figure 4). We speculate that this resemblance can be explained by the fact that, when specific features or objects are prevalent in an image, larger patches are more tolerant regarding the exact position of these features or objects. For example, when people observe two faces in an image, one on the left side and one on the right side, the exact pixel positions of the faces are not critical for symmetry perception in our approach, as long as the faces have roughly corresponding positions with respect to the left/right symmetry axis.

Although the higher layers seem to resemble human symmetry perception of the CD album covers best, we cannot unconditionally recommend to use higher-layer features for getting the best results with other types of stimuli. Higher-layer features are not well understood yet, despite intense research [16,28,29]. Yosinski et al. [25] investigated how transferable learned features are between different tasks and found that the features from the first two layers only can be considered truly generic. Higher-layer features tend to be specific to the set of images that were used during training; this specificity may potentially limit their usefulness when novel images are encoded by the CNNs. Although we did not observe such a negative effect in our study, this potential problem should be kept in mind.

In order to evaluate the correlation between subjective ratings and calculated symmetry values, we measured Spearman's rank (non-parametric) correlation. Thus, we did not exactly replicate the behavioral measures, but predicted their relative strength. We observed that quadratic and cubic models fit the relation between our measure and the subjective ratings better than a linear model, which indicates that the relation between the two measures is not strictly linear. In other words, our algorithm does not match the exact subjective ratings that one would get from human observers. Rather, the algorithm predicts the relative subjective impression of symmetry in sets of images. This correspondence is strongest when symmetry is either very prominent or almost absent. With intermediate degrees of symmetry, human observers tend to agree less on how symmetric an image is (Figure 6). At the same time, the correspondence with the calculated values is less precise (Figure 5).

5. Conclusions

We propose a novel computational method that was developed to predict human left/right symmetry ratings for complex, non-geometrical images, as exemplified by CD album covers. The aim of the model is to closely match subjective symmetry as judged by human observers. For this purpose, we used filters learned by CNNs because they are akin to receptive fields in the early human visual system and get more and more abstract at higher layers of the CNNs. In order to evaluate our method, we compared the results from the computational model with subjective ratings by 20 participants who assessed left/right symmetry in a dataset of 300 different album covers. We evaluated different model configurations by calculating the correlation between the computationally obtained results and the ratings by humans.

Results demonstrate that our algorithm outperforms a recently proposed method for measuring continuous symmetry in an image by comparing pixel intensities [12]. Moreover, the correlation increased from 0.80 to 0.90 when we used filters from higher layers that focus on more abstract features. However, it remains to be established whether our approach also works for images other than album covers. For arbitrary images, we recommend to use second-layer features because they are known to be more universal than higher-layer features and lead to better results than first-layer features in our study.

In future research, we will use the proposed symmetry measure to study the role of symmetry in aesthetic perception, for example, by applying the measure to images of visual artworks and photographs.

Acknowledgments: The authors are grateful to Maria Grebenkina for providing the digital collection of CD album covers, and to members of the group for suggestions and discussions. This work was supported by funds from the Institute of Anatomy I, University of Jena School of Medicine.

Author Contributions: Anselm Brachmann and Christoph Redies conceived and designed the experiments; Anselm Brachmann performed the experiments and analyzed the data; Anselm Brachmann and Christoph Redies wrote the paper.

Conflicts of Interest: The authors declare no conflict of interest. The funding sponsors had no role in the design of the study; in the collection, analyses, or interpretation of data; in the writing of the manuscript, and in the decision to publish the results.

References

1. Bronshtein, I.; Semendyayev, K.; Musiol, G.; Mühlig, H. *Handbook of Mathematics*; Springer: Berlin/Heidelberg, Germany, 2015.
2. Wagemans, J. Detection of visual symmetries. *Spat. Vis.* **1995**, *9*, 9–32.
3. Grammer, K.; Thornhill, R. Human (Homo sapiens) facial attractiveness and sexual selection: The role of symmetry and averageness. *J. Comp. Psychol.* **1994**, *108*, 233.
4. Møller, A.P.; Swaddle, J.P. *Asymmetry, Developmental Stability and Evolution*; Oxford University Press: Oxford, UK, 1997.
5. Tinio, P.; Smith, J. *The Cambridge Handbook of the Psychology of Aesthetics and the Arts*; Cambridge Handbooks in Psychology; Cambridge University Press: Cambridge, UK, 2014.
6. Zaidel, D.W.; Aarde, S.M.; Baig, K. Appearance of symmetry, beauty, and health in human faces. *Brain Cogn.* **2005**, *57*, 261–263.
7. Jacobsen, T.; Höfel, L. Aesthetic judgments of novel graphic patterns: Analyses of individual judgments. *Percept. Motor Skills* **2002**, *95*, 755–766.
8. Liu, Y.; Hel-Or, H.; Kaplan, C.S.; Kaplan, C.S.; Van Gool, L. Computational symmetry in computer vision and computer graphics. *Found. Trends® Comput. Grap. Vis.* **2010**, *5*, 1–195.
9. Chen, P.-C.; Hays, J.; Lee, S.; Park, M.; Liu, Y. A quantitative evaluation of symmetry detection algorithms. In *Technical Report CMU-RI-TR-07-36*; Carnegie Mellon University: Pittsburgh, PA, USA, 2007.
10. Liu, J.; Slota, G.; Zheng, G.; Wu, Z.; Park, M.; Lee, S.; Rauschert, I.; Liu, Y. Symmetry detection from realworld images competition 2013: Summary and results. In Proceedings of the 2013 IEEE Conference on Computer Vision and Pattern Recognition Workshops, Portland, OR, USA, 25–27 June 2013; pp. 200–205.
11. Zabrodsky, H.; Peleg, S.; Avnir, D. Symmetry as a continuous feature. *IEEE Trans. Pattern Anal. Mach. Intell.* **1995**, *17*, 1154–1166.
12. Den Heijer, E. Evolving symmetric and balanced art. In *Computational Intelligence*; Springer: Berlin, Germany, 2015; pp. 33–47.
13. Shaker, F.; Monadjemi, A. A new symmetry measure based on gabor filters. In Proceedings of the 2015 23rd Iranian Conference on Electrical Engineering, Tehran, Iran, 10–14 May 2015; pp. 705–710.
14. Wurtz, R.; Kandel, E. Central visual pathway. In *Principles of Neural Science*, 4th ed.; Kandel, E., Schwartz, J., Jessell, T., Eds.; McGraw-Hill: New York, NY, USA, 2000; pp. 523–547.

15. Lennie, P. Color vision. In *Principles of Neural Science*, 4th ed.; ER, K., Schwartz, J., Jessell, T., Eds.; McGraw-Hill: New York, NY, USA, 2000; pp. 572–589.

16. Yosinski, J.; Clune, J.; Nguyen, A.; Fuchs, T.; Lipson, H. Understanding neural networks through deep visualization. In Proceedings of the Deep Learning Workshop, International Conference on Machine Learning (ICML), Lille, France, 10–11 July 2015.

17. LeCun, Y.; Bengio, Y. Convolutional networks for images, speech, and time series. In *The Handbook of Brain Theory and Neural Networks*; Massachusetts Institute of Technology (MIT) Press: Cambridge, MA, USA, 1995; pp. 255–258.

18. Lecun, Y.; Bottou, L.; Bengio, Y.; Haffner, P. Gradient-based learning applied to document recognition. *Proc. IEEE* **1998**, *86*, 2278–2324.

19. Krizhevsky, A.; Sutskever, I.; Hinton, G.E. Imagenet classification with deep convolutional neural networks. In *Advances in Neural Information Processing Systems*; Massachusetts Institute of Technology (MIT) Press: Cambridge, MA, USA, 2012; pp. 1097–1105.

20. Simonyan, K.; Zisserman, A. Very deep convolutional networks for large-scale image recognition. *Comput. Sci. arXiv* **2014**, arXiv:1409.1556.

21. Karpathy, A.; Fei-Fei, L. Deep visual-semantic alignments for generating image descriptions. In Proceedings of the IEEE Conference on Computer Vision and Pattern Recognition, Boston, MA, USA, 7–12 June 2015; pp. 3128–3137.

22. Gatys, L.A.; Ecker, A.S.; Bethge, M. Texture synthesis and the controlled generation of natural stimuli using convolutional neural networks. *Comput. Sci. arXiv* **2015**, arXiv:1505.07376.

23. Abdel-Hamid, O.; Mohamed, A.R.; Jiang, H.; Deng, L.; Penn, G.; Yu, D. Convolutional neural networks for speech recognition. *IEEE/ACM Trans. Audio Speech Lang. Process.* **2014**, *22*, 1533–1545.

24. Jia, Y.; Shelhamer, E.; Donahue, J.; Karayev, S.; Long, J.; Girshick, R.; Guadarrama, S.; Darrell, T. Caffe: convolutional architecture for fast feature embedding. In Proceedings of the 22nd Association of Computing Machinery (ACM) international conference on Multimedia, Orlando, FL, USA, 3–7 November 2014; pp. 675–678.

25. Yosinski, J.; Clune, J.; Bengio, Y.; Lipson, H. How transferable are features in deep neural networks? *Comput. Sci. arXiv* **2014**, arXiv:1411.1792.

26. D'Agostino, R.B. An omnibus test of normality for moderate and large size samples. *Biometrika* **1971**, *58*, 341–348.

27. Marčelja, S. Mathematical description of the responses of simple cortical cells. *J. Opt. Soc. Am.* **1980**, *70*, 1297–1300.

28. Zeiler, M.; Fergus, R. Visualizing and understanding convolutional networks. In Proceedings of the European Conference on Computer Vision, Zurich, Switzerland, 6–12 September 2014; pp. 818–833.

29. Mahendran, A.; Vedaldi, A. Understanding deep image representations by inverting them. In Proceedings of the 2015 IEEE Conference on Computer Vision and Pattern Recognition (CVPR), Boston, MA, USA, 7–12 June 2015; pp. 5188–5196.

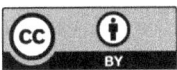

symmetry

MDPI

Article

The Conformal Camera in Modeling Active Binocular Vision

Jacek Turski

Department of Mathematics and Statistics, University of Houston-Downtown, Houston, TX 77002, USA; TurskiJ@uhd.edu or TurskiJ@gmail.com; Tel.: +1-713-349-9934

Academic Editor: Lewis Griffin
Received: 25 July 2016; Accepted: 25 August 2016; Published: 31 August 2016

Abstract: Primate vision is an active process that constructs a stable internal representation of the 3D world based on 2D sensory inputs that are inherently unstable due to incessant eye movements. We present here a mathematical framework for processing visual information for a biologically-mediated active vision stereo system with asymmetric conformal cameras. This model utilizes the geometric analysis on the Riemann sphere developed in the group-theoretic framework of the conformal camera, thus far only applicable in modeling monocular vision. The asymmetric conformal camera model constructed here includes the fovea's asymmetric displacement on the retina and the eye's natural crystalline lens tilt and decentration, as observed in ophthalmological diagnostics. We extend the group-theoretic framework underlying the conformal camera to the stereo system with asymmetric conformal cameras. Our numerical simulation shows that the theoretical horopter curves in this stereo system are conics that well approximate the empirical longitudinal horopters of the primate vision system.

Keywords: active vision; the conformal camera; the Riemann sphere; Möbius geometry; complex projective geometry; projective Fourier transform; retinotopy; binocular vision; horopter

---

1. Introduction

Primates must explore the environment with saccades and smooth pursuit eye movements because acuity in primate foveate vision is limited to a visual angle of a mere two degrees. With about four saccades/s, the high-acuity fovea can be successively fixated on the scene's salient and behaviorally-relevant parts at a speed of up to 900 deg/s. Smooth pursuit at up to 100 deg/s keeps the fovea focused on slowly-moving objects, while a combination of smooth pursuit and saccades tracks objects moving either unpredictably or faster than 30 deg/s.

In the primate brain, most of the neurons processing visual information encode the position of objects in gaze-centered coordinates, that is in the frame attached at the fovea in retino-cortical maps. Although this retinotopic information is constantly changing due to the eye's incessant movements, our perception appears stable. Thus, primate vision must be thought of as the outcome of an active process that constructs a clear and stable internal representation of the 3D world based on a combination of unstable sensory inputs and oculomotor signals.

Our computational methodology based on the conformal camera underlying geometric analysis of the Riemann sphere, developed in [1–3], addresses some of the challenges in modeling active vision. Most notably, by modeling the external scene projected on the retina of a rotating eye with the correspondingly updated retino-cortical maps, it can provide us with efficient algorithms capable of maintaining visual stability when imaging with an anthropomorphic camera head mounted on a moving platform replicating human eye movements [4–6].

In this paper, we first review the conformal camera's group-theoretic framework, which, till now, has only been formulated for modeling monocular vision. Then, we discuss the extension of this framework to a model of stereo vision that conforms to the physiological data of primate eyes. We divide the presented material into the prior and recent work and the original contributions.

1.1. Prior and Recent Work

This paper is organized in two parts. The first consists of Sections 2–4 that reviews our prior and recent work. In Section 2, the image projective transformations in the conformal camera are given by the Möbius group $\mathbf{PSL}(2, \mathbb{C})$ acting by linear fractional mappings on the camera's image plane identified with the Riemann sphere. The group $\mathbf{PSL}(2, \mathbb{C})$ establishes the group of holomorphic automorphisms of the complex structure on the Riemann sphere [7]. The invariants under these automorphisms furnish both Möbius geometry [8] and complex projective geometry [9].

Section 3 introduces both the continuous and discrete projective Fourier transforms. The group of image projective transformations in the conformal camera is the simplest semisimple group. Since representations on semisimple groups have a well-understood mathematical theory, we can provide the conformal camera that possesses its own Fourier analysis, a direction in the representation theory of the semisimple Lie groups [10]. The projective Fourier transform (PFT) is constructed by restricting Fourier analysis on the group $\mathbf{SL}(2, \mathbb{C})$, the double cover of $\mathbf{PSL}(2, \mathbb{C})$, to the image plane of the conformal camera. We stress that the complex projective geometry underlying the conformal camera contrasts with the real projective geometry usually used in computational vision, which does not possess meaningful Fourier analysis on its group of motions.

Next, in Section 4, we discuss the conformal camera's relevance to the computational aspects of anthropomorphic vision. We start here with a discussion of the conformal camera's relevance to early and intermediate-level vision. Then, we discuss the modeling of retinotopy with the conformal camera. We point out that the discrete PFT (DPFT) is computable by a fast Fourier transform algorithm (FFT) in the log-polar coordinates that approximate the retino-cortical maps of the visual and oculomotor pathways. These retinotopic maps are believed to be fundamental to the primate's cortical computations for processing visual and oculomotor information [11].

The DPFT of an integrable image is constructed after the image is regularized by removing a disk around the logarithmic singularity. This disk represents the foveal region. Then, we discuss the numerical implementation of the DPFT in image processing. Although the foveal vision is indispensable for our overal visual proficiency, it is rather less important to the proper functioning of the active vision that is mainly supported by peripheral processes [12].

We conclude this section by discussing the conformal camera's geometric analysis used in the development of efficient algorithms supporting the stability of visual information for a robotic eye mounted on the moving platform that replicates human smooth pursuit and saccadic eye movements [4,6].

1.2. Original Contributions

The second part of this paper studies the extension of our modeling with the conformal camera to binocular vision. In Section 5, after we review the background of biological stereo vision, we explain how the conformal camera can model the stereo system with a simplified version of the schematic eye, one with a spherical eyeball and rotational symmetry about the optical axis. In contrast to this simplified eye model, the fovea center in the primate's eye is supratemporal on the retina, and the visual axis that connects the fixation point with the fovea center is angled about 5.2 degrees nasally to the optical axis.

In Section 6, we develop the asymmetric conformal camera model of the eye that includes both the fovea's asymmetric displacement and the lens' tilt and decentration observed in ophthalmological diagnostics. From the group-theoretic framework of the asymmetric conformal camera, we conclude that tilting and translating the image plane is like putting 'conformal glasses' on the standard conformal camera. Finally, in Section 7, we demonstrate, by a numerical simulation in GeoGebra, that the resulting horizontal horopter curves can be seen as conics that well approximate the empirical horopters, as originally postulated in [13].

1.3. Related Work

Directly related to our work is the modeling done by Schwartz' group [14,15]. Each of both approaches uses a different complex logarithmic function for modeling human retinotopy. Later in Section 4.3, we compare these two models. In addition to complex logarithmic mappings, different foveated mappings have been proposed in biologically-mediated image processing, for example [16,17].

There are also other less directly related approaches. In [18], the depth reconstruction from water drops is developed and evaluated. The three key steps used are: the water-drop 3D shape reconstruction, depth estimation using stereo and water-drop image rectification. However, the lack of high resolution images of water drops degraded the overall performance of the depth estimation.

Maybe the most interesting work is presented in [19], which develops the catadioptric camera that used a planar spherical mirror array. This reference, in particular, considered digital refocusing for artistic depth of field effects in wide-angle scenes and wide-angle dense depth estimation. In another setup, the spherical mirrors in the array were replaced with refractive spheres, and the image captured by looking through a planar array of refractive acrylic balls was shown in [19]. We wonder if this setup could model the vision systems based on the insects' compound eyes. One can possibly arrange the refractive spheres' array on the convex surface to produce the wraparound vision of insects.

2. The Conformal Camera

The conformal camera with the underlying geometric and computational framework was proposed in [1].

2.1. Stereographic Projection

The conformal camera consists of a unit sphere S^2 that models the retina and a plane $\mathbb{C}$ through the sphere's center O where the image processing takes place. The spatial points are centrally projected onto both the sphere and the image plane through the nodal point N, chosen on the sphere such that the line interval ON is perpendicular to the image plane; see Figure 1.

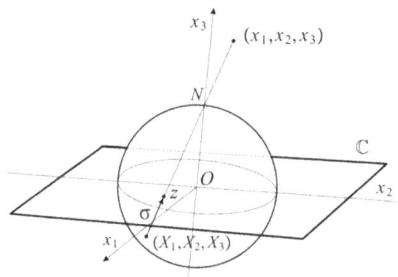

Figure 1. The conformal camera as the eye model. The points in the object space are centrally projected into the sphere. The sphere and the center of projection N represent the eye's retina and nodal point. The 'image' entity is given by stereographic projection σ from the sphere to the plane $\mathbb{C}$. Because σ is conformal and maps circles to circles (see the text), it preserves the 'retinal illuminance', that is the pixels. This image representation is appropriate for efficient computational processing.

The camera's orientation in space is described by a positively-oriented orthonormal frame (e_1, e_2, e_3), such that $e_3 = \overrightarrow{ON}$. The frame is attached to the camera's center O, giving spatial coordinates (x_1, x_2, x_3). The image plane $x_3 = 0$ is parametrized with complex coordinates $x_1 + ix_2$. Then, the projection into the image plane $\mathbb{C}$ is given by:

$$j(x_1, x_2, x_3) = z = \frac{x_1 + ix_2}{1 - x_3}. \tag{1}$$

The restriction of (1) to the sphere $S^2 \setminus \{N\}$ defines stereographic projection $\sigma = j|_{S^2}$. In this definition, the mapping σ is extended by $\sigma(N) = \infty$ with the point ∞ appended to the image plane $\mathbb{C}$, identifying the sphere S^2 with the extended image plane $\hat{\mathbb{C}} = \mathbb{C} \cup \{\infty\}$. With this identification, $\hat{\mathbb{C}}$ is known as the Riemann sphere. Stereographic projection σ is conformal, that is the mapping σ preserves the angle of two intersecting curves. In addition, stereographic projection maps circles in the sphere that do not contain N to a circle in the plane and maps a circle passing through N to a line that can be considered a circle through ∞ [20].

2.2. The Group of Image Projective Transformations

A stationary planar object, or a planar surface of a 3D object, shown in Figure 2 as a black rectangular region in the scene, is projected into the image plane in the initial gaze (Gaze 1) of the conformal camera. The gaze change from Gaze 1 to Gaze 2 is shown in Figure 2 as a horizontal rotation ϕ.

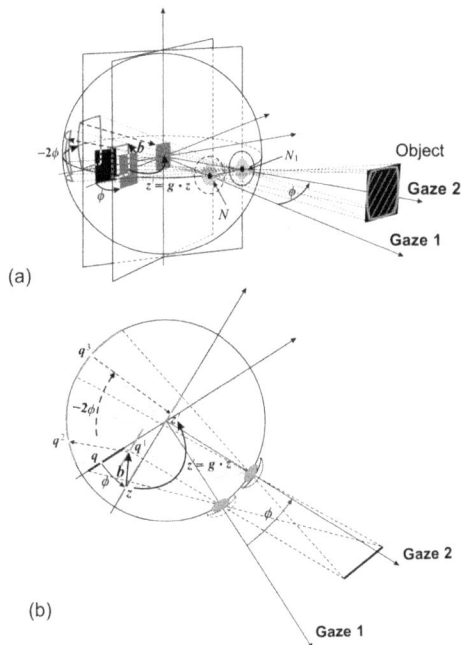

(a)

(b)

Figure 2. (**a**) When the camera gaze is rotated by ϕ, the image projective transformation is given here in the rotated image plane by the g-transformation that results from the composition of two basic image transformations. The first involves the image that is translated by the vector (**b**) and projected back into the image plane. The second transformation is given in terms of the image projected into the sphere, rotated by -2ϕ, and projected back into the image plane. The image transformation adds the conformal distortions, schematically shown by the transformed image's back projection into the plane containing the planar object. (**b**) The camera and scene are shown in the view seen when looking from above. Here, the sequence of transformations $q \mapsto z \mapsto q^1 \mapsto q^2 \mapsto q^3 \mapsto z' = g \cdot z$ explains the image projective transformation.

The image transformations resulting from the gaze change are compositions of the two basic transformations that are schematically shown in Figure 2 in the rotated image plane. Alternatively, these transformations can be formulated in the initial image plane [6].

The first basic image transformation, the h-transformation, is rendered by translating the object's projected image by $\mathbf{b} = \langle b_1, b_2, b_3 \rangle$ and then projecting it centrally through the rotated nodal point N_1 back into the image plane (stereographic projection σ in Figure 1). It is given by the following mapping:

$$h(b_1 b_2, b_3) \cdot z = \frac{z + b_1 + ib_2}{1 - b_3} = \frac{\delta z + \gamma \delta}{1/\delta} = \begin{bmatrix} \delta & \gamma \delta \\ 0 & 1/\delta \end{bmatrix} \cdot z \tag{2}$$

where $\delta = (1 - b_3)^{-1/2}$ and $\gamma = b_1 + ib_2$. The last equality in (2) defines the linear-fractional mapping in terms of the matrix h.

The second basic image transformation resulting from the gaze rotation with the angle ϕ is denoted as the k-transformation. This transformation is defined by projecting the output from the h-transformation into the sphere through the center of projection N_1, rotating it with the sphere by the angle -2ϕ and then projecting it back to the (rotated) image plane. Here, the gaze rotation with ϕ results in the sphere rotation by -2ϕ by the central angle theorem. In general, the image transformation corresponding to the gaze rotation by the Euler angles (ψ, ϕ, ψ') is the following k-transformation:

$$k(\psi, -2\phi, \psi') \cdot z = \frac{\alpha z + \beta}{-\overline{\beta} z + \overline{\alpha}} = \begin{bmatrix} \alpha & \beta \\ -\overline{\beta} & \overline{\alpha} \end{bmatrix} \cdot z, \tag{3}$$

where $\alpha = e^{-i(\psi+\psi')/2} \cos \phi$ and $\beta = -e^{-i(\psi-\psi')/2} \sin \phi$.

In the k-transformation, rotation angles can be assumed to be known, for they are used by the biological vision system to program the eye movements that fixate targets. We have shown in [5] how to estimate the intended gaze rotation from the image of the target. The h-transformation is given in terms of the unknown vector $\mathbf{b} = \langle b_1, b_2, b_3 \rangle$.

The composition of the basic transformations in (2) and (3),

$$\begin{aligned} g \cdot z &= k(\psi, -2\phi, \psi') \cdot [h(b_1 b_2, b_3) \cdot z] \\ &= [k(\psi, -2\phi, \psi') h(b_1 b_2, b_3)] \cdot z, \end{aligned} \tag{4}$$

can be done with the multiplication of matrices, as shown in the second line of (4).

Because the mappings (4) are conformal, they introduce the conformal distortions shown in Figure 2 by the back-projected gray-shaded region outlined on the object in the scene. Although these distortions could be removed with minimal computational cost [1,3], we do not, because they are useful in visual information processing [5].

In the language of groups, $h(b_1, b_2, b_3) \in \mathbf{A}\widetilde{\mathbf{N}}$, where:

$$\mathbf{A} = \left\{ \begin{bmatrix} \delta & 0 \\ 0 & \delta^{-1} \end{bmatrix} : \delta > 0 \right\} \text{ and } \widetilde{\mathbf{N}} = \left\{ \begin{bmatrix} 1 & \gamma \\ 0 & 1 \end{bmatrix} : \gamma \in \mathbb{C} \right\} \tag{5}$$

and $k(\psi, -2\phi, \psi') \in \mathbf{SU}(2)$, where:

$$\mathbf{SU}(2) = \left\{ \begin{bmatrix} \alpha & \beta \\ -\overline{\beta} & \overline{\alpha} \end{bmatrix} : |\alpha|^2 + |\beta|^2 = 1 \right\}$$

is the double cover of the group of rotations $\mathbf{SO}(3)$ [21]. Thus, $\mathbf{SU}(2)$ is isomorphic to the group of unit quaternions.

The polar decomposition $\mathbf{SL}(2, \mathbb{C}) = \mathbf{SU}(2)\mathbf{A}\mathbf{SU}(2)$, where:

$$\mathbf{SL}(2,\mathbb{C}) = \left\{ \begin{bmatrix} a & b \\ c & d \end{bmatrix} : ad - bc = 1 \right\},$$

implies that the finite iterations of h- and k-transformations generate the action of $\mathbf{SL}(2,\mathbb{C})$ on the Riemann sphere $\hat{\mathbb{C}}$ by linear-fractional mappings:

$$\begin{bmatrix} a & b \\ c & d \end{bmatrix} \cdot z = \frac{az + b}{cz + d} \tag{6}$$

such that:

$$\begin{bmatrix} a & b \\ c & d \end{bmatrix} \cdot \infty = a/c, \quad \begin{bmatrix} a & b \\ c & d \end{bmatrix} \cdot (-d/c) = \infty \text{ if } c \neq 0, \text{ and } \begin{bmatrix} a & b \\ 0 & d \end{bmatrix} \cdot \infty = \infty.$$

An image intensity function f's projective transformations are given by the following action:

$$f(z) \longmapsto f\left(g^{-1} \cdot z \right) = f\left(\frac{dz - c}{-bz + a} \right), \quad g = \begin{bmatrix} a & b \\ c & d \end{bmatrix} \in \mathbf{PSL}(2,\mathbb{C}) \tag{7}$$

where we need the quotient group:

$$\mathbf{PSL}(2,\mathbb{C}) = \mathbf{SL}(2,\mathbb{C})/\{\pm Id\}$$

to identify matrices $\pm g$ because $g \cdot z = (-g) \cdot z$.

2.3. Geometry of the Image Plane

The group $\mathbf{PSL}(2,\mathbb{C})$ with the action (6) is known as the Möbius group of holomorphic automorphisms on the Riemann sphere $\hat{\mathbb{C}}$ that gives the complex, or analytic, structure on $\hat{\mathbb{C}}$ [7]. In the Kleinian view of geometry, known as the Erlanger program, Möbius geometry is the study of invariants under the group of holomorphic automorphisms [8]. Further, the group $\mathbf{PSL}(2,\mathbb{C})$ also defines the projective geometry of a one-dimensional complex space [9], giving us the isomorphism of the complex projective line and the Riemann sphere. This means that the conformal camera synthesizes geometric and analytic, or numerical, structures to provide a unique computational environment that is geometrically precise and numerically efficient.

The image plane of the conformal camera does not admit a distance that is invariant under image projective transformations. Consequently, the geometry of the camera does not possess a Riemann metric. For instance, there are no geodesics and curvature. However, because linear-fractional transformations map circles to circles, circles may play the role of geodesics, with the inverse of the circle's radius playing the role of curvature. This makes the conformal camera relevant to the intermediate-level vision computational aspects of natural scene understanding, later discussed in Section 4.2.

3. Fourier Analysis on the Projective Group

3.1. Group Representations and Fourier Analysis

The main role of the theory of group representation, in relation to Fourier analysis, is to decompose the space of square-integrable functions defined on a set the group acts naturally on in terms of the irreducible unitary representations; the simplest homomorphisms of the group into the set of unitary linear operators on a Hilbert space.

In this decomposition, the generalized Fourier transform plays the same role on any group as the classical Fourier transform does on the additive group of real numbers. In this classical case of Fourier transform, the irreducible unitary representations are homomorphisms of the additive group into the multiplicative group of complex numbers of modulus one, or the circle group. These homomorphisms are given by the complex exponential functions present in the standard Fourier integral [22].

Because group theory underlies geometry through Klein's Erlanger program that classifies most of geometries by the corresponding groups of transformations, this geometric Fourier analysis emphasizes the covariance of the decompositions with respect to the geometric transformations.

The group $\mathbf{SL}(2,\mathbb{C})$ is the simplest of semisimple groups that have a well-understood representation theory initiated by Gelfand's school and completed by Harish-Chandra [23].

Therefore, the conformal camera possesses its own Fourier analysis well adapted to image projective transformations given by the group $\mathbf{SL}(2,\mathbb{C})$ acting on the Hilbert space of square-integrable functions on the image plane $\widehat{\mathbb{C}}$ [2,3].

3.2. Projective Fourier Transform

The projective Fourier analysis has been constructed by restricting geometric Fourier analysis on $\mathbf{SL}(2,\mathbb{C})$ to the image plane of the conformal camera (see Section 7 in [2]). The resulting projective Fourier transform (PFT) of a given image intensity function f is the following:

$$\hat{f}(s,k) = \frac{i}{2} \int f(z)|z|^{-is-1} \left(\frac{z}{|z|}\right)^{-k} dz d\bar{z}, \tag{8}$$

where $(s,k) \in \mathbf{R} \times \mathbf{Z}$, and, if $z = x_1 + ix_2$, then $(i/2)dz d\bar{z} = dx_1 dx_2$. In log-polar coordinates (u,θ) given by $\ln re^{i\theta} = \ln r + i\theta = u + i\theta$, (8) takes on the form of the standard Fourier integral:

$$\hat{f}(s,k) = \int f(e^{u+i\theta})e^u e^{-i(us+\theta k)} du d\theta. \tag{9}$$

Inverting it, we obtain the representation of the image intensity function in the (u,θ)-coordinates,

$$e^u f(u,\theta) = \frac{1}{(2\pi)^2} \sum_{k=-\infty}^{\infty} \int \hat{f}(s,k)e^{i(us+\theta k)} ds,$$

where $f(u,\theta) = f(e^{u+i\theta})$. We stress that although the functions f and f have the same values at the corresponding points, they are defined on different spaces; the function f is defined on the log-polar space (the cortical visual area), while f is defined on the image plane (the retina).

The construction of the discrete PFT is aided by fact that, despite the logarithmic singularity of log-polar coordinates, an image f that is integrable on $\mathbb{C} \setminus \{0\}$ has finite PFT:

$$|\hat{f}(s,k)| \leq \int_0^{2\pi} \int_{-\infty}^{u_1} f(e^{u+i\theta})e^u du d\theta = \int_0^{2\pi} \int_0^{r_1} f(re^{i\theta}) dr d\theta < \infty. \tag{10}$$

3.3. Non-Compact and Compact Realizations of PFT

It should be noted that the one-dimensional PFT was constructed from the infinite dimensional Fourier transform on $\mathbf{SL}(2,\mathbb{C})$ in the non-compact picture of irreducible unitary representations of group $\mathbf{SL}(2,\mathbb{C})$; see [2]. Later in [3], the second, finite dimensional projective Fourier transform was constructed in the compact picture of irreducible unitary representations of group $\mathbf{SL}(2,\mathbb{C})$. Both pictures have been used to study group representations in semisimple representation theory; each picture simplifies representations by emphasizing different aspects without the loss of information; see [10].

The functions $\Pi_{k,s}(z) = |z|^{is} \left(\frac{z}{|z|}\right)^k$ in the projective Fourier transform (8) play the role of exponentials in the standard Fourier transform. In the language of group representation theory, one-dimensional representations $\Pi_{k,s}(z)$ are the only unitary representations of the Borel subgroup $\mathbf{B} = \mathbf{MAN}$ of $\mathbf{SL}(2,\mathbb{C})$, where:

$$\mathbf{M} = \left\{ \begin{bmatrix} e^{i\theta} & 0 \\ 0 & e^{-i\theta} \end{bmatrix} \right\}, \ \mathbf{N} = \tilde{\mathbf{N}}^T.$$

In contrast, all of the nontrivial irreducible unitary representations of $\mathbf{SL}(2,\mathbb{C})$ are infinite-dimensional. Now, the group $\mathbf{B}$ 'exhausts' the projective group $\mathbf{SL}(2,\mathbb{C})$ by Gauss decomposition $\mathbf{SL}(2,\mathbb{C}) \doteq \tilde{\mathbf{N}}\mathbf{B}$, where '$\doteq$' means that equality holds up to a lower dimensional subset of the zero measure, that is almost everywhere, and $\tilde{\mathbf{N}}$ in (5) represents Euclidean translations under the action (6). These facts justify the use of the name 'projective Fourier transform' and allow us to develop numerically-efficient implementations of this transform in image processing well adapted to projective transformations [2].

3.4. Discrete Projective Fourier Transform

It follows from (10) that we can remove a disk $|z| \leq r_a$ to regularize f, such that the support of $f(u, \theta)$ is contained within $(\ln r_a, \ln r_b) \times [0, 2\pi)$, and approximate the integral in (9) by a double Riemann sum with equally-spaced partition points:

$$(u_k, \theta_l) = (\ln r_a + \delta k, \frac{2\pi}{N} l), \tag{11}$$

where $0 \leq k \leq M - 1, 0 \leq l \leq N - 1$ and $\delta = T/M$ with $T = \ln(r_b/r_a)$. We can obtain (see [2] for details) the discrete projective Fourier transform (DPFT),

$$\hat{f}_{m,n} = \sum_{k=0}^{M-1} \sum_{l=0}^{N-1} f_{k,l} e^{u_k} e^{-i2\pi mk/M} e^{-i2\pi nl/N} \tag{12}$$

and its inverse,

$$f_{k,l} = \frac{1}{MN} \sum_{m=0}^{M-1} \sum_{n=0}^{N-1} \hat{f}_{m,n} e^{-u_k} e^{i2\pi mk/M} e^{i2\pi nl/N}, \tag{13}$$

where $f_{k,l} = (2\pi T/MN)f(e^{u_k} e^{i\theta_l})$ are image plane samples and $f_{k,l} = (2\pi T/MN)f(u_k, \theta_l)$ are log-polar samples. Both expressions (12) and (13) can be computed efficiently by FFT.

4. Discussion: Biologically-Mediated Vision

4.1. Imaging with the Conformal Camera

The action of the group of image projective transformations on the image function is given without precise relation to the object; recall the definition of the h-transformation in (2). Even for horizontal rotations of the conformal camera, vector b needs to be defined. However, this vector does not need to be defined when imaging with the conformal camera is applied to processing visual information during saccades [4]. On the other hand, for processing visual information during smooth pursuit with the conformal camera, the analytical expression for the vector b was derived in [6] by using the objects' relative motions. Later in Section 4.5, we review the results obtained in [4,6] that make possible the development of algorithmic steps for processing visual information in an anthropomorphic camera head mounted on the moving platform that replicates human eye movements.

Moreover, the imaging with the conformal camera must be considered only for 'planar' objects, that is the planar surfaces of 3D objects. To justify this requirement, we note that only the most basic features are extracted from the impinged visual information on the retina before being sent to the areas of the brain used for processing. Thus, the initial image of the centrally-projected scene is comprised of numerous brightness and color spots from many different locations in space and does not contain explicit information about the perceptual organization of the scene [24]. What is initially perceived is a small number of objects' surfaces segmented from the background and each other [25]. The object's

3D attributes and the scene's spatial organizations are acquired when 2D projections on the retina are processed by numerous cortical areas downstream the visual pathway. This processing extracts the monocular information (texture gradients, relative size, linear and aerial perspectives, shadows and motion parallax) and, when two eyes see the scene, the binocular information (depth and shape).

4.2. Intermediate-Level Vision

Intermediate-level vision is made up of perceptual analyses carried out by the brain and is responsible for our ability to identify objects when they are partially occluded and our ability to perceive an object to be the same even as size and perspective changes.

For more comprehensive discussion of the relevance of the conformal camera to computational aspects of intermediate vision we refer to [4]. Here, following this reference, we only mention how the fact that the conformal camera's image plane geometry does not possess the invarient distance, is not preventing intermediate-level shape recognition. The brain employs two basic intermediate-level vision descriptors in identifying global objects: the medial axis transformation [26] and the curvature extrema [27]. The medial axis, which the visual system extracts as a skeletal description of objects [28], can be defined as the set of the centers of the maximal circles inscribed inside the contour. The curvatures at the corresponding points of the contour are given by the inverse radii of the circles.

Since circles are preserved under image projective transformations, the intermediate-level descriptors are preserved during the conformal camera's movements. We conclude that imaging with the conformal camera should be relevant to modeling primate visual perception that is supported by intermediate-level vision processes.

4.3. DPFT in Modeling Retinotopy

Information from the visual field, sampled and processed by the retina, arrives to the midbrain's superior colliculus (SC) and, via the lateral geniculate nucleus (LGN), to the primary visual cortex (V1). Both SC and V1 contain retinotopic maps. These retinotopic maps can be characterized by the following principle (e.g., [29]): for the contralateral visual field, retinotopy transforms the retinal polar coordinates centered at the fovea to the cortical coordinates given by the perpendicular polar and eccentricity axes. Further, the amount of cortical tissue dedicated to the representation of a unit distance on the retina, the magnification factor, is inversely related to its eccentricity, implying that foveal regions are characterized by a large cortical magnification, with the extrafoveal region scaled logarithmically with eccentricity [29].

As the retinal image changes during gaze rotations, the retinotopic map in V1 undergoes the corresponding changes that form the input for subsequent topographically-organized visual areas.

The mappings $w = \ln(z \pm a) - \ln a$ give an accepted approximation of the retinotopic structure in V1 and SC areas [15,30], where $a > 0$ removes logarithmic singularity and $\pm a$ indicates either the left or right brain hemisphere, depending on its sign. On the other hand, the DPFT that provides the data model for image representation can be efficiently computed by FFT in log-polar coordinates given by the complex logarithmic mapping $w = \ln z$. Thus, this logarithmic mapping must be used in our model to approximate retinotopy.

However, both complex logarithmic mappings give similar approximations for the peripheral region. In fact, for $|z| \ll a$, $\ln(z \pm a) - \ln a$ is well approximated by $\pm z/a$, while for $|z| \gg a$, it is dominated by $\ln z$. Moreover, to construct discrete sampling for DPFT, the image is regularized by removing a disk $|z| \leq r_a$, which represents the foveal region that contains the singularity of $\ln z$ at $z = 0$. Although it may seem at first that our model is compromised by the loss of a foveal region of about a 2 deg central angle, our next discussion demonstrates how the opposite may be true.

From the basic properties of $\ln z$,

$$\ln(e^{i\phi}z) = \ln z + i\phi, \quad \ln(\rho z) = \ln z + \ln \rho,$$

it follows that the rotation and dilation transformations of an intensity function in exp-polar coordinates $f(e^u e^{i\theta})$ correspond to simple translations of the log-polar image $\mathfrak{f}(u, \theta)$ via:

$$f(e^{i\phi} e^u e^{i\theta}) = f\left(e^u e^{i(\theta+\phi)}\right) = \mathfrak{f}(u, \theta + \phi)$$

and:

$$f(\rho e^u e^{i\theta}) = f(e^{u+v} e^{i\theta}) = \mathfrak{f}(u + v, \theta).$$

The functions f and $\mathfrak{f}$ were introduced in Section 3.2.

These distinctive features of $\ln z$ are useful in the development of image identification and recognition algorithms. The Schwartz model of retinotopy, therefore, results in the destruction of these properties so critical to computational vision.

Further, psychophysiological evidence suggests the difference in the functional roles that fovea and periphery play in vision. These different roles, very likely, involve different image processing principles [31,32]. An example of the separation in foveal and peripheral processing is explained in [31] in the context of curve balls in baseball. Often, batters report that balls undergo a dramatic and nearly discontinuous shift in their position as they dive in a downward path near home plate. This shift in the ball's position occurs when the image of the ball passes the boundary on the retina between these two regions. The authors argue in [31] that this phenomenon is a result of the differences between foveal and peripheral processing.

We finally mention the computational advantages of representing images in terms of the PFT rather than in terms of the exponential chirp transform (ECT) developed by the Schwartz research group in [14]. The ECT is constructed by making the substitution:

$$(x, y) = (e^u \cos \theta, e^u \sin \theta) \tag{14}$$

in the standard 2D Fourier integral. Because the Jacobian of the transformation (14) is translation-invariant, this substitution makes the ECT well adapted to translations in Cartesian coordinates. There is then a clear dissonance between the nonuniform retinal image sampling grid and this shift invariance of the ECT. On the other hand, the PFT is a genuine Fourier transform constructed from irreducible unitary representations of the group of image projective transformations. Further, the change of variables by:

$$u = \ln r \tag{15}$$

transforms the PFT into the standard Fourier integral. Thus, the discrete PFT is computable by FFT in log-polar coordinates that approximate the retinotopy.

The difference between (14) and (15) implies that the PFT does not experience the problem of exponentially-growing frequencies, like the ECT does, and for a band-limited original image, there is no difficulty with the Nyquist sampling condition in log-polar space [2,3].

4.4. Numerical Implementation of DPFT

The DPFT approximation was obtained using the rectangular sampling grid (u_k, θ_l) in (11), corresponding, under the mapping:

$$u_k + i\theta_l \longmapsto z_{k,l} = e^{u_k + i\theta_l} = r_k e^{i\theta_l},$$

to a nonuniform sampling grid with equal sectors:

$$\alpha = \theta_{l+1} - \theta_l = \frac{2\pi}{N}, l = 0, 1, ..., N - 1$$

and exponentially-increasing radii:

$$\rho_k = r_{k+1} - r_k = e^{u_{k+1}} - e^{u_k} = e^{u_k}(e^\delta - 1) = r_k(e^\delta - 1), k = 0, 1, ..., M - 1,$$

where $\delta = u_{k+1} - u_k$ is the spacing $\delta = T/M$ and $r_0 = r_a$ is the radius of the disc that has been removed to regularize the logarithmic singularity of $u = \ln r$.

For completeness of this discussion, we recall our calculations in [4]. To do this, we assume that we have been given a picture of the size $A \times B$ displayed with K dots per unit length. In addition, we assume that the retinal coordinates' origin is the picture's center. The central disc of radius r_0 represents the foveal region of a uniform sampling grid with the number of the pixels N_f, given by $\pi r_0^2 = N_f/K^2$. The number of sectors is obtained from the condition $2\pi(r_0 + r_1)/2 \approx N(1/K)$, where $N = [2\pi r_0 K + \pi]$. Here, $[a]$ is the closest integer to a. To obtain the number of rings M, we assume that $\rho_0 = r_0(e^\delta - 1) = 1/K$ and $r_b = r_M = r_0 e^{M\delta}$. We can take either $r_b = (1/K)\min(A, B)/2$ or $r_b = (1/K)\sqrt{A^2 + B^2}/2$. Thus, $\delta = \ln[(1 + 1/r_0 K]$ and $M = (1/\delta)\ln(r_b/r_0)$.

Example 1. *We let $A \times B = 512 \times 512$ and $K = 4$ per mm, so that the physical dimensions in mm are 128×128 and $r_b = 128\sqrt{2}/2 = 90.5$. Furthermore, we let $N_f = 296$, so that $r_0 = 2.427$ and $N = 64$. Finally, $\delta = \ln(10.7084/9.7084) \approx 0.09804$ and $(1/0.09804)\ln(90.5/2.427) \approx M = 37$. The sampling grid consists of points in polar coordinates: $(r_k + \rho_{k+1}/2, \theta_l + \pi/64) = (2.552 e^{k0.09804}, (2l + 1)\pi/64)$, $k = 0, 1, ..., 36, l = 0, 1, ..., 63$.*

In this example, the original image has 262,144 pixels, whereas both foveal and peripheral representations of the image contain only 2,664 pixels. Thus, there are about 100-times more pixels in the original image than in the image sampled in log-polar coordinates. To compare, light carrying visual information about the external world is initially sampled by about 125 million photoreceptors. When processed by the retinal circuitry, this visual information converges on about 1.5 million ganglion cell axons that carry the output from the eye.

4.5. Visual Information during Robotic Eye Movements

There are significant differences in the way visual information in a robotic eye with the silicon retina is processed during smooth pursuit and saccades. When a robotic eye is tracking a slowly-moving target by stabilizing its image on the high-acuity central region of a silicon retina, the image of the stationary background is sweeping across the retina in the opposite direction. The sensory information used in maintaining perceptual stability includes the retinal motion information and the extraretinal information, such as intended eye movements or short-time memory of previous movements [33]. On the other hand, the high saccadic rotational speed markedly restricts the use of visual information during eye movements between fixations. Therefore, the discrete difference between the visual information at the initial gaze position and at the saccade's target must be used in the perisaccadic image processing to support perceptual stability. Identification of the visuosaccadic pathway [34] supports the idea that the brain uses a copy of the oculomotor command of the impending saccade, referred to as the efference copy, to shift transiently neuronal activities of stimuli to their future location before the eyes' saccade takes them there. This shift gives access to the visual information at the saccade target before the saccade is executed. It is believed that this predictive remapping mechanism contributes to visual stability [35].

4.5.1. Visual Information during Smooth Pursuit

During smooth pursuit, anticipatory planning is needed for perceptual stability of an autonomous robot. In [6], the stationary background's image transformations during the horizontal gaze rotations are obtained using the relative motions of the background with respect to the conformal camera.

Figure 3 shows the horizontal intersection of the conformal camera and the scene. It explains how the vector **b** is defined in terms of the relative motions of the line segment PQ, the horizontal intersection of the planar object.

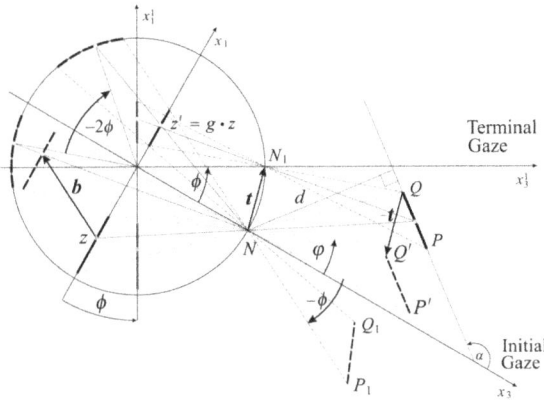

Figure 3. When the camera gaze is rotated by ϕ, the image projective transformation is given by the g-transformation where $g = kh$ is the result of the composition of the line segment PQ relative movements. Since the gaze rotation induces the nodal point translation by $\mathbf{t}$, the object PQ relative movements in the scene are composed of the translation by $-\mathbf{t}$ corresponding to the translation of the image by **b** (i.e., the h-transformation) and the rotation by $-\phi$ corresponding to the sphere rotation by -2ϕ (i.e., the k-transformation).

Under this assumption, we derived in [6] the geometrically-exact expression for the vector **b** (Equations (14) and (15) in [6]) that specifies the h transformation during the horizontal gaze rotation. We model the gaze change during the tracking movement as a sequence of small-angle horizontal rotations ($\phi_m, m = 1, 2, 3, ...$).

In order to derive the anticipatory background's image transformations for a known tracking sequence of gaze rotations, we approximate of vector **b** to the first order in ϕ,

$$\mathbf{b} = \pm \frac{\phi}{d} \langle \sin \alpha, 0, \cos \alpha \rangle, \tag{16}$$

where α gives the orientation relative to the initial coordinate system of the line containing the line segment PQ and d is the distance to this line from the nodal point; see Figure 3. Furthermore, in the above approximation, the upper sign is for $\alpha > \varphi$, and the lower sign is for $\alpha < \varphi$. Since the α and d fix this horizontal line, the approximation (16) does not depend on the planar object size and where on its plane it is located.

The derivation of the vector **b** in (16) is the main result that allows for the given sequence of gaze rotations ($\phi_m, m = 1, 2, 3, ...$) to obtain the corresponding sequence of projective transformations ($g_m, m = 1, 2, 3...$) that are useful for maintaining perceptual stability. Taking the iteration of the smooth pursuit's transformations g_m, we obtain the background object's image projective transformations given in terms of the gaze rotations ϕ_m, the orientation angle α and the distance d. We refer to [6] for the complete discussion.

Since the gaze rotations are assumed known in order to execute robotic eye rotations and both α and d can be estimated, our modeling of the visual information during smooth pursuit of the conformal camera can support the anticipatory image processing. This can be used to support the stability of of visual information during tracking movements by an anthropomorphic camera needed for an autonomous robot efficient interaction with the real world, in real time.

4.5.2. Visual Information during Saccades

The model of perisaccadic perception in [4] is based on the model suggested in [36] that an efference copy of the impending eye movement, generated by SC, is used to briefly shift activity of some visual neurons toward the cortical fovea. This shift remaps the presaccadic neuronal activity to their future postsaccadic locations around the saccade target. Because the shifts occurs in logarithmic coordinates approximating retinotopy, the model can also explain the phenomenon of the mislocalization of briefly-flashed probes around the saccade's onset, as observed by humans in laboratory experiments [37].

We outline here the steps in modeling perisaccadic predictive image processing and refer to [4] for a more detailed discussion. The scene with the upcoming saccade target at the point T is projected into the image plane of the conformal camera and sampled according to the distribution of the photoreceptor/ganglion cells:

$$f_{m,n} = (2\pi T/MN)f(e^{u_m}e^{i\theta_n}). \tag{17}$$

Next, DPFT $f_{k,l}$ in (12) is computed by FFT in log-polar coordinates (u_k, θ_l). The inverse DPFT (13) computed again by FFT renders the image cortical representation:

$$f_{k,l} = (2\pi T/MN)f(u_k, \theta_l). \tag{18}$$

A short time before the saccade's onset and during the saccade movement that redirects the gaze line from F to T, log-polar (cortical) coordinates are remapped by shifting the frame centered at the neuronal activity of the stimuli around T to the future foveal location when eyes fixate on T. The salient part of the image is then shifted by $(h\delta, -j\gamma)$ toward the cortical fovea. This neural process is modeled by the standard Fourier transform shift property applied to the inverse DPFT,

$$f_{m+h,n-j} = \frac{1}{MN}\sum_{k=0}^{M-1}\sum_{l=0}^{N-1}\left(e^{i2\pi hk/M}e^{-i2\pi jl/N}\hat{f}_{k,l}e^{-(u_k+h\delta)}e^{i2\pi mk/M}e^{i2\pi nl/N}\right),$$

which can be computed by FFT.

Finally, the perisaccadic compression observed in laboratory experiments is obtained by transforming the cortical image representation to the visual field representation:

$$
\begin{aligned}
f_{m+h,n-j} &= (2\pi T/MN)f(u_m + h\delta, \theta_n - j\gamma) \\
&= (2\pi T/MN)f(e^{u_m+h\delta}e^{i[\theta_n-j\gamma]}) \\
&= (2\pi T/MN)f(e^{h\delta}r_m e^{i[\theta_n-j\gamma]}),
\end{aligned}
$$

where $\gamma = 2\pi/N$. We see that under the the shift of the coordinate system (u_m, θ_n) by $(h\delta, -j\gamma)$, the original position $r_m e^{i\theta_n}$ is transformed to $e^{-h\delta}r_m e^{i(\theta_n-j\gamma)}$. The multiplication of r_m by $e^{-h\delta}$ results in the compression of the scene around the saccade target T.

5. Binocular Vision and the Conformal Camera

Each of our two eyes receives a slightly different retinal projection of a scene due to their lateral separation from each other. Nevertheless, we experience our visual world as if it were seen from just one viewpoint. The two disparate 2D retinal images are fused into one image that gives us the impression of a 3D space. The locus of points in space that are seen singularly is known as the horopter, and the perceived direction that represents the visual axes of the two eyes is often referred to as the cyclopean axis.

The small differences in the images on the the right and left eyes, resulting from their separation, is referred as binocular disparity, or stereopsis. When the eyes fixate on a point, any other point in a scene that lies either in front or behind the horopter curve, subtends different angle on each retina between the image and the center of the fovea. This difference defines retinal disparity, which provides a cue for the object's depth from an observer's point of fixation. Then, the relative disparity is defined as the difference in retinal disparities for a pair of points. The relative disparity provides a cue for the perception of 3D structure, components of which include relative depth and shape. Relative disparity is usually assumed to not depend on the eyes' positions [38].

Conventional geometric theory of binocular projections is incorrect in identifying the geometric horopter with the Vieth–Müller circle. This two-century old theory incorrectly assumes that the eye's optical node coincides with the eyeball's rotational center, yet it still influences theoretical developments in binocular vision. Anatomically-correct binocular projection geometry was recently presented in [39].

The main results in [39] are the following: (1) the Vieth–Müller circle is the isovergence circle that is not the geometric horopter; and (2) relative disparity depends on eye position when the nodal point is at the anatomically-correct location. Moreover, calculations for typical viewing distances show that such changes in relative disparity are within binocular acuity limits [40]. During fixation, the eyes continually jitter, drift and make micro-saccades, and we hypothesize in [39] that the small changes in perceived size and shape during these eye movements may be needed, not only for perceptual benefits, such as 'breaking camouflage', but also for the aesthetic benefit of stereopsis [41].

The geometric horopter in [39] corresponds to a simplified version of the schematic eye, also called a reduced eye. In this model, the two nodal points coincide at the refractive surface's center of curvature. The light from the fixation point travels through the nodal point to the center of the fovea, a path referred to as the visual axis. The optical axis coincides with the visual axis when the fovea center is assumed to coincide with the posterior pole. This model of the reduced eye complies with the conformal camera's imaging framework discussed in Section 2, resulting in the conformal camera that is capable of modeling stereo vision.

Still, the reduced eye model remains an idealization. The eyeball is not perfectly spherical, and when it rotates in the socket, the center of rotation slightly moves. Although these aspects may affect the eye optics quality, for example myopia occurs if the eyeball is too long, we do not consider them in this study.

In contrast to the reduced eye model, the eye's fovea center is supratemporal on the retina, and the visual axis is angled about 5.2 degrees nasally to the optical axis. This angle is called the α angle. Moreover, ophthalmological diagnostics have shown that even in normal eyes with good visual acuity, a small amount of lens misalignments relative to the optic axis do exist [42,43].

The importance of the eyes' asymmetry follows from two facts. The first is well-known: the empirical longitudinal horopter deviates from the circular curves that form the geometric horopters. This so-called Hering–Hillebrand horopter deviation, shown in Figure 4, can be explained by asymmetry in the spatial positions of the corresponding elements in the two eyes. Two retinal elements, each one in a different eye, are corresponding if they invoke a single percept when stimulated. The second fact is the claim recently made in [44] that the natural crystalline lens tilt and decentration in humans is inclined to compensate for various types of aberration.

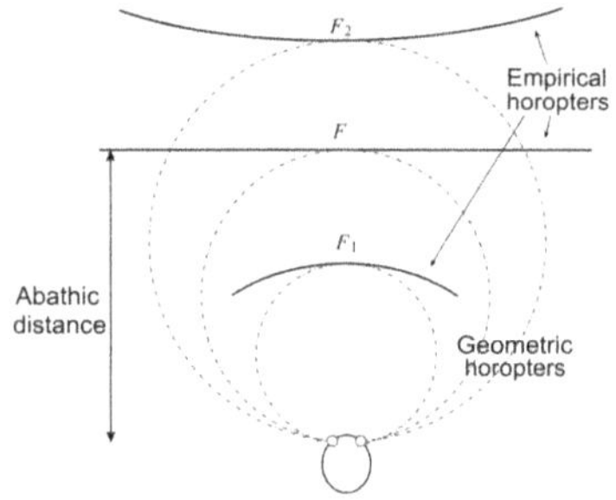

Figure 4. Empirical longitudinal horopters are shown schematically for symmetric convergence points. Abathic distance is defined here as the distance from the line connecting the eye centers to the fixation point *F* at which the horopter is a straight line.

6. The Asymmetric Conformal Camera

To model the eye with both the tilt and decentration of the natural crystalline lens, we present in this section the asymmetric conformal camera. Although the optical axis should best approximate the lost symmetry in the alignment of the eye's components, we assume that this axis is the line passing through the nodal point and the spherical eyeball's rotation center.

The modified conformal camera is obtained by rotating the image plane about the x_2-axis by the angle β and then translating the origin by z_0, as shown in Figure 5. We refer to Figure 5 for the notation used in the remaining part of the paper. The immediate requirement is that the visual axis passing through the nodal point and point z_0 forms the angle $\alpha = 5.2°$ with the optical axis.

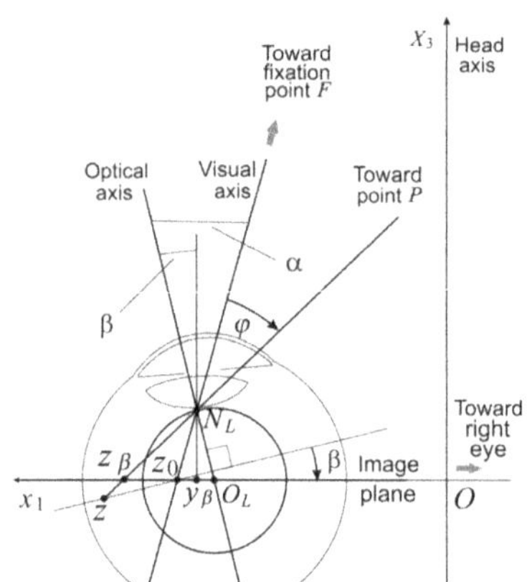

Figure 5. The eye model with an asymmetrically-displaced fovea and a tilted and decentered lens outlined with thin (1 pt) curves. The asymmetric conformal camera is outlined with thick (2 pt) curves. The stereo system is obtained if the left camera is reflected in the head axis X_3. Each camera's image plane, shown here for the left eye, is perpendicular to the head axis, such that the horopter curve is a straight line passing through the fixation point *F* at the abathic distance from origin *O*.

However, because the nodal point is identified with the 'north pole' of the stereographic projection, the point $N(0,0,1)$, we place the nodal point 1 cm from the eye rotation center to simplify the discussion. This discrepancy with the physiological distance of 0.6 cm can be easily corrected. The angles $\alpha = 5.2°$

and β give the fovea an asymmetric displacement of $\widehat{fp} = 1.63$ mm and the lens decentration $y_\beta = \sin \beta$.

The points on the image plane have coordinates relative to the plane origin O_L. The projection $\zeta_\beta = z_\beta - z_0$ of the space point on the tilted image plane with the 'foveal' center at z_0 can be expressed in terms of the projection z on the original image plane, allowing us to find the transformation between image planes. To this end, we note that $|y_\beta N_L| = \cos \beta$.

Then, from the right triangles $\Delta z_0 y_\beta N_L$ and $\Delta z_\beta y_\beta N_L$, we get:

$$\frac{z_0 - y_\beta}{\cos \beta} = \tan(\alpha - \beta)$$

and:

$$\frac{z_\beta - y_\beta}{\cos \beta} = \tan(\varphi + \alpha - \beta).$$

Solving those last two formulas for $z_0 - y_\beta$ and $z_\beta - y_\beta$, and taking the difference, we obtain:

$$u_\beta = z_\beta - z_0 = \cos \beta \left[\tan(\varphi + \alpha - \beta) - \tan(\alpha - \beta) \right]$$
$$= \cos \beta \left[\frac{\tan(\varphi + \alpha) - \tan \beta}{1 + \tan(\varphi + \alpha) \tan \beta} - \frac{\tan(\alpha - \beta) \left[1 + \tan(\varphi + \alpha) \tan \beta \right]}{1 + \tan(\varphi + \alpha) \tan \beta} \right]. \tag{19}$$

Next, from the right triangle $\Delta z C_L N_L$, we have:

$$z = \tan(\varphi + \alpha). \tag{20}$$

Introducing (20) to (19), we obtain:

$$\zeta_\beta = \cos \beta \left[\frac{z - \tan \beta}{1 + z \tan \beta} - \frac{\tan(\alpha - \beta) \left[1 + z \tan \beta \right]}{1 + z \tan \beta} \right]$$
$$= \frac{z \left[\cos \beta - \sin \beta \tan(\alpha - \beta) \right] - \cos \beta \tan(\alpha - \beta)}{z \tan \beta + 1},$$

which can be expressed by the following linear fractional action:

$$\zeta_\beta = \begin{bmatrix} \frac{\cos \beta - \sin \beta \tan(\alpha - \beta)}{\cos^{1/2} \beta} & -\cos^{1/2} \beta \tan(\alpha - \beta) \\ \frac{\sin \beta}{\cos^{3/2} \beta} & \frac{1}{\cos^{1/2} \beta} \end{bmatrix} \cdot z$$
$$= \frac{\frac{\cos \beta - \sin \beta \tan(\alpha - \beta)}{\cos^{1/2} \beta} z - \cos^{1/2} \beta \tan(\alpha - \beta)}{\frac{\sin \beta}{\cos^{3/2} \beta} z + \frac{1}{\cos^{1/2} \beta}}. \tag{21}$$

We call the matrix in (21) by m_β, so that $\zeta_\beta = m_\beta \cdot z$. If $z' = g \cdot z$ and $\zeta'_\beta = m_\beta \cdot z'$, then $m_\beta \cdot z' = m_\beta g m_\beta^{-1} m_\beta \cdot z$ shows that:

$$\zeta'_\beta = g_\beta \cdot \zeta_\beta \quad \text{where} \quad g_\beta = m_\beta g m_\beta^{-1}.$$

We have just derived the conjugate map of g by m_β,

$$\mathbf{SL}(2, \mathbb{C}) \ni g \longmapsto g_\beta = m_\beta g m_\beta^{-1} \in \mathbf{SL}(2, \mathbb{C}), \tag{22}$$

which satisfies:

$$(g_1)_\beta (g_2)_\beta = m_\beta g_1 m_\beta^{-1} m_\beta g_2 m_\beta^{-1} = m_\beta g_1 g_2 m_\beta^{-1} = (g_1 g_2)_\beta \tag{23}$$

and:

$$(g_\beta)^{-1} = \left(m_\beta g m_\beta^{-1}\right)^{-1} = m_\beta g^{-1} m_\beta^{-1} = (g^{-1})_\beta. \tag{24}$$

The map (22) is the inner automorphism of the group $\mathbf{SL}(2, \mathbb{C})$. This inner automorphism maps the group of image projective transformations onto itself by using the image projective transformation m_β that represents the camera's asymmetry.

Since g and g_β have the same algebraic properties by (23) and (24), they behave geometrically in the same way. For instance, the *kh*-transformation discussed in Section 1, which gives the image transformation from the conformal camera gaze change, is preserved under the conjugation because $(kh)_\beta = k_\beta h_\beta$. Thus, we can work with the asymmetric conformal camera as we did with the standard conformal camera.

To this end, given the image intensity function $f : D \to \mathbb{R}$ in the standard conformal camera, we define the image intensity function:

$$f_\beta : m_\beta(D) \to \mathbb{R}$$

on the image plane as follows: $f_\beta(z_\beta) = f(m_\beta^{-1} \cdot z_\beta) = f(z)$. Then,

$$T_g f(z) = f(g^{-1} \cdot z) = f(m_\beta^{-1} m_\beta g^{-1} m_\beta^{-1} m_\beta \cdot z) = f_\beta(g_\beta^{-1} \cdot z_\beta) = T_{g_\beta} f_\beta(z_\beta).$$

The relation between g and g_β can be expressed in the following commutative diagram:

$$
\begin{array}{ccc}
\widehat{\mathbb{C}} & \xrightarrow{\;g\;} & \widehat{\mathbb{C}} \\
m_\beta \downarrow & & \downarrow m_\beta \\
\widehat{\mathbb{C}} & \xrightarrow{\;g_\beta\;} & \widehat{\mathbb{C}}
\end{array}
$$

where the transformation m_β can be considered a coordinate transformation. Then, the conjugate $g_\beta = m_\beta g m_\beta^{-1}$ has the form corresponding to base changes in linear algebra. To see this, we let a linear map be represented by matrices M and N in two different bases. Then, $N = PMP^{-1}$, where P is the base change matrix.

The result of tilting and translating the image plane does not affect the conformal camera's geometric and computational frameworks; this can be phrased as putting 'conformal glasses' on the camera.

7. Discussion: Modeling Empirical Horopters

Two points, each in one of the two eyes' retinas, are considered corresponding if they give the same perceived visual direction. The circular shape of the geometric horopter is the consequence of a simple geometric assumption on corresponding points: two retinal points, onto which a non-fixated point in space is projected through each of the two nodal points, are corresponding if the angles subtended at the two eyes with fixation lines are equal.

If one relaxes this assumption by assuming that corresponding points in the temporal direction from the center of the fovea towards the periphery are compressed as compared with corresponding points in the nasal direction, the geometric horizontal horopter curves are no longer circular; see Figure 2.16 in [45].

The asymmetric conformal camera is defined by rotating the image plane by the angle β about the eye's axis, the vertical axis to the horizontal visual plane and translating the plane origin by z_0 in the temporal direction (cf. Figure 5). In doing this, we demand that the angle between the fixation axis passing through the nodal point and point z_0 and the optical axis passing through the nodal point and spherical eyeball center of rotation is the angle $\alpha = 5.2°$. Here, z_0 is the stereographic projection of the fovea center f.

Now, a simple geometric fact follows: when equally-spaced points on the rotated image plane are projected into the sphere with the nodal point N_L as the center of projection, their images on the sphere are compressed in the temporal direction from f, as compared with the nasal direction.

In this section, we study the horizontal horopter curves of the stereo system with asymmetric conformal cameras by back projecting the pairs of corresponding points from the uniformly-distributed points on the camera's image plane to the object space. From [13], we expected that the horopters would be approximated by conics. To test this, we choose six points for each fixation: five points to give a unique conic curve and the sixth point to verify that this is indeed the horopter conic. One of these six points is the fixation point that is always on the horopter. Further, the nodal points and the point that does not project to the image plane, projecting instead to ∞, are taken as the points on the horopter, except for when the horopter is a straight line. When the horopter is a straight line, we need only three points.

To do this, we fix the camera's parameters as follows. The abathic distance is the fixation point's distance when the horopter is a straight line; see Figure 4. This occurs when the fixation point of the two eye models provides two image planes that are perpendicular to the head axis. This orientation of the eyes with the abathic distance at the fixation point is shown in Figure 5 if this figure is completed by adding the right eye as the reflection of the left eye about the head axis X_3. Then, the abathic distance for the eye radius of 1 cm, with a given α, β and the ocular separation a, can be easily expressed as:

$$d_\beta = \frac{\cos\beta\left[\frac{a}{2}\cos(\alpha-\beta)+\sin\alpha\right]}{\sin\alpha - \sin\beta\cos(\alpha-\beta)}. \tag{25}$$

We use in (25) the physiologically-accurate values of $\alpha = 5.2°$ and $a = 6.5$ cm. Then, assuming the values of β in the range $-0.1° \le \beta \le 4.2°$ we find, using (25), the observed abathic distance values in humans in the range 35 cm $\le d_\beta \le$ 190 cm with an average value of $d_{3.3°} = 100$ cm. The assumed values of the angle β are in the range of the crystalline lens tilt's angle, as measured in healthy human eyes [42].

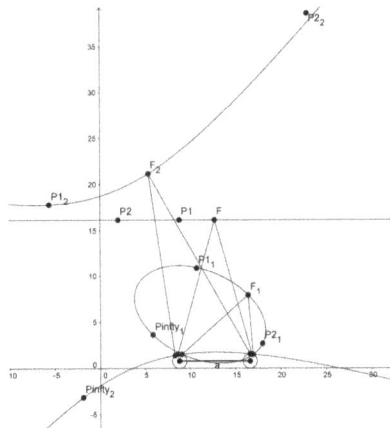

Figure 6. The graphs of the three horizontal horopters, the ellipse for fixation F_1 (163.7, 79.5), the straight line for fixation F (126.8, 161.4) and the hyperbola for fixation F_2 (53.4, 211.5), with coordinates given in millimeters. The eye radius is 7.9 mm; the interocular distance is 78.0 mm, $\alpha = 16°$ and $\beta = 10°$. For each of the fixations F_i, $i = 1, 2$, the six points were obtained by back projecting the corresponding points. These six points included the fixation point, the two nodal points, the point $Pinfty_i$ that projects to ∞ and two additional points, $P1_i$ and $P2_i$. Five of these points were used to obtain the conics, and the sixth point was used for the verification. The straight-line horopter is for the fixation point at the abathic distance and is given by three points, F, P_1 and P_2.

In the simulation with GeoGebra, we use different values for our parameters than those that would be used in the human binocular system. In order to display horopters with three different shapes, ellipse, straight line and hyperbola, in one graphical window output, we take the eye radius of 7.9 mm, the interocular distance of 78 mm, $\alpha = 16°$ and $\beta = 10°$. The graphs of the horopters obtained in GeoGebra are shown in Figure 6. The fixation points are given in the caption of this figure.

We note that the hyperbola has two branches, one passing through the fixation point and the other passing through the nodal points. GeoGebra also computed the conics' equations:

the ellipse:
$$-7.9x^2 - 7.2xy - 14.9y^2 + 216.9x + 253.5y = 1566.0,$$

the line:
$$y = 161.4,$$

and the hyperbola:
$$4.8x^2 + 12.0xy - 12.8y^2 - 144.6x + 216.4y = -447.4.$$

The main purpose of the simulation with GeoGebra is to study qualitatively the shape of the horizontal horopters for the proposed binocular model to see how they are related to the empirical horopters. As we demonstrated before, our binocular model accounts for the typical characteristics of the human binocular system, such as the shape of horopter curves and the abathic distance. Most notably, the simulation with GeoGebra shows that the horopters given by the stereo system with eyes modeled by the asymmetric conformal cameras are well approximated by conical curves. It was proposed by Ogle in [13] that primates' empirical horopters should be approximated by such conics.

8. Conclusions

The first part of the paper reviewed the conformal camera's geometric analysis developed by the author in the group-theoretic framework [1–3]. We identified the semisimple group $\mathbf{SL}(2,\mathbb{C})$ as the group of image transformations during the conformal camera's gaze rotations. This group is the double cover of $\mathbf{PSL}(2,\mathbb{C})$, the group that gives both the complex structure on the Riemann sphere and the one-dimensional complex geometry. This duality synthesizes the analytic and geometric structures.

Representation theory on semisimple groups, one of the greatest achievements of 20th century mathematics, allows the conformal camera to possess its own Fourier analysis. The projective Fourier transform was constructed by restricting Fourier analysis on the group $\mathbf{SL}(2,\mathbb{C})$ to the image plane of the conformal camera. The image representation in terms of the discrete projective Fourier transform can be efficiently computed by a fast Fourier transform algorithm in the log-polar coordinates. These coordinates approximate the retino-cortical maps of the visual pathways. This means that the projective Fourier transform is well adapted to both image transformations produced by the conformal camera's gaze change and to the correspondingly updated log-polar maps.

The first part of the paper was concluded with a discussion of the conformal camera's relevance to the computational aspects of anthropomorphic vision. First, we discussed the relevance of imaging with the conformal camera to early and intermediate-level vision. Then, we compared the conformal camera model of retinotopy with the accepted Schwartz model and pointed out the conformal camera's advantages in biologically-mediated image processing. We also discussed numerical implementation of the discrete projective Fourier transform. In this implementation, the log-polar image contained 100-times less pixels than the original image, comparable to the ratio of 125 million photoreceptors sampling incoming visual information to 1.5 million of ganglion cell axons carrying the output from the eye to the brain. Finally, we briefly reviewed image processing for stability during the conformal camera tracking and saccadic movements.

The model with the conformal camera was developed to process visual information in an anthropomorphic camera head mounted on a moving platform replicating human eye movements.

It was demonstrated in the author's previous studies that this model is capable of supporting the stability of foveate vision when the environment is explored with about four saccadic eye movements per second and when the eye executes smooth pursuit eye movements. Previously, this model only considered aspects of monocular vision.

In the second part of the paper, binocular vision was reviewed and the stereo extension of the conformal camera's group-theoretic framework was presented. We did this for the eye model that includes the asymmetrically-displaced fovea on the retina and the tilted and decentered natural crystalline lens. We concluded this part showing, with a numerical simulation, that the resultant horopters are conics that well approximate the empirical horopters.

The geometry of the conical horopters in the stereo system with asymmetric conformal cameras requires further study. In the near future, the spatial orientation and shape of the conic curves need to be derived in terms of the perceived direction and the parameters of asymmetry. This will allow the development of disparity maps for the stereo system with asymmetric conformal cameras.

Acknowledgments: The author thanks the reviewers for helpful comments. The research presented in this paper was supported in part by NSF Grant CCR-9901957.

Conflicts of Interest: The author declares no conflict of interest.

Abbreviations

The following abbreviations are used in this manuscript:

PFT	projective Fourier transform
DPFT	discrete projective Fourier transform
FFT	fast Fourier transform
SC	superior colliculus
LGN	lateral geniculate nucleus
V1	primary visual cortex
ECT	exponential chirp transform

References

1. Turski, J. Projective Fourier analysis for patterns. *Pattern Recognit.* **2000**, *33*, 2033–2043.
2. Turski, J. Geometric Fourier Analysis of the Conformal Camera for Active Vision. *SIAM Rev.* **2004**, *46*, 230–255.
3. Turski, J. Geometric Fourier Analysis for Computational Vision. *J. Fourier Anal. Appl.* **2005**, *11*, 1–23.
4. Turski, J. Robotic Vision with the Conformal Camera: Modeling Perisaccadic Perception. *J. Robot.* **2010**, doi:10.1155/2010/130285.
5. Turski, J. Imaging with the Conformal Camera. In *Proc IPCVIPR*; CSREA Press: Las Vegas, NV, USA, 2012; Volume 2, pp. 1–7.
6. Turski, J. Modeling of Active Vision During Smooth Pursuit of a Robotic Eye. *Electron. Imaging* **2016**, *10*, 1–8.
7. Jones, G.; Singerman, D. *Complex Functions*; Cambridge University Press: Cambridge, UK, 1987.
8. Henle, M. *Modern Geometries. The Analytical Approach*; Prentice Hall: Upper Saddle River, NJ, USA, 1997.
9. Berger, M. *Geometry I*; Springer: New York, NY, USA, 1987.
10. Knapp, A.W. *Representation Theory of Semisimple Groups: An Overview Based on Examples*; Princeton University Press: Princeton, NJ, USA, 1986.
11. Kaas, J.H. Topographic Maps are Fundamental to Sensory Processing. *Brain Res. Bull.* **1997**, *44*, 107–112.
12. Larson, A.M.; Loschky, L.C. The contributions of central versus peripheral vision to scene gist recognition. *J. Vis.* **2009**, *9*, 1–16.
13. Ogle, K.N. Analytical treatment of the longitudinal horopter. *J. Opt. Soc. Am.* **1932**, *22*, 665–728.
14. Bonmassar, G.; Schwartz, E.L. Space-variant Fourier analysis: The Exponential Chirp transform. *IEEE Trans. Pattern Anal.* **1997**, *19*, 1080–1089.
15. Schwartz, E.L. Computational anatomy and functional architecture of striate cortex. *Vis. Res.* **1980**, *20*, 645–669.

16. Balasuriya, L.S.; Siebert, J.P. An artificial retina with a selforganized retina receptive field tessellation. In Proceedings of the AISB 2003 Symposium: Biologically Inspired Machine Vison, Theory and Applications, Aberystwyth, UK, 7–11 April 2003; pp. 34–42.

17. Bulduc, M.; Levine, M.D. A review of bilogically motivated space-variant data reduction models for robotic vision. *Comput. Vis. Image Underst.* **1998**, *689*, 170–184.

18. You, S.; Tan, R.T.; Kawakami, R.; Mukaigawa, Y.; Ikeuch, K. Waterdrops Stereo. Available online: https://arxiv.org/pdf/1604.00730.pdf (accessed on 4 April 2016).

19. Taguchi, Y.; Agrawal, A.; Veeraraghavan, A.; Ramalingam, S.; Raskar, R. Axial-Cones: Modeling Spherical Catadioptric Cameras for Wide-Angle Light Field Rendering. *ACM Trans. Graph.* **2010**, *29*, doi:10.1145/1882261.1866194.

20. Needham, T. *Visual Complex Analysis*; Oxford University Press: New York, NY, USA, 2002.

21. Altmann, S.L. *Rotations, Quaternions and Double Groups*; Oxford University Press: Oxford, UK; New York, NY, USA, 1986.

22. Sally, P.J., Jr. Harmonic analysis and group representations. In *Studies in Harmonic Analysis*; Ash, J.M., Ed.; Mathematical Association of America: Washington, DC, USA, 1976; Volume 13, pp. 224–256.

23. Herb, R.A. An Elementary Introduction to Harish-Chandra's Work. In *Mathematical Legacy of Harish-Chandra—A Celebration of Representation Theory and Harmonic Analysis*; Doran, R.S., Varadarajan, V.S., Eds.; AMS: Providence, RI, USA, 2000; Volume 68, pp. 59–75.

24. Shapley, R. Early vision is early in time. *Neuron* **2007**, *56*, 755–756.

25. Roelfsema, P.R.; Tolboom, M.; Khayat, P.S. Different Processing Phases for Features, Figures, and Selective Attention in the Primary Visual Cortex. *Neuron* **2007**, *56*, 785–792.

26. Blum, H. Biological shape and visual science. *J. Theor. Biol.* **1973**, *38*, 205–287.

27. Hoffman, D.D.; Richards, W.A. Parts of recognition. *Cognition* **1984**, *18*, 65–96.

28. Kovacs, I.; Julesz, B. Perceptual sensitivity maps within globally defined visual shapes. *Nature* **1994**, *370*, 644–646.

29. Engel, S.A.; Glover, G.H.; Wendell, B.A. Retinotopic organization in human visual cortex and the spatial precision of MRI. *Cerabral Cortex.* **1997**, *7*, 181–192.

30. Tabareau, N.; Bennequin, N.D.; Berthoz, A.; Slotine, J.-J. Geometry of the superior colliculic mapping and efficient oculomotor computation. *Biol. Cybern.* **2007**, *97*, 279–292.

31. Shapiro, A.; Lu, Z.-L.; Huang, C.-B.; Knight, E.; Ennis, R. Transitions between Central and Peripheral Vision Create Spatial/Temporal Distortions: A Hypothesis Concerning the Perceived Break of the Curveball. *PLoS ONE* **2010**, *5*, doi:10.1371/journal.pone.0013296.

32. Xing, J.; Heeger, D.J. Center-surround interaction in foveal and peripheral vision. *Vis. Res.* **2000**, *40*, 3065–3072.

33. Newsome, W.T.; Wurtz, R.H.; Komatsu, H. Relation of cortical areas MT and MST to pursuit eye movements. II. Differentiation of retinal from extraretinal imputes. *J. Neurophysiol.* **1988**, *60*, 604–620.

34. Sommer, M.A.; Wurtz, R.H. A pathway in primate brain for internal monitoring of movements. *Science* **2002**, *296*, 1480–1482.

35. Hall, N.J.; Colby, C.L. Remapping for visual stability. *Philos. Trans. R. Soc.* **2010**, *366*, 528–539.

36. VanRullen, R. A simple translation in cortical log-coordinates may account for the pattern of saccadic localization errors. *Biol. Cybern.* **2004**, *91*, 131–137.

37. Ross, J.; Morrone, M.C.; Goldberg, M.E.; Burr, D.C. Changes in visual perception at the time of saccades. *Trend Neurosci.* **2001**, *24*, 113–121.

38. Marr, D. *Vision*; Freeman: New York, NY, USA, 1985.

39. Turski, J. On Binocular Vision: The Geometric Horopter and Cyclopean Eye. *Vis. Res.* **2016**, *119*, 73–81.

40. Wilcox, L.M.; Harris, J.M. Fundamentals of stereopsis. In *Encyclopedia of the Eye*; Dartt, D.A., Besharse, J.C., Dana, R., Eds.; Academic Press: New York, NY, USA, 2007; Volume 2, pp. 164–171.

41. Ponce, C.R.; Born, R.T. Stereopsis. *Curr. Biol.* **2008**, *18*, R845–R850.

42. Chang, Y.; Wu, H.-M.; Lin, Y.-F. The axial misalignment between ocular lens and cornea observed by MRI (I)—At fixed accommodative state. *Vis. Res.* **2007**, *47*, 71–84.

43. Mester, U.; Tand, S.; Kaymak, H. Decentration and tilt of a single-piece aspheric intraocular lens compared with the lens position in young phakic eyes. *J. Cataract Refract. Surg.* **2009**, *35*, 485–490.

44. Artal, P.; Guirao, A.; Berrio, E.; Williams, D.R. Compensation of corneal aberrations by the internal optics in the human eye. *J. Vis.* **2001**, *1*, 1–8.

45. Howard, I.P.; Rogers, B.J. *Binocular Vision and Stereopsis*; University Press Scholarship Online: Oxford, UK, 2008; doi:10.1093/acprof:oso/9780195084764.001.0001.

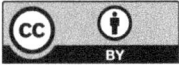

symmetry

MDPI

Article

Modeling Bottom-Up Visual Attention Using Dihedral Group D_4 [†]

Puneet Sharma

Department of Engineering & Safety (IIS-IVT), UiT-The Arctic University of Norway, Tromsø-9037, Norway; er.puneetsharma@gmail.com; Tel.: +47-776-60391

†   This paper is an extended version of my paper published in 11th International Symposium on Visual Computing (ISVC 2015).

Academic Editors: Marco Bertamini and Lewis Griffin
Received: 27 April 2016; Accepted: 9 August 2016; Published: 15 August 2016

Abstract: In this paper, first, we briefly describe the dihedral group D_4 that serves as the basis for calculating saliency in our proposed model. Second, our saliency model makes two major changes in a latest state-of-the-art model known as group-based asymmetry. First, based on the properties of the dihedral group D_4, we simplify the asymmetry calculations associated with the measurement of saliency. This results is an algorithm that reduces the number of calculations by at least half that makes it the fastest among the six best algorithms used in this research article. Second, in order to maximize the information across different chromatic and multi-resolution features, the color image space is de-correlated. We evaluate our algorithm against 10 state-of-the-art saliency models. Our results show that by using optimal parameters for a given dataset, our proposed model can outperform the best saliency algorithm in the literature. However, as the differences among the (few) best saliency models are small, we would like to suggest that our proposed model is among the best and the fastest among the best. Finally, as a part of future work, we suggest that our proposed approach on saliency can be extended to include three-dimensional image data.

Keywords: image analysis; saliency

1. Introduction

While searching for a person on a busy street, we look at people while neglecting other aspects of the scene, such as road signs, buildings and cars. However, in the absence of the given task, we would pay attention to different features of the same scene. In the literature [1], it is described as a combination of two different mechanisms: top-down and bottom-up.

Top-down pertains to how a target object is defined or described in the scene; for instance, while searching for a person, we would start by selecting all people in the scene as likely candidates and disregard the candidates that do not match the features of the target person until the correct person is found. To model this, we need a description of the scene in terms of all of the objects, and the unique features associated with each object, such that the uniqueness of the features can be used for distinguishing similar objects from one another. Given the sheer number of man-made and natural objects in our daily lives and the ambiguity associated with the definition of an object itself makes the modeling of top-down mechanisms perplexing. To this end, recent attempts have been made by [2,3] using machine learning-based methods.

Bottom-up (also known as visual saliency) mechanisms are associated with the attributes of a scene that draw our attention to a particular location. These low-level image attributes include: motion, color, contrast and brightness [4]. Bottom-up mechanisms are involuntary and faster compared to top-down ones [1]. For instance, a red object among green objects and an object placed horizontally among vertical objects are some stimuli that would automatically capture our attention in the environment.

Owing to the limited number of low-level image attributes, modeling visual saliency is relatively less complex.

In the past two decades, modeling visual saliency has generated much interest in the research community. In addition to contributing towards the understanding of human vision, it has also paved the way for a number of computer and machine vision applications. These applications include: image and video compression [5–8], robot localization [9,10], image retrieval [11], image and video quality assessment [12,13], dynamic lighting [14], advertisement [15], artistic image rendering [16] and human-robot interaction [17,18]. In salient object detection, the applications include: target detection [19], image segmentation [20,21] and image resizing [22,23].

In a recent study by Alsam et al. [24,25], it was proposed that asymmetry can be used as a measure of saliency. In order to calculate the asymmetry of an image region, the authors used dihedral group D_4, which is the symmetry group of the square. D_4 consists of eight group elements, namely rotation by 0, 90, 180 and 270 degrees and reflection about the horizontal, vertical and two diagonal axes. The saliency maps obtained from their algorithm show good correspondence with the saliency maps calculated from the classic visual saliency model by Itti et al. [26].

Inspired by the fact that bottom-up calculations are fast, in this paper, we use the symmetries present in the dihedral group D_4 to make the calculations associated with the D_4 group elements simpler and faster to implement. In doing so, we modify the saliency model proposed by Alsam et al. [24,25]. For details, please see Section 3.

Next, we are motivated by the study by Garcia-Diaz et al. [27], which implies that in order to quantify distinct information in a scene, our visual system de-correlates its chromatic and multi-resolution features. Based on this, we perform the de-correlation of the input color image by calculating its principal components (details in Section 3.3).

2. Theory

A dihedral group D_n is the group of symmetries of an n-sided regular polygon, i.e., all sides have the same length, and all angles are equal. D_n has n rotational symmetries and n reflection symmetries. In other words, it has n axes of symmetry and 2n different symmetries [28]. For instance, the polygons for $n = 3, 4, 5$ and 6 and the associated reflection symmetries are shown in Figure 1. Here, we can see that when n is odd, each axis of symmetry connects the vertex with the midpoint of the opposite side. When n is even, there are $n/2$ symmetry axes connecting the midpoints of opposite sides and $n/2$ symmetry axes connecting opposite vertices.

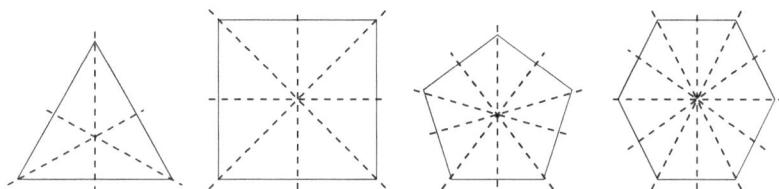

Figure 1. Polygons for n = 3, 4, 5 and 6 and the associated reflection symmetries. Here, we can see that when *n* is odd, each axis of symmetry connects the vertex with the midpoint of the opposite side. When *n* is even, there are *n*/2 symmetry axes connecting the midpoints of opposite sides and *n*/2 symmetry axes connecting opposite vertices.

A group is a set G together with a binary operation $*$ on its elements. This operation $*$ must behave such that:

(i)   G must be closed under $*$, that is for every pair of elements g_1, g_2 in G, we must have that $g_1 * g_2$ is again an element in G.

(ii)   The operation $*$ must be associative, that is for all elements g_1, g_2, g_3 in G, we must have that:

$$g_1 * (g_2 * g_3) = (g_1 * g_2) * g_3.$$

(iii)   There is an element e in G, called the identity element, such that for all $g \in G$, we have that:

$$e * g = g = g * e.$$

(iv)   For every element g in G, there is an element g^{-1} in G, called the inverse of g, such that:

$$g * g^{-1} = e = g^{-1} * g.$$

2.1. The Group D_4

In this paper, we are interested in D_4, the symmetry group of the square. The ease of computational complexity associated with dividing an image grid into square regions and the fact that the D_4 group has shown promising results in various computer vision applications [29–33] motivated us to use this group for our proposed algorithm.

The group D_4 has eight elements, four rotational symmetries and four reflection symmetries. The rotations are $0°$, $90°$, $180°$ and $270°$, and the reflections are defined along the four axes shown in Figure 1. We refer to these elements as $\sigma_0, \sigma_1, \ldots, \sigma_7$. Note that the identity element is rotation by $0°$ and that for each element, there is another element that has the opposite effect on the square, as required in the definition of a group. The group operation is the composition of two such transformations. As an example of one of the group elements, consider Figure 2, where we demonstrate rotation by $90°$ counterclockwise on a square with labeled corners.

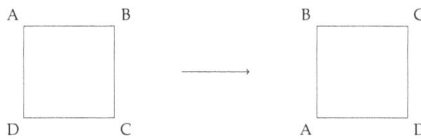

Figure 2. Rotation of the square by $90°$ counterclockwise.

3. Method

3.1. Background

Alsam et al. [24,25] proposed a saliency model that uses asymmetry as a measure of saliency. In order to calculate saliency, the input image is decomposed into non-overlapping square blocks (as shown at the top-left in Figure 3), and for each block, the absolute difference between the block itself and the result of the D_4 group elements acting on the block is calculated. As shown at the bottom-right in Figure 3, the asymmetry values of the square blocks pertaining to uniform regions are close to zero. The sum of the absolute differences (also known as the L_1 norm) for each block is used as a measure of the asymmetry for the block. The asymmetry values for all of the blocks are then collected in an image matrix and scaled up to the size of the original image using bilinear interpolation. In order to capture both the local and the global salient details in an image, three different image resolutions are used. All maps are combined linearly to get a single saliency map.

In their algorithm, the asymmetry of a square region is calculated as follows: M (i.e., the square block) is defined as an $n \times n$-matrix and σ_i as one of the eight group elements of D_4. The eight elements are the rotations along $0°$, $90°$, $180°$ and $270°$ and the reflections along the horizontal, vertical and two diagonal axes of the square. As an example, the eight group transformations pertaining to a square block of the image are shown in Figure 3. Asymmetry of M by σ_i is denoted by $A(M)$ to be,

$$A(M) = \sum_{i=0}^{7} ||M - \sigma_i M||_1, \tag{1}$$

where $||_1$ represents the L_1 norm. Instead of calculating asymmetry values associated with each group element and followed by their sum, we propose that the algorithm can run faster if the calculations in Equation (1) are made simpler. For this, we propose a fast implementation of these operations pertaining to the D_4 group elements.

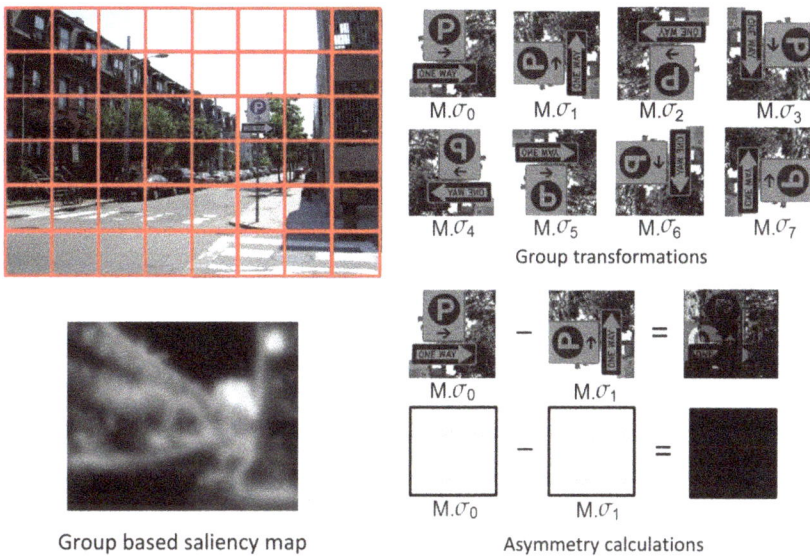

Figure 3. Original group-based algorithm proposed by Alsam et al. [24,25], the figure shows an example image (from [16]) along with the associated saliency map. The figure on the top-right shows the eight group transformations pertaining to a square block of an image. Bottom-right figures show the asymmetry calculations for square blocks pertaining to uniform and non-uniform regions. We can see that for uniform regions, this value is close to zero. Please note that bright locations represent higher values, and dark locations represent low values.

3.2. Fast Implementation of the Group Operations

Let us assume M as a 4 by 4 matrix,

$$M = \begin{bmatrix} \alpha_1 & a & b & \beta_1 \\ c & \alpha_2 & \beta_2 & d \\ e & \gamma_2 & \delta_2 & f \\ \gamma_1 & g & h & \delta_1 \end{bmatrix}$$

The asymmetry $A(M)$ of the matrix M is measured as the sum of the absolute differences of the different permutations of the matrix entries pertaining to the D_4 group elements and the original. The total number of such differences is determined to be 40. As the calculations associated with absolute differences are repeated for the rotation and reflection elements of the dihedral group D_4, our objective is to find the factors associated with these repeated differences.

For our calculations, we divide the set of matrix entries into two computational categories: the diagonal entries (highlighted in yellow) and the rest of the entries of M. Please note that these calculations can be generalized to any matrix of size n by n, given that n is even.

For the rest of the entries, first, we can look at $|a - b|$. This element will only be possible if we flip the matrix about the vertical axis. This will result in two parts in the sum, $|a - b|$ and $|b - a|$, giving a factor 2. Here, a and b represent a reflection symmetric pair, and all other reflection symmetric pairs will behave in the same way. Now, let us focus on $|a - d|$. This represents a rotational symmetric pair. Rotating the matrix counterclockwise will move d onto the position of a giving a part $|a - d|$ in the sum. Rotating clockwise gives us $|d - a|$. As these differences are not plausible in any other way, this gives us a factor of 2. All other rotational symmetric pairs will behave in the same way. This means that the asymmetry for the rest of the entries can be calculated as follows:

$$2|a - b| + 2|a - c| + 2|a - d| + \cdots + 2|g - h|. \tag{2}$$

For the diagonal entries, we can see that they exhibit both rotation and reflection symmetries. For instance, we can move β to the place of α and α to β with one reflection and two rotations. This gives us a factor of 4. The asymmetry of one set of diagonal entries can be calculated as follows:

$$4|\alpha - \beta| + 4|\alpha - \gamma| + 4|\alpha - \delta| + 4|\beta - \gamma| + 4|\beta - \delta| + 4|\gamma - \delta|. \tag{3}$$

The asymmetry for both diagonal entries and the rest is represented as,

$$
\begin{aligned}
A(M) \quad = \quad & 4|\alpha_1 - \beta_1| + 4|\alpha_1 - \gamma_1| + \cdots + 4|\gamma_1 - \delta_1| \\
& +4|\alpha_2 - \beta_2| + 4|\alpha_2 - \gamma_2| + \cdots + 4|\gamma_2 - \delta_2| \\
& +2|a - b| + 2|a - c| + \cdots + 2|g - h|.
\end{aligned} \tag{4}
$$

As shown in Equation (4), the asymmetry calculations associated with the matrix M are reduced to a quarter for the diagonal entries and one-half for the rest of the entries. This makes the proposed algorithm at least twice as fast.

3.3. De-Correlation of Color Image Channels

De-correlation of color image channels is done as follows: First, using bilinear interpolation, we create three resolutions (original, half and quarter) of the RGB color image. In order to collect all of the information in a matrix, the (half and one-quarter) resolutions are rescaled to the size of original. This gives us a matrix I of size w by h by n, where w is the width of the original, h is the height and n is the number of channels ($3 \times 3 = 9$).

Second, by rearranging the matrix entries of I, we create a two-dimensional matrix A of size $w \times h$ by n. We do normalization of A around the mean as,

$$B = A - \mu, \tag{5}$$

where μ is the mean for each of the channels, and B is $w \times h$ by n.

Third, we calculate the correlation matrix of B as,

$$C = B^T B, \tag{6}$$

where the size of C is n by n.

Fourth, the Eigen decomposition of a symmetric matrix is represented as,

$$C = VDV^T, \tag{7}$$

where V is a square matrix whose columns are eigenvectors of C and D is the diagonal matrix whose diagonal entries are the corresponding eigenvalues.

Finally, the image channels are transformed into eigenvector space (also known as principal components) as:

$$E = V^T(A - \mu), \tag{8}$$

where E is the transformed space matrix, which is rearranged to get back the de-correlated channels.

3.4. Implementation of the Algorithm

First, the input color image is rescaled to half the original resolution. Second, by using the de-correlation procedure described in Section 3.3 on the resulting image, we get 9 de-correlated multi-resolution and chromatic channels. Third, a fixed block size (e.g., 12) is selected, as discussed later in Section 4.6; this choice is governed by the dataset. If the rows and columns of the de-correlated channels are not divisible by the block size, then they are padded with neighboring information along the right and bottom corners. Finally, the saliency map is generated by using the procedure outlined in Section 3.2. The code is open source and is available at Matlab Central for the research community.

4. Comparing Different Saliency Models

The performance of visual saliency algorithms is usually judged by how well the two-dimensional saliency maps can predict the human eye fixations for a given image. Center-bias is a key factor that can influence the evaluation of saliency algorithms [34].

4.1. Center-Bias

While viewing images, observers tend to look at the center regions more as compared to peripheral regions. As a result of that, a majority of fixations fall at the image center. This effect is known as center-bias and is well documented in vision studies [35,36]. The two main reasons for this are: first, the tendency of photographers to place the objects at the center of the image; second, the viewing strategy employed by observers, i.e., to look at center locations more in order to acquire the most information about a scene [37]. The presence of center-bias in fixations makes it difficult to analyze the correspondence between the fixated regions and the salient image regions.

4.2. Shuffled AUC Metric

The shuffled AUC metric was proposed by Tatler et al. [35] and later used by Zhang et al. [38] to mitigate the effect of center-bias in fixations. The shuffled AUC metric is a variant of AUC [39], which is known as the area under the receiver operating characteristic curve. For a detailed description of AUC, please see the study by Fawcett [39].

To calculate the shuffled AUC metric for a given image and one observer, the locations fixated by the observer are associated with the positive class (in a manner similar to the regular AUC metric); however, the locations for the negative class are selected randomly from the fixated locations of other unrelated images, such that they do not coincide with the locations from the positive class. Similar to the regular AUC, the shuffled AUC metric gives us a scalar value in the interval [0,1]. If the value is one then it indicates that the saliency model is perfect in predicting fixations. If shuffled $AUC <= 0.5$, then it implies that the performance of the saliency model is not better than a random classifier or chance prediction.

4.3. Dataset

For the analysis, we used the eye tracking database from the study by Judd et al. [16]. The database consists of 1003 images selected randomly from different categories and different geographical locations. In the eye tracking experiment [16], these images were shown to fifteen different users under free viewing conditions for a period of 3 s each. In the database, a majority of the images are 1024 pixels in width and 768 pixels in height. These landscape images were specifically used in the evaluation.

4.4. Saliency Models

For our comparison, eleven state-of-the-art saliency models, namely, **AIM** by Bruce and Tsotsos [40], **AWS** by Garcia-Diaz et al. [27], **Erdem** by Erdem and Erdem [22], **Hou** by Hou and Zhang [41], **Spec** by Schauerte and Stiefelhagen [42], **GBA** by Alsam et al. [24,25], **fast GBA** proposed in this paper ($S_f = 0.5$, $N_r = 3$, $b = 22$; for details, please see Section 4.6), **GBVS** by Harel et al. [43], **Itti** by Itti et al. [26], **Judd** by Judd et al. [16] and **LG** by Borji and Itti [44] are used. In line with the study by Borji et al. [45], two models are selected to provide a baseline for the evaluation. **Gauss** is defined as a two-dimensional Gaussian blob at the center of the image. Different radii of the Gaussian blob are tested, and the radius that corresponds best with human eye fixations is selected.

The **IO** model is based on the fact that an observer's fixations can be predicted best by the fixations of other observers viewing the same image. In this model, the map for an observer is calculated as follows: first, the fixations corresponding to a given image from all of the observers except the one under consideration are averaged into a single two-dimensional map. Having done that, the fixations are spread by smoothing the map using a Gaussian filter. The IO model gives us an upper bound on the level of correspondence that is expected between the saliency models and the fixations. Figure 4 shows a test image and the associated saliency maps from different saliency algorithms.

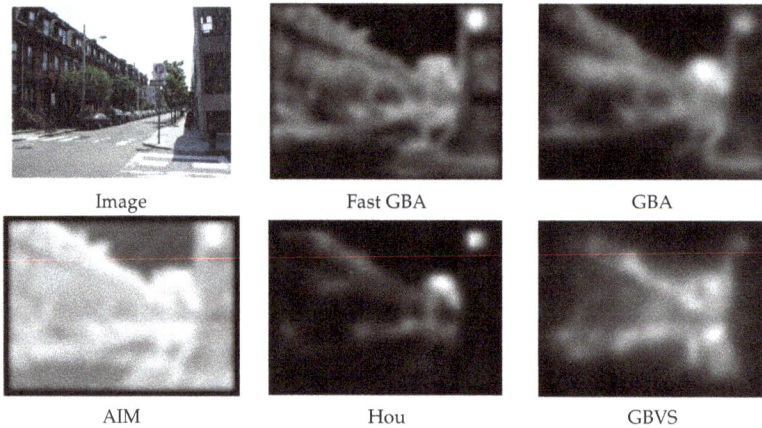

| Image | Fast GBA | GBA |
| AIM | Hou | GBVS |

Figure 4. *Cont.*

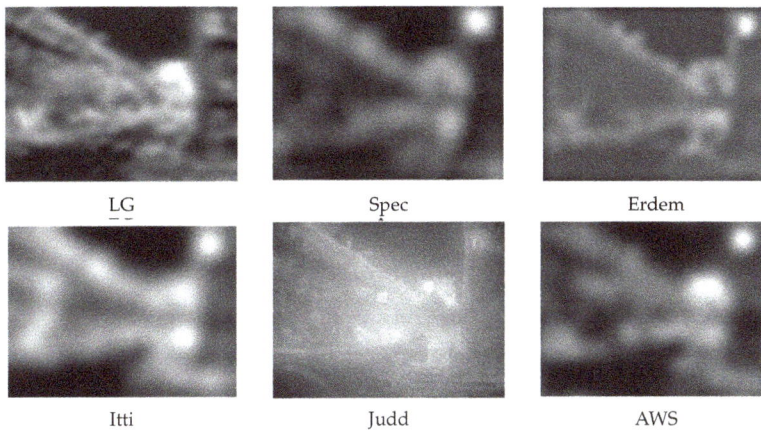

Figure 4. Figure shows a test image (from the database [16]) and the associated saliency maps from different saliency algorithms used in the paper.

4.5. Ranking among the Saliency Models

We compare the ranking of saliency models using the shuffled AUC metric. From the results in Figure 5, we note that, first, the Gauss model is ranked the worst indicating that the shuffled AUC metric counters the effects associated with the center-bias. Second, the AWS model is ranked the best followed by the proposed fast GBA model. It is important to note that a majority of the state-of-the-art saliency models, such as Itti, Hou, Spec, GBA, fast GBA LG, Erdem, AIM and AWS, are quite close to each other in terms of their performance.

Next, we compare the average run times (for 463 landscape images) of the saliency models that rank at the same or better than Itti, i.e., the classic saliency model. For a better visualization, we use the natural logarithm of the average run times. For this, we used MATLAB R2015 on a 64-bit windows PC with a 3.16-GHz Intel processor and 4 GB RAM. From Figure 6, we observe that the algorithms Hou, and Spec are the fastest. However, among the top six algorithms, the proposed fast GBA model is the fastest. Furthermore, it shows that Fast GBA is nearly 31-times faster than the original GBA algorithm. It is important to note that the original GBA algorithm is crude in implementation, i.e., the eight group transformations are performed iteratively and kept in the memory. In the fast GBA model, reducing the computational complexity (by employing the steps mentioned in Section 3.2) also reduces the memory and software complexity of the proposed model, which is reflected in the results.

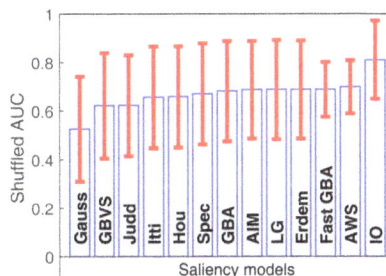

Figure 5. Ranking of different saliency models using the shuffled AUC metric. The results are obtained from the fixation data of 463 landscape images and fifteen observers.

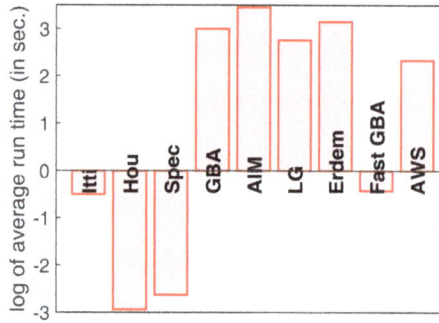

Figure 6. Average run time across 463 landscape images for different saliency models: Itti = 0.60, Hou = 0.05, Spec = 0.07, GBA = 20.13, AIM = 31.75, LG = 15.70, Erdem = 23.35, Fast GBA = 0.65, AWS = 10.27. All run times are in seconds. For a better visualization, we use the natural logarithm of the average run times.

4.6. Optimizing the Proposed Fast GBA Model

The performance of the proposed model is influenced by the choice of parameters, such as block size, which depends on the size of an average image in the database used for testing. To find the optimal parameters for our algorithm, we use three variables: image scaling factor S_f (which rescales the original image in order to reduce the number of calculations), block size b and number of resolutions N_r (different resolutions to capture local and global details). For this analysis, we use $S_f = 0.5$ (half size) and $S_f = 1$, b in the range [12, 50], and $N_r = 1, 2$ and 3. The results obtained by using the shuffled AUC metric for the three variables are shown in the first row of Figure 7. The figure on the top-left shows the shuffled AUC values for $S_f = 0.5$, with the red, green and blue lines depicting N_r as 1, 2 and 3, respectively, while the figure on the top-right shows the shuffled AUC values for $S_f = 1$. In the second row of Figure 7, we depict the average run time of the algorithm for the different values of S_f, b and N_r. The results indicate that: First, increasing the number of resolutions improves the performance of the proposed model. Second, based on the figures in the second row, we note that using $S_f = 0.5$ (i.e., working with an image of half the original resolution) reduces the run time to less than one second. Third, we observe (in the figure on the top-right) that the shuffled AUC values for our algorithm exceed the values obtained from the AWS model (i.e., the best saliency model, represented by the black dashed line) for the following parameters: $S_f = 1$, $N_r = 3$, $b = 14, 22, 34, 46$, and $S_f = 1$, $N_r = 2$, $b = 46$. In other words, using the optimal parameters (mentioned above), our proposed model outranks the best saliency model in the literature; however, we believe that the differences between the top 5 algorithms (AIM, LG, Erdem, fast GBA and AWS) are too small to rank one as the best over the rest. Fourth, from the figure on the bottom-right, we note that using the optimal parameters increases the run time to a few seconds (a minimum of 1.7 to a maximum of 4.7 s), which are still faster than the run time of the AWS model (i.e., 10.2 s). Please note that in order to highlight the intrinsic nature of the fast GBA model, no GPU computing was employed.

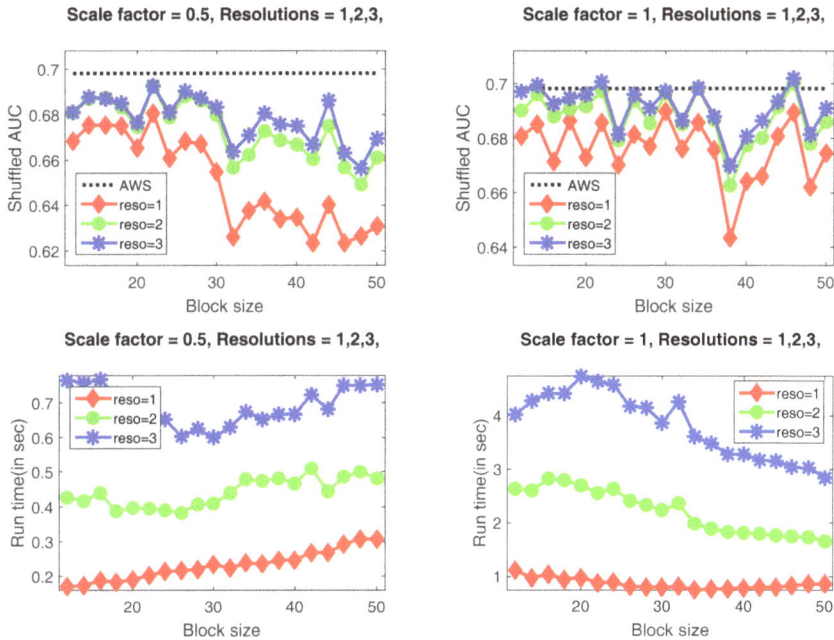

Figure 7. The results obtained by using the shuffled AUC metric for the three variables are shown in the first row. The figure on the top-left shows the shuffled AUC values for $S_f = 0.5$, with the red, green and blue lines depicting N_r as 1, 2 and 3 respectively, while, the figure on the top-right shows the shuffled AUC values for $S_f = 1$. In the second row, we show the average run time of the algorithm for the different values of S_f, b and N_r.

4.7. Impact of De-Correlation on the Performance of the Proposed Fast GBA Model

To observe if de-correlation of color image channels (mentioned in Section 3.3) influences the performance of group-based saliency models, we performed an analysis on two versions of the GBA by Alsam et al. [24,25] and the proposed fast GBA models. In the first versions of both algorithms, we used the color space from the original GBA algorithm (luminance channel, red-green and blue-yellow color opponency channels). In other words, the first versions do not use de-correlated color space. In the second versions, we used the de-correlated color space (from Section 3.3).

Using the shuffled AUC metric (as shown in Figure 8), the results show that the GBA-Decorr and fast GBA-Decorr models give quite similar values when implemented without de-correlation, and a similar trend is exhibited by the GBA + Decorr and Fast GBA + Decorr models, which are implemented using de-correlated color space. For all algorithms, we used the following parameters: $S_f = 0.5$, $N_r = 3$, $b = 22$. Our results suggest that using de-correlation of the color image channels improves the performance of group-based saliency models. Furthermore, this implies that other saliency models can also benefit from using a de-correlated color space.

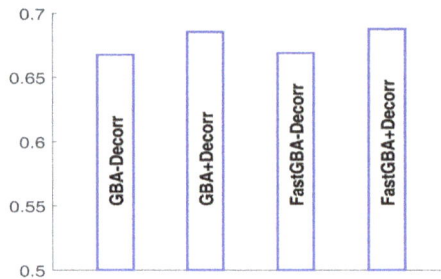

Figure 8. GBA-Decorr and fast GBA-Decorr models give quite similar values when implemented without de-correlation, and a similar trend is exhibited by the GBA + Decorr and fast GBA + Decorr models, which are implemented using de-correlated color space. For all algorithms, we used the following parameters $S_f = 0.5$, $N_r = 3$, $b = 22$. The results are obtained from the fixation data of 463 landscape images and fifteen observers using the shuffled AUC metric.

5. Future Work

We believe that our proposed approach on saliency can be extended to include three-dimensional image data (such as magnetic resonance imaging). In order to calculate saliency for three-dimensional data, we can use the symmetry groups for a cube.

A cube has 48 symmetries that can be represented by the transformations of products of the groups S_4 and S_2. S_2 is the symmetric group of degree two and has two elements: the identity and the permutation interchanging the two points [28]. S_4 is a symmetric group of degree four, i.e., all permutations on a set of size four [28]. This group has 24 elements that are obtained by rotations about opposite faces, opposite diagonals and opposite edges of the cube. For instance, Figure 9 shows the different rotational symmetries of the cube. We note that from the rotations along opposite diagonals, faces and edges, we get 8, 9 and 6 elements, respectively. These elements along with the identity form the 24 elements of the S_4 group.

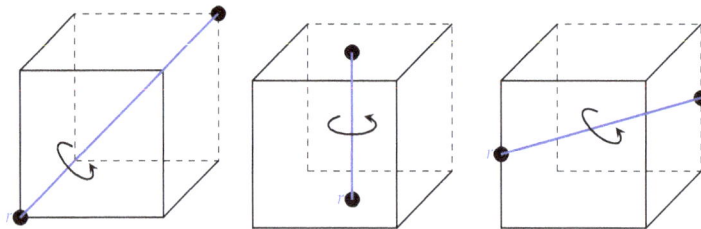

Figure 9. (Left) Number of axes with opposite diagonals like this = 4. We can rotate by 120 or 240 degrees around these axes. These operations give eight elements. (Center) Number of axes with opposite faces like this = 3. We can either rotate by 90, 180 or 270 degrees around these axes. These operations give nine elements. (Right) Number of axes with opposite edges like this = 6. We can rotate by 180 degrees around these axes. These operations give six elements.

Saliency for three-dimensional image data can be calculated by employing the same procedure as discussed in Section 3, but instead of computing in two-dimensional space using the D_4 group, we can calculate it in three-dimensional space using the $S_4 \times S_2$ transformations. For example, after dividing the three-dimensional scene into uniform sized cubes, we can rotate and reflect a cube and record the values associated with the transformations. The recorded values can be collected in a matrix and rescaled along each of the three planes, i.e., X-Y, Y-Z, Z-X, to get a three-dimensional feature map. The resulting feature maps corresponding to the 48 elements can be combined to get a representation of saliency for the three-dimensional scene. This is left as future work, and we hope that this will help future researchers to venture towards three-dimensional saliency.

6. Conclusions

In this article, first, we briefly describe the dihedral group D_4 that is used for calculating saliency in our proposed model. Second, our saliency model makes the two following changes in a latest state-of-the-art model known as group-based asymmetry: first, based on the properties of the dihedral group D_4, we simplify the asymmetry calculations associated with the measurement of saliency. This results is an algorithm that reduces the number of calculations by at least half that makes it the fastest among the six best algorithms used in this research article. Two, in order to maximize the information across different chromatic and multi-resolution features, the color image space is de-correlated. We evaluate our algorithm against 10 state-of-the-art saliency models. Our results clearly show that by using optimal parameters for a given dataset our proposed model can outperform the best saliency algorithm in the literature. However, as the differences among the (few) best saliency models are small, we would like to suggest that our proposed model is among the best and the fastest among the best. In the end, as a part of future work, we suggest that our proposed approach on saliency can be extended to include three-dimensional image data.

Conflicts of Interest: The author declare no conflict of interest.

References

1. Suder, K.; Worgotter, F. The control of low-level information flow in the visual system. *Rev. Neurosci.* **2000**, *11*, 127–146.
2. Yang, J.; Yang, M.H. Top-down visual saliency via joint CRF and dictionary learning. In Proceedings of the 2012 IEEE Conference on Computer Vision and Pattern Recognition (CVPR), Providence, RI, USA, 16–21 June 2012; pp. 2296–2303.
3. He, S.; Lau, R.W.; Yang, Q. Exemplar-Driven Top-Down Saliency Detection via Deep Association. In Proceedings of the IEEE Conference on Computer Vision and Pattern Recognition, Las Vegas, NV, USA, 27–30 June 2016.
4. Koch, C.; Ullman, S. Shifts in selective visual attention: Towards the underlying neural circuitry. *Hum. Neurobiol.* **1985**, *4*, 219–227.
5. Itti, L. Automatic Foveation for Video Compression Using a Neurobiological Model of Visual Attention. *IEEE Trans. Image Process.* **2004**, *13*, 1304–1318.
6. Yu, S.X.; Lisin, D.A. Image Compression based on Visual Saliency at Individual Scales. In Proceedings of the 5th International Symposium on Advances in Visual Computing Part I, Las Vegas, NV, USA, 30 November–2 December 2009; pp. 157–166.
7. Alsam, A.; Rivertz, H.; Sharma, P. What the Eye Did Not See—A Fusion Approach to Image Coding. In *Advances in Visual Computing*; Bebis, G., Boyle, R., Parvin, B., Koracin, D., Fowlkes, C., Wang, S., Choi, M.H., Mantler, S., Schulze, J., Acevedo, D., Eds.; Lecture Notes in Computer Science; Springer: Berlin/Heidelberg, Germany, 2012; Volume 7432, pp. 199–208.
8. Alsam, A.; Rivertz, H.J.; Sharma, P. What the eye did not see–A fusion approach to image coding. *Int. J. Artif. Intell. Tools* **2013**, *22*, 1360014.
9. Siagian, C.; Itti, L. Biologically-Inspired Robotics Vision Monte-Carlo Localization in the Outdoor Environment. In Proceedings of the IEEE International Conference on Intelligent Robots and Systems, San Diego, CA, USA, 29 October–2 November 2007.
10. Frintrop, S.; Jensfelt, P.; Christensen, H.I. Attentional Landmark Selection for Visual SLAM. In Proceedings of the IEEE/RSJ International Conference on Intelligent Robots and Systems, Beijing, China, 9–15 October 2006.
11. Kadir, T.; Brady, M. Saliency, Scale and Image Description. *Int. J. Comput. Vis.* **2001**, *45*, 83–105.

12. Feng, X.; Liu, T.; Yang, D.; Wang, Y. Saliency based objective quality assessment of decoded video affected by packet losses. In Proceedings of the 15th IEEE International Conference on Image Processing, San Diego, CA, USA, 12–15 October 2008; pp. 2560–2563.

13. Ma, Q.; Zhang, L. Saliency-Based Image Quality Assessment Criterion. In *Advanced Intelligent Computing Theories and Applications. With Aspects of Theoretical and Methodological Issues*; Huang, D.S., Wunsch, D.C.I., Levine, D., Jo, K.H., Eds.; Lecture Notes in Computer Science; Springer: Berlin/Heidelberg, Germany, 2008; Volume 5226, pp. 1124–1133.

14. El-Nasr, M.; Vasilakos, A.; Rao, C.; Zupko, J. Dynamic Intelligent Lighting for Directing Visual Attention in Interactive 3-D Scenes. *IEEE Trans. Comput. Intell. AI Games* **2009**, *1*, 145–153.

15. Rosenholtz, R.; Dorai, A.; Freeman, R. Do predictions of visual perception aid design? *ACM Trans. Appl. Percept.* **2011**, *8*, 12:1–12:20.

16. Judd, T.; Ehinger, K.; Durand, F.; Torralba, A. Learning to predict where humans look. In Proceedings of the 2009 IEEE International Conference on Computer Vision (ICCV), Kyoto, Japan, 27 September–4 October 2009; pp. 2106–2113.

17. Breazeal, C.; Scassellati, B. A Context-Dependent Attention System for a Social Robot; In Proceedings of the International Joint Conference on Artificial Intelligence (IJCAI), Stockholm, Sweden, 31 July–6 August 1999; pp. 1146–1153.

18. Ajallooeian, M.; Borji, A.; Araabi, B.; Ahmadabadi, M.; Moradi, H. An application to interactive robotic marionette playing based on saliency maps. In Proceedings of the 18th IEEE International Symposium on Robot and Human Interactive Communication, Toyama, Japan, 27 September–2 October 2009; pp. 841–847.

19. Itti, L.; Koch, C. A saliency-based search mechanism for overt and covert shifts of visual attention. *Vis. Res.* **2000**, *40*, 1489–1506.

20. Liu, T.; Sun, J.; Zheng, N.N.; Tang, X.; Shum, H.Y. Learning to Detect A Salient Object. In Proceedings of the 2007 IEEE Conference on Computer Vision and Pattern Recognition, Minneapolis, MN, USA, 18–23 June 2007.

21. Achanta, R.; Estrada, F.; Wils, P.; Süsstrunk, S. Salient region detection and segmentation. In Proceedings of the 6th International Conference on Computer Vision Systems, Santorini, Greece, 12–15 May 2008; pp. 66–75.

22. Erdem, E.; Erdem, A. Visual saliency estimation by nonlinearly integrating features using region covariances. *J. Vis.* **2013**, *13*, 1–20.

23. He, S.; Lau, R.W.H.; Liu, W.; Huang, Z.; Yang, Q. SuperCNN: A Superpixelwise Convolutional Neural Network for Salient Object Detection. *Int. J. Comput. Vis.* **2015**, *115*, 330–344.

24. Alsam, A.; Sharma, P.; Wrålsen, A. Asymmetry as a Measure of Visual Saliency. *Lecture Notes in Computer Science (LNCS)*; Springer-Verlag: Berlin/Heidelberg, Germany, 2013; Volume 7944, pp. 591–600.

25. Alsam, A.; Sharma, P.; Wrålsen, A. Calculating saliency using the dihedral group D4. *J. Imaging Sci. Technol.* **2014**, *58*, 10504:1–10504:12.

26. Itti, L.; Koch, C.; Niebur, E. A Model of Saliency-Based Visual Attention for Rapid Scene Analysis. *IEEE Trans. Pattern Anal. Mach. Intell.* **1998**, *20*, 1254–1259.

27. Garcia-Diaz, A.; Fdez-Vidal, X.R.; Pardo, X.M.; Dosil, R. Saliency from hierarchical adaptation through decorrelation and variance normalization. *Image Vis. Comput.* **2012**, *30*, 51–64.

28. Dummit, D.S.; Foote, R.M. *Abstract Algebra*, 3rd ed; John Wiley & Sons: Hoboken, NJ, USA, 2004.

29. Lenz, R. Using representations of the dihedral groups in the design of early vision filters. In Proceedings of the IEEE International Conference on Acoustics, Speech, and Signal Processing (ICASSP-93), Minneapolis, MN, USA, 27–30 April 1993; pp. 165–168.

30. Lenz, R. Investigation of Receptive Fields Using Representations of the Dihedral Groups. *J. Vis. Commun. Image Represent.* **1995**, *6*, 209–227.

31. Foote, R.; Mirchandani, G.; Rockmore, D.N.; Healy, D.; Olson, T. A wreath product group approach to signal and image processing. I. Multiresolution analysis. *IEEE Trans. Signal Process.* **2000**, *48*, 102–132.

32. Chang, W.Y. Image Processing with Wreath Products. Master's Thesis, Harvey Mudd College, Claremont, CA, USA, 2004.

33. Lenz, R.; Bui, T.H.; Takase, K. A group theoretical toolbox for color image operators. In Proceedings of the IEEE International Conference on Image Processing, Genoa, Italy, 11–14 September 2005; Volume 3, pp. 557–560.

34. Sharma, P. Evaluating visual saliency algorithms: Past, present and future. *J. Imaging Sci. Technol.* **2015**, *59*, 50501:1–50501:17.
35. Tatler, B.W.; Baddeley, R.J.; Gilchrist, I.D. Visual correlates of fixation selection: Effects of scale and time. *Vis. Res.* **2005**, *45*, 643–659.
36. Tatler, B.W. The central fixation bias in scene viewing: Selecting an optimal viewing position independently of motor biases and image feature distributions. *J. Vis.* **2007**, *7*, 1–17.
37. Tseng, P.H.; Carmi, R.; Cameron, I.G.M.; Munoz, D.P.; Itti, L. Quantifying center bias of observers in free viewing of dynamic natural scenes. *J. Vis.* **2009**, *9*, 1–16.
38. Zhang, L.; Tong, M.H.; Marks, T.K.; Shan, H.; Cottrell, G.W. SUN: A Bayesian framework for saliency using natural statistics. *J. Vis.* **2008**, *8*, 1–20.
39. Fawcett, T. ROC Graphs with Instance-Varying Costs. *Pattern Recognit. Lett.* **2004**, *27*, 882–891.
40. Bruce, N.D.B.; Tsotsos, J.K. Saliency Based on Information Maximization. In Proceedings of the Neural Information Processing Systems conference (NIPS 2005), Vancouver, BC, Canada, 5–10 December 2005; pp. 155–162.
41. Hou, X.; Zhang, L. Computer Vision and Pattern Recognition. In Proceedings of the IEEE Conference on Saliency Detection: A Spectral Residual Approach, Minneapolis, MN, USA, 17–22 June 2007; pp. 1–8.
42. Schauerte, B.; Stiefelhagen, R. Predicting Human Gaze using Quaternion DCT Image Signature Saliency and Face Detection. In Proceedings of the IEEE Workshop on the Applications of Computer Vision (WACV), Breckenridge, CO, USA, 9–11 January 2012.
43. Harel, J.; Koch, C.; Perona, P. Graph-Based Visual Saliency. In *Proceedings of Neural Information Processing Systems (NIPS)*; MIT Press: Cambridge, MA, USA, 2006; pp. 545–552.
44. Borji, A.; Itti, L. Exploiting Local and Global Patch Rarities for Saliency Detection. In Proceedings of the IEEE Conference on Computer Vision and Pattern Recognition (CVPR), Providence, RI, USA, 18–20 June 2012; pp. 1–8.
45. Borji, A.; Sihite, D.N.; Itti, L. Quantitative Analysis of Human-Model Agreement in Visual Saliency Modeling: A Comparative Study. *IEEE Trans. Image Process.* **2013**, *22*, 55–69.

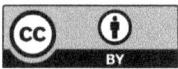

symmetry

MDPI

Article

Relationship between Fractal Dimension and Spectral Scaling Decay Rate in Computer-Generated Fractals

Alexander J. Bies [1],*, Cooper R. Boydston [2], Richard P. Taylor [2] and Margaret E. Sereno [1]

[1] Department of Psychology, University of Oregon, Eugene, OR 97405, USA; msereno@uoregon.edu
[2] Department of Physics, University of Oregon, Eugene, OR 97405, USA; nashua56@gmail.com (C.R.B.); rpt@uoregon.edu (R.P.T.)
* Correspondence: alexanderbies@gmail.com or bies@uoregon.edu; Tel.: +1-812-457-7965

Academic Editor: Marco Bertamini
Received: 11 April 2016; Accepted: 12 July 2016; Published: 19 July 2016

Abstract: Two measures are commonly used to describe scale-invariant complexity in images: fractal dimension (D) and power spectrum decay rate (β). Although a relationship between these measures has been derived mathematically, empirical validation across measurements is lacking. Here, we determine the relationship between D and β for 1- and 2-dimensional fractals. We find that for 1-dimensional fractals, measurements of D and β obey the derived relationship. Similarly, in 2-dimensional fractals, measurements along any straight-line path across the fractal's surface obey the mathematically derived relationship. However, the standard approach of vision researchers is to measure β of the surface after 2-dimensional Fourier decomposition rather than along a straight-line path. This surface technique provides measurements of β that do not obey the mathematically derived relationship with D. Instead, this method produces values of β that imply that the fractal's surface is much smoother than the measurements along the straight lines indicate. To facilitate communication across disciplines, we provide empirically derived equations for relating each measure of β to D. Finally, we discuss implications for future research on topics including stress reduction and the perception of motion in the context of a generalized equation relating β to D.

Keywords: fractal patterns; scale-invariance; fractal dimension; spectral scaling; midpoint displacement; Fourier noise; Fourier decomposition

1. Introduction

Researchers from diverse disciplines ranging from physics to psychology have converged on the question of how to quantify the scaling symmetry of natural objects. In one camp, fractals researchers describe objects such as clouds, coastlines, mountain ridgelines, and trees using a scale-invariant power law to measure the rate at which structure appears as the scale of measurement decreases [1–6], though debates continue regarding which power-laws, if any, best describe natural phenomena [7–11]. The following equation is a common example:

$$N \sim L^{-D} \tag{1}$$

where N is the extent to which the fractal fills space as measured at scale L [1,4]. The power law's exponent D is called the fractal dimension.

Consider Figure 1a,b, which plots a fractal terrain in x, y, and z space, as a demonstration of how D relates to the object's Euclidean dimension E. The topological dimension of this surface is $E = 2$ and it is embedded in a space of $E = 3$. Its fractal dimension, $D_{(Surface)}$, lies in the range between these two Euclidean dimensions: $2 < D_{(Surface)} < 3$. Taking a vertical slice through this terrain (i.e., taking its intersection with the xz or yz plane) creates a fractal "mountain" profile (see Figure 1c) quantified by $D_{(Mountain\ Edge)} = D_{(Surface)} - 1$. Similarly, taking a horizontal slice creates a fractal "coastline" (see Figure 1d) with $D_{(Coastal\ Edge)} = D_{(Mountain\ Edge)}$. To measure $D_{(Surface)}$, mathematicians and natural scientists typically determine $D_{(Mountain\ Edge)}$ or $D_{(Coastal\ Edge)}$ (and then add 1) because the measurements involved are easier and faster to implement than for measurements of $D_{(Surface)}$.

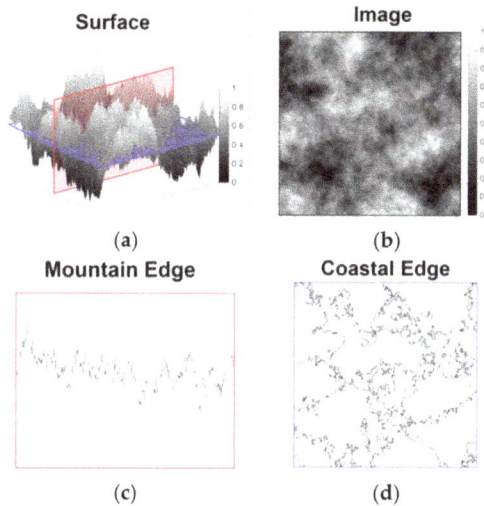

Figure 1. Plots of a fractal terrain with $D = 2.5$ and its intersection with axial planes; (a) "Surface" plot of a fractal terrain; (b) intensity "image" of the terrain; (c) "mountain edge" profile of an "*xz*-slice" or "*yz*-slice" of the terrain; (d) "coastal edge" of an "*xy*-slice" of the terrain.

Vision researchers similarly use a power law to capture the scale-invariant properties of the fractal. However, they typically focus on the power spectrum decay rate (β) of the terrain's intensity image [12–21]. This intensity image is generated by converting the terrain height into either grayscale variations (high is white, black is low) to create a grayscale map (see Figure 1b) or color variations to create a "heat map". The following power law then characterizes the fractal structure in these maps and has, in particular, proved useful for quantifying the spectral scaling decay rate of grayscale images of natural scenes:

$$S_V(f) = 1/(cf^{\beta}) \tag{2}$$

where $S_V(f)$ is the spectral density (power), f is the spatial frequency, and β and c are constants.

Voss [5] considered the Hurst exponent H, which by definition is related to D as follows:

$$D = E + 1 - H \tag{3}$$

where E is the Euclidean topological dimension. H and D lie in the following ranges: $0 < H < 1$, $E < D < E + 1$. He then derived the relationship between H and β for a fractional Brownian function:

$$\beta = 2H + 1 \tag{4}$$

where $1 < \beta < 3$. Accordingly, Voss [5] stated that an approximation of the relationship for "the statistically self-affine fractional Brownian function $V_H(x)$, with x in an E-dimensional Euclidian space, which has a fractal dimension D and spectral density $S_V(f) \propto 1/f^{\beta}$, for the fluctuations along a straight line path in any direction in E-space" is provided by the equation

$$D = E + (3 - \beta)/2 \tag{5}$$

However, through this definition, Voss [5] stipulates a different measure of β than that typically used by vision researchers. The definition specifies the measure of β be taken along the intersection of the fractal with a plane parallel to the z-axis—a mountain edge—and measuring the spectral decay of the 1-dimensional trace—a mountain profile. Thus, β in Equations (4) and (5) are what we will hereafter call $β_{(Mountain\ Edge)}$.

The relationship highlighted in Equation (5) between D and $β_{(Mountain\ Edge)}$ has not been observed empirically for either 1-dimensional ($E = 1$, $D ⩽ 2$) or 2-dimensional ($E = 2$, $D ⩽ 3$) fractals. To experimentally discern this relationship, we use two methods for generating fractals—namely, midpoint displacement fractals (in which D serves as the input parameter) and fractal Fourier noise (in which β is the input). We find that, when measured along a straight-line path, the relationship described by Voss [5] holds for fractals with both $E = 1$ and 2. However, the relationship described by Voss [5] does not extend to the observed relationship between measurements of D and β when β is measured by the standard method of vision researchers (in a 2-dimensional Fourier space, which we will hereafter call $β_{(Surface)}$). A new equation that extends the relationship between D and β to multi-dimensional Fourier spaces has the potential to enhance discourse among mathematicians, who are experts in the geometry of fractals, physicists, who are experts in surfaces and textures, and vision scientists, who are experts in animals' sensation and perception of geometric shapes, surfaces, and textures.

Further consideration of the relationship between D and β is both important and timely because new studies are being performed using fractals to investigate a variety of behaviors including aesthetics [22–27], navigation [28], object pareidolia (perceiving coherent forms in noise) [29,30], sensitivity [24], and associated neural mechanisms [31–33]. This is especially important in aesthetics research, where there have been claims of universality in preference for patterns of moderately low complexity [23,26,34–37]. To test this hypothesis, it is necessary to be able to translate the units of measurement of researchers who alternately use D [22,25,26,28,29,31,33–40], β [14,24,30,32,41–46], or, infrequently, both [23,27]. The crux of the problem, perhaps, is that D is a general parameter that quantifies complexity in a variety of patterns, whereas β is limited (at least in practice) in its ability to quantify some patterns' complexity. For example, Fourier analysis is poorly suited to describe the complexity of patterns including strange attractors and some line fractals (e.g., dragon fractals and Koch snowflakes), which have been used by vision researchers to study aesthetics [25,31,34,35] and perceived complexity [47]. This provides a strong impetus to convert to D when forming general conclusions. Still, there is a great deal of utility in presenting fractal noise patterns that are defined in terms of β as visual stimuli, precisely because they mimic the statistics of natural scenes [12,13,15–21]. Here, we provide the basis for translation between the parameters D and β in a general equation that follows from empirical analysis of the relationships between measures of D and β.

2. Materials and Methods

Midpoint displacement and Fourier noise fractals were generated and analyzed in MATLAB version 2015b.

2.1. Midpoint Displacement Fractals

Sets of random midpoint displacement fractal lines (see Section 2.1.1) and images (see Section 2.1.2) were generated using an algorithm described by Fournier, Fussel, and Carpenter [2], which allowed us to specify D.

2.1.1. One-Dimensional Midpoint Displacement Fractals

To generate each 1-dimensional midpoint displacement fractal as a trace, a vertex, V, was added to the midpoint of an initial set of two endpoints and displaced vertically by a value randomly selected from a Gaussian distribution, with $σ = 1$, that was scaled by a factor of $2^{-2(3 - D)(R + 1)}$, where D is the fractal dimension and R is the current level of recursion. This process is shown schematically for an exact midpoint displacement fractal that is not affected by random perturbations in Figure 2. As in the schematic, the scaling factor of the fractals generated for this study was held constant for each vertex at a given level of recursion, and changed with each level of recursion. The vertices at each recursion served as endpoints in the next level of recursion for R recursions in order to generate time-series data.

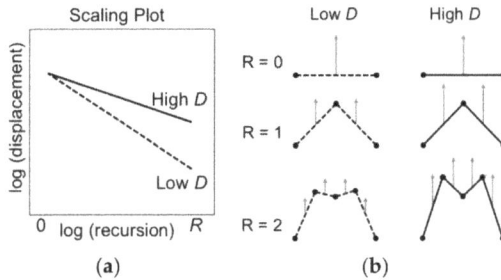

Figure 2. Illustration of the generation of 1-dimensional midpoint displacement fractals. (**a**) Cartoon graph of a scaling plot in log–log coordinates that determines the rate of scaling of midpoint displacements across recursions for high (solid line) and low (dashed line) D fractals; (**b**) Schematics of recursions 0–2 are shown for low (dashed line) and high (solid line) D exact midpoint displacement fractals. Gray arrows indicate displacements that occur with each recursion in (b).

We retained the random values used for vertical displacement to generate sets of fractals that varied in D but retained the structure introduced at each level of recursion (see Figure 3).

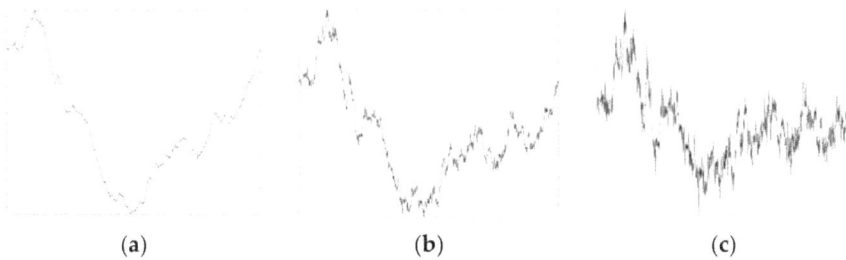

Figure 3. Plots of 1-dimensional statistical midpoint displacement fractals. (**a**–**c**) Fractal traces that vary in D, such that D = 1.2, 1.5, and 1.8, are generated from a single set of random numbers that contribute to the variable length and direction of displacement of the midpoints at each recursion.

2.1.2. Two-Dimensional Midpoint Displacement Fractals

To generate each 2-dimensional midpoint displacement fractal as an image, a vertex, V, was added to the midpoint of an initial set of four edge points and displaced according to the generation rules described in Section 2.1.1 (see illustration of the generation process in Figure 4). The vertices at each recursion served as edges in the next level of recursion for n recursions in order to generate gray-scale intensity images.

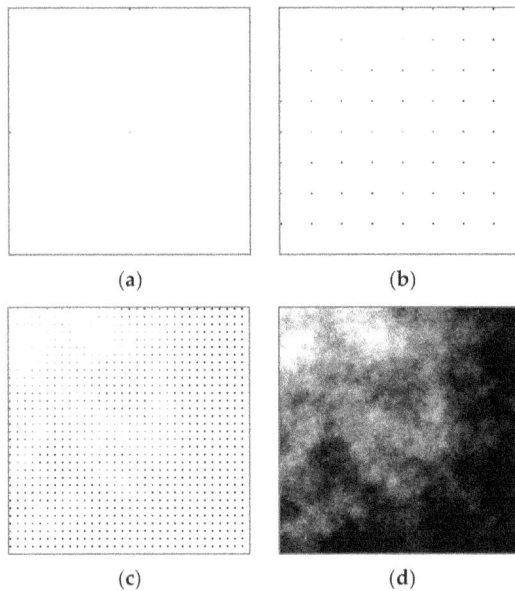

Figure 4. Illustration of the generation of a 2-dimensional midpoint displacement fractal as the heights (indicated by grayscale intensity) of particular points are specified over eight recursions. (**a–d**) The second, fourth, sixth, and final recursions are shown. In (**a–c**), white space indicates points for which height has not yet been specified.

We retained the random values used for vertical displacement to generate sets of fractal terrains that varied in D but retained consistent large-scale structures (see Figure 5).

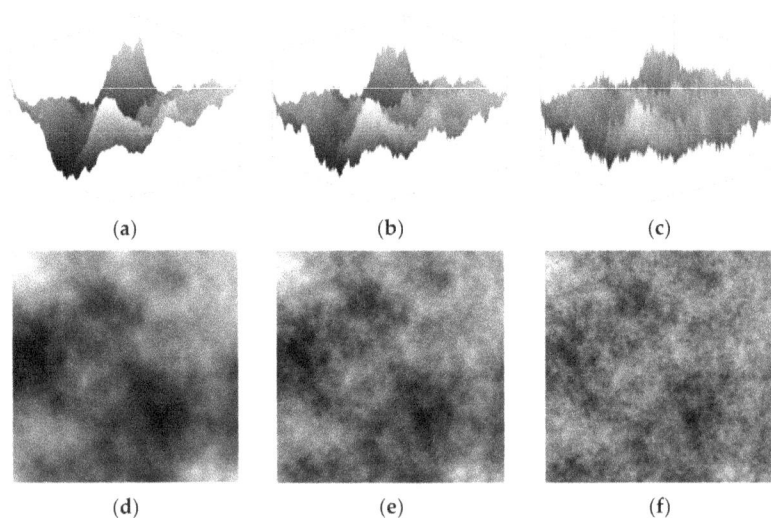

Figure 5. Plots of 2-dimensional midpoint displacement fractals. (**a–c**) Surface plots of fractals generated from a single set of random numbers that vary in D, such that $D = 1.2, 1.5$, and 1.8; (**d–f**) Grayscale intensity map images of the surface plots in (**a–c**).

2.2. One- and Two-Dimensional Fractal Fourier Noise

Sets of fractal noise were generated using an algorithm described by Saupe [3], which allowed us to specify β.

For an image of size x by y pixels, an x by y amplitude matrix is created in which amplitude is specified for each spatial frequency by applying Equation (2). Each frequency is then assigned a phase specified by a phase matrix of size x by y, which consists of numbers that are randomly selected from a Gaussian distribution. The amplitude and phase matrices are then subjected to an inverse Fourier transform to generate a time series (if x or $y = 1$) or an image (if x and $y > 1$). The resulting fractals have scaling properties defined by their respective input β values (see Figures 6 and 7).

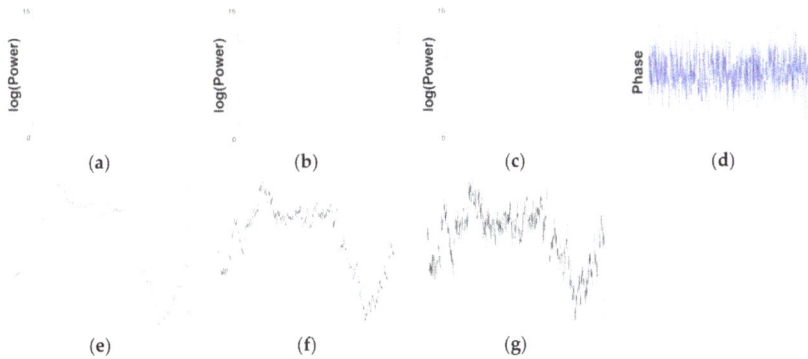

Figure 6. Generation of 1-dimensional Fourier noise fractals. (**a–c**) Power (*y*-axis) as a function of frequency (*x*-axis) for $β_{(Input)}$ = 2.6, 2, and 1.4; (**d**) Set of random phases (*y*-axis) as a function of frequency (*x*-axis); (**e–g**) fractal traces resulting from the pairing of the phases in panel (**d**) with power spectra from (**a–c**) respectively.

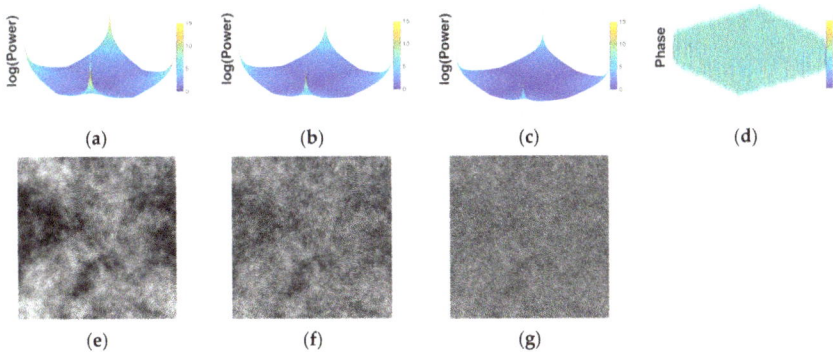

Figure 7. Generation of 2-dimensional Fourier noise fractals. (**a–c**) Power (*z*-axis) as a function of frequency in *xy* coordinates for $β_{(Input)}$ = 2.6, 2, and 1.4; (**d**) Set of random phases (*z*-axis) as a function of frequency in *xy* coordinates; (**e–g**) fractal terrains resulting from the pairing of the phases in panel (**d**) with power spectra from (**a–c**) respectively.

As with the midpoint displacement fractals, we retained the matrices of random numbers used to determine the phases of each spatial frequency (see Figures 6d and 7d) to generate sets of fractal noise images that differed only in their spectral scaling. One-dimensional fractal time series were generated from phase maps with amplitude series that varied in the specified β, $β_{(input)}$ (see Figure 6e–g).

Values of $\beta_{(input)}$ were paired with phase maps to create 2-dimensional fractal images as well (see Figure 7e–g).

2.3. Measurement of the Box Counting Dimension

2.3.1. Box Counting Analysis of 1-Dimensional Fractals: $D_{(Mountain\ Edge)}$

Box counting was performed on the intersection of 1-dimensional fractals with a horizontal line at the trace's median height. For the 2-dimensional fractal images, a fractal dust set was formed by taking the intersection of the height values of each row of the image with a line intersecting the median height. This dust set was used to compute the box counting dimension through the use of custom Matlab scripts. Briefly, for each box size with side length L, from the length of the fractal to a single pixel in steps of $L/2$ for a total of n steps, the image is covered with a set of boxes, and the number of boxes that contain any non-zero quantity of points is counted. The box counts of pairs of neighboring grid scales from $L/(2^3)$ to $L/(2^{n-3})$ were averaged to compute D, while the counts from the grid scales outside this range (the larger and smaller boxes, where $n = \{0, 1, 2, n-2, n-1,$ and $n\}$), were not used. The embedding dimension of the series of points is 1, but the embedding dimension of the fractal mountain edge is 2, so we averaged these values of D, computed for pairs of grid sizes, and added 1 to report the fractal dimension of the 1-dimensional fractals, $D_{(Mountain\ Edge)}$, which span the range $1 < D_{(Mountain\ Edge)} < 2$.

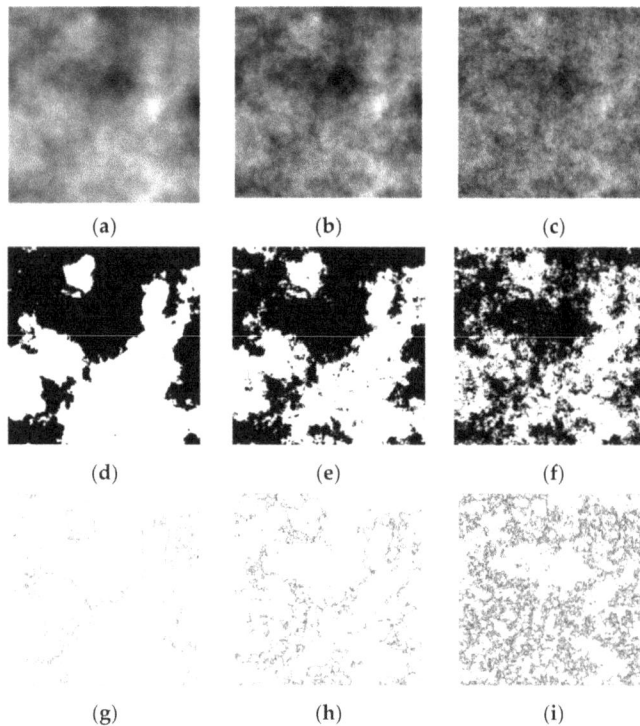

Figure 8. Edge extraction procedure for 2-dimensional midpoint displacement fractals. (**a**–**c**) Grayscale intensity map images of fractals generated from a single set of random numbers that vary in D, such that $D = 1.2$, 1.5, and 1.8; (**d**–**f**) Binary images resulting from the threshold procedure applied to the terrains shown in (**a**–**c**); (**g**–**i**) Coastal edges extracted from the binary images shown in (**d**–**f**).

2.3.2. Box Counting Analysis of *xy* Slices of 2-Dimensional Fractal Coastlines: $D_{(Coastal\ Edge)}$

To isolate the coastal edge of a fractal terrain, the median intensity value of the intensity image was selected as the level at which a binary threshold procedure was applied with the Matlab command *im2bw*. The median, in particular, was selected because it is the level at which all of the resultant binary images have roughly equivalent black and white regions across the range of *D*. The edge of the binary images was extracted with the Matlab command *bwperim*. Figure 8 provides examples of the edge extraction process. This particular luminance edge—extracted from the coastal edge images and shown in Figure 8g–i —served as the set on which box counting was performed.

Box counting was performed on the coastal edge images as described in Section 2.3.1, with the exception that the boxes were applied as a grid over the image. Here, the embedding dimension is 2, so for the coastal edge images we report the measured values of D, $D_{(Coastal\ Edge)}$, which span the range $1 < D_{(Coastal\ Edge)} < 2$.

2.4. Fourier Decomposition and Measurement of β

2.4.1. Spectral Scaling Analysis of 1-Dimensional Fractals: $\beta_{(Mountain\ Edge)}$

Fractal traces (see examples in Figures 3 and 6e–g) were decomposed with a 1-dimensional Fast Fourier Transform. The square of the real-valued component was retained. Power was plotted against frequency in log–log coordinates, and the slope of a least squares regression line was retained as an empirical measure of the spectral decay rate, $\beta_{(Mountain\ Edge)}$, of the time series.

2.4.2. Spectral Scaling Analysis of 2-Dimensional Fractal Intensity Images: $\beta_{(Surface)}$

Each image was decomposed with a 2-dimensional Fast Fourier Transform. The lowest frequency components were centered, and the square of the real-valued component was retained and transformed into polar coordinates. For each polar angle, power was plotted against frequency in log-log coordinates, and the average was retained as an empirical measure of the spectral decay rate, $\beta_{(Surface)}$, of the image (see Figure 9a–c).

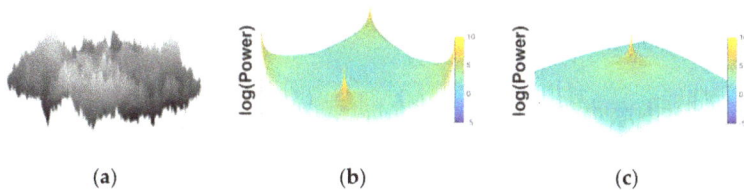

(a)   (b)   (c)

Figure 9. Fourier decomposition of 2-dimensional fractals. (**a**) Fractal surface generated with the inverse Fourier method; (**b**) Power spectrum of the Fourier decomposition of the terrain shown in (**a**); (**c**) Power spectrum shown in (**b**) with low spatial frequencies centered.

3. Results

3.1. Relationship between $D_{(Mountain\ Edge)}$ and $\beta_{(Mountain\ Edge)}$ for 1-Dimensional Fractals

We first analyzed 1-dimensional midpoint displacement and Fourier noise fractals to validate our measures and test Voss's approximation of the relationship between D and β for 1-dimensional fractals. To validate our box counting measure, values of D ranging from 1 to 2 in steps of 0.05 were used to generate 100 sets of midpoint fractals of length 2^{20}. The measurement technique described in Section 2.3.1 over-estimates D by a progressively smaller amount as D approaches 2, as shown in Figure 10a. This is a minor measurement error. Accordingly, the best linear fit, $D_{(Input)} = 0.91 + 0.16 \times D_{(Mountain\ Edge)}$, for which $R^2 = 0.97$ (Figure 10a, black line), deviates from the unity line (Figure 10a, blue line) by only a small amount.

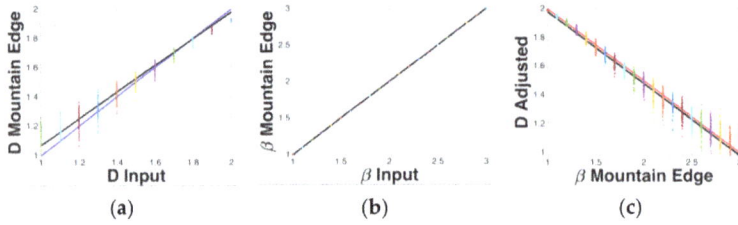

Figure 10. 1-dimensional fractal measurements. (**a**) Midpoint displacement fractals' $D_{(Mountain\ Edge)}$ measurements plotted against their $D_{(Input)}$ values; (**b**) Fourier noise fractals' $\beta_{(Mountain\ Edge)}$ measurements plotted against their $\beta_{(Input)}$ values; (**c**) Fourier noise fractals' $D_{(Mountain\ Edge)}$ measurements, adjusted by the linear fit from panel (**a**), plotted against their $\beta_{(Mountain\ Edge)}$ measurements. In each panel, the best linear fit for the data is shown with a black line. In panels (**a**,**b**), unity is represented by the blue line. In panel (**c**), Voss's approximation (Equation (5)) is represented by the red line. Data are colored to distinguish adjacent input values such that each datum's color is determined by $D_{(Input)}$ in panel (**a**) and $\beta_{(Input)}$ in panels (**b**,**c**).

To validate our spectral scaling rate measure, values of β ranging from 1 to 3 in steps of 0.1 were used to generate 100 sets of fractal Fourier noise of length 2^{20}. The measurement technique described in Section 2.4.1 does well at approximating β (as shown in Figure 10b), with the best linear fit, $\beta_{(Input)} = 0.0003 + 0.9999 \times \beta_{(Mountain\ Edge)}$, for which $R^2 = 1.00$ (Figure 10b, black line), overlapped by the unity line (Figure 10b, blue line).

These measures reliably reflect their input parameters, so we determined the extent to which these empirical measurements are consistent with Voss's approximation, Equation (5). Because our box counting technique results in a small measurement error across the range of dimension, we adjusted the measured D values of the fractal Fourier noise by substituting $D_{(Mountain\ Edge)}$ into the experimentally determined regression equation stated above in this section and computing the expected $D_{(Input)}$, which we call $D_{(Adjusted)}$ (as shown in Figure 10c). The best linear fit—$D_{(Adjusted)} = 2.48 - 0.50 \times \beta_{(Mountain\ Edge)}$—for which $R^2 = 0.97$ (Figure 10c, black line), is close to Voss's approximation (Equation (5)), given $E = 1$ (Figure 10c, red line). We conclude that Voss's approximation for fractals with $E < D < E + 1$ and $1 < \beta < 3$ is accurate when $E = 1$. We also note that the difference between Equation (5) and our regression equation is inconsequential, and both overlap our measurements across the range of D and β.

3.2. Relation of $D_{(Mountain\ Edge)}$ and $D_{(Coastal\ Edge)}$ for 2-Dimensional Fractals

Voss [5] generalized the relationship between D and β to n-dimensional spaces in Equation (5), so we next consider the case of $E = 2$, the dimensional space of our visual field. To do so, we first generated 100 sets of midpoint displacement fractals with values of D ranging from 2 to 3 in steps of 0.05 with side length 2^{11}. For each fractal, the dimension of the mountain profile was measured according to the technique described in Section 2.3.1. These measures of $D_{(Mountain\ Edge)}$ were averaged together for each image. Again, this under- and over-estimates D by a progressively larger amount as D approaches 2 and 1, respectively, as shown in Figure 11a. The best linear fit—$D_{(Input)} = 0.38 + 0.77 \times D_{(Mountain\ Edge)}$, for which $R^2 = 0.87$ (Figure 11a, black line)—deviates from the unity line (Figure 11a, blue line) in a manner similar to that observed for 1-dimensional fractals. When the coastal edge of the image was measured according to the technique described in Section 2.3.2, we observe a similar trend, with the best linear fit—$D_{(Input)} = 0.28 + 0.81 \times D_{(Coastal\ Edge)}$, for which $R^2 = 0.97$ (Figure 11b, black line)—deviating from the unity line (Figure 11b, blue line) in a manner similar to that observed for the dust measurement technique. These measures of D, averaged mountain edges and coastal edge values, are reasonable approximations of each other, with the best linear fit $D_{(Mountain\ Edge)} = 0.07 + 0.93 \times D_{(Coastal\ Edge)}$, for which $R^2 = 0.86$ (Figure 11c). Both of these measures provide an accurate means by which to compute the fractal dimension of an image.

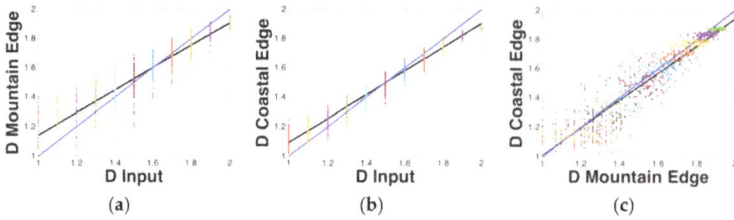

Figure 11. 2-dimensional fractal D measurements. (**a**) Midpoint displacement fractals' $D_{(Mountain\ Edge)}$ measurements plotted against their $D_{(Input)}$ values; (**b**) Midpoint displacement fractals' $D_{(Coastal\ Edge)}$ measurements plotted against their $D_{(Input)}$ values; (**c**) Midpoint displacement fractals' $D_{(Coastal\ Edge)}$ measurements plotted against their $D_{(Mountain\ Edge)}$ measurements. In each panel, unity is represented by the blue line, while the best linear fit for the data is represented by the black line. Data are colored to distinguish adjacent input values such that each datum's color is determined by $D_{(Input)}$ in panels (a–c).

3.3. Relation of $\beta_{(Mountain\ Edge)}$ and $\beta_{(Surface)}$ for 2-Dimensional Fractals

Having found that our measures of D were consistent with each other, we aimed to test their relation to β. To this end, we generated 100 sets of fractal Fourier noise images with values of $\beta_{(Input)}$ ranging from 1 to 3, in steps of 0.1, with side length 2^{11} pixels. Measuring the spectral decay of a 2-dimensional Fourier analysis as described in Section 2.4.2 provides measured $\beta_{(Surface)}$ values that are consistent with the specified input $\beta_{(Input)}$ values, with the best linear fit $\beta_{(Surface)} = 0.12 + 0.95 \times \beta_{(Input)}$, for which $R^2 = 0.9999$ (see Figure 12a). Having verified the generation process with an analysis in native space, we measured the β of these 2-dimensional fractals along a straight line path, $\beta_{(Mountain\ Edge)}$. We averaged the $\beta_{(Mountain\ Edge)}$ measurements for each row of each image, as described in Section 2.4.1, to allow us to follow the definition put forth by Voss [5]. We found that these values of $\beta_{(Mountain\ Edge)}$ differ from the specified input β values (see Figure 12b), with an offset as evidenced by the best linear fit $\beta_{(Mountain\ Edge)} = -0.39 + 0.82 \times \beta_{(Input)}$, for which $R^2 = 0.998$ (Figure 12b, black line).

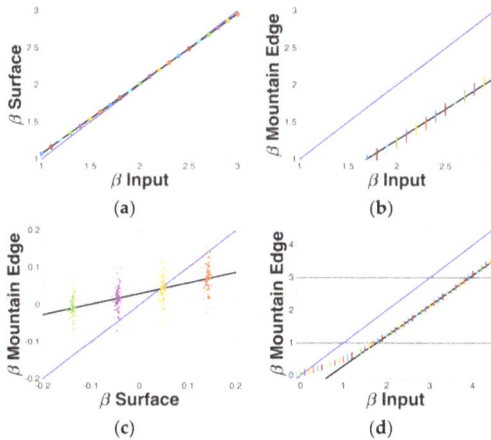

Figure 12. 2-dimensional fractal β measurements. (**a**) Fourier noise fractals' $\beta_{(Surface)}$ measurements plotted against their β input values; (**b**) Fourier noise fractals' $\beta_{(Mountain\ Edge)}$ measurements plotted against their $\beta_{(Input)}$ values; (**c**) Fourier noise fractals' $\beta_{(Mountain\ Edge)}$ measurements plotted against their $\beta_{(Surface)}$ measurements, showing that the measures converge at $\beta = 0$; (**d**) Fourier noise fractals' $\beta_{(Mountain\ Edge)}$ measurements plotted against their $\beta_{(Input)}$ values. In each panel, unity is represented by the blue line, while the best linear fit for the data is represented by the black line. Data are colored to distinguish adjacent input values such that each datum's color is determined by $\beta_{(Input)}$ in panels (a–d).

We visually inspected the mountain profiles to confirm that their frequency content was indeed different from that implied by $\beta_{(Input)}$. We found that the mountain profile from a fractal terrain with an arbitrary value of $\beta_{(Surface)}$, β_i, is rougher (i.e., has a larger contribution of fine structure) than a mountain profile from a 1-dimensional fractal with $\beta_{(Mountain\ Edge)} = \beta_i$ (see Figure 13). We then took measurements for an ensemble of 100 random phase maps around $\beta = 0$, which show that our measures converge when there is equal power across frequencies (see Figure 12c). An exploratory analysis on a new set of images with $0 \leqslant \beta_{(Input)} \leqslant 4.5$ allowed us to empirically determine that fractal Fourier noise terrains with $\beta_{(Input)}$ values in the range $1.8 < \beta_{(Input)} < 3.8$ consistently give $\beta_{(Mountain\ Edge)}$ values in the range $1 < \beta_{(Mountain\ Edge)} < 3$ (see Figure 12d). We found that $\beta_{(Input)}$ and $\beta_{(Mountain\ Edge)}$ are relatable by the regression equation $\beta_{(Mountain\ Edge)} = -0.64 + 0.93 \times \beta_{(Input)}$, for which $R^2 = 0.997$ (Figure 12d, black line), across the range $1 < \beta_{(Mountain)} < 3$ and $1.8 < \beta_{(Input)} < 3.8$.

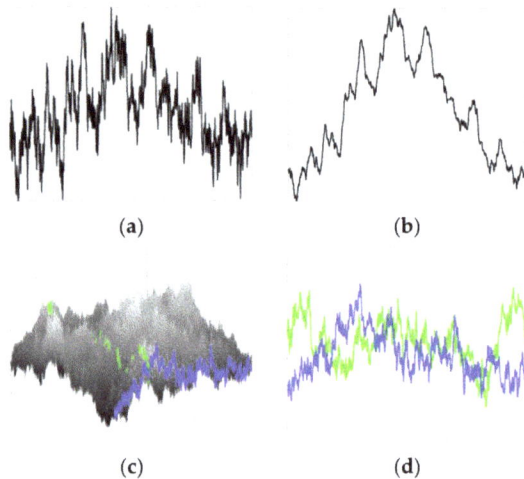

Figure 13. Mountain profiles from 1 and 2-dimensional fractal Fourier noise. (**a**) 1-dimensional fractal with $\beta_{(Input)} = 1.5$; (**b**) 1-dimensional fractal with $\beta_{Input} = 2.5$; (**c**) 2-dimensional fractal with $\beta_{(Input)} = 2.5$; (**d**) 1-dimensional fractal mountain edges from the terrain in (c).

An important validation of our analysis techniques is that $\beta_{(Mountain\ Edge)}$ and $\beta_{(Surface)}$ approximately converge at $\beta = 0$ (as expected), because for white noise, there is equal power across frequencies. This would be trivial if the two measures followed the unity line (Figure 12d, blue line), but certifies that our otherwise non-equivalent measures accurately describe white noise. We note that our β values exhibit slight measurement errors, such that classical Brownian traces ($\beta_{(Mountain\ Edge)} = 2$, $\beta_{(Surface)} = 3$) have empirically determined means of (2.14, 2.95). In the absence of measurement error, the empirically determined range $1.8 < \beta_{(Input)} < 3.8$ would be $2 < \beta_{(Surface)} < 4$.

3.4. Relation of β to D for 2-Dimensional Fractals

To relate the two measures of β to D, we generated another 100 sets of fractal Fourier noise with values of $\beta_{(Input)}$ ranging from 0 to 5 in steps of 0.1 with side length 2^{11} pixels.

3.4.1. Relation of $\beta_{(Mountain\ Edge)}$ to $D_{(Coastal\ Edge)}$ of 2-Dimensional Fractals

First, we investigated the extension of Voss's [5] approximation to $E = 2$ by determining the relationship between $D_{(Coastal\ Edge)}$ and $\beta_{(Mountain\ Edge)}$. We performed the Fourier analysis described in Section 2.4.1 on each row of each image, and measured the rows' fractal dimension with the technique described in Section 2.3.2. The relationship between these measures is described by a best linear fit—$\beta_{(Mountain\ Edge)} = 5.18 - 2.00 \times D_{(Coastal\ Edge)}$, for which $R^2 = 0.99$ (Figure 14a, black line)—which approximates Voss's [5] equation (Figure 14a, red line, which is Equation (5)). This confirms Voss's [5] assertion that measuring along a straight-line path will provide measures of D and β that are related by Equation (5).

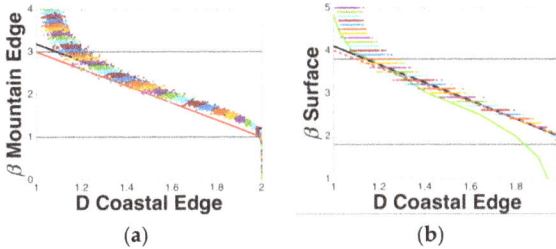

Figure 14. 2-dimensional fractal measurements of Fourier noise (**a,b**). (**a**) Fourier noise fractals' $\beta_{(Mountain\ Edge)}$ measurements plotted against their $D_{(Coastal\ Edge)}$ measurements; (**b**) Fourier noise fractals' $\beta_{(Surface)}$ measurements plotted against their $D_{(Coastal\ Edge)}$ measurements. In each panel, the best linear fit for the data within the region that was shown to exhibit fractal scaling (identified with gray lines) is shown with a black line. In panel (a), Voss's [5] equation (Equation (5)) is shown with a red line. In panel (b), Spehar & Taylor's [23] data is shown with a green line and our extension of Voss's [5] equation (Equation (11)) is shown with a red dashed line. Data are colored to distinguish adjacent input values such that each datum's color is determined by $\beta_{(Input)}$ in panels (a,b).

3.4.2. Relation of $\beta_{(Surface)}$ to $D_{(Coastal\ Edge)}$ for 2-Dimensional Fractals

We next measured β using the method described in Section 2.4.2, $\beta_{(Surface)}$, which captures the radial scaling properties of the images. When plotted against $D_{(Coastal\ Edge)}$, we observe that the relationship between these measures is described by a best linear fit, $\beta_{(Surface)} = 6.24 - 2.14 \times D_{(Coastal\ Edge)}$, for which $R^2 = 0.99$ (Figure 14b, black line). The observed relationship agrees with the data from a smaller set of images previously reported by Spehar and Taylor [23] (Figure 14b, green line). Significantly, this observed relationship between $\beta_{(Surface)}$ and $D_{(Coastal\ Edge)}$ agrees with Equation (11) which we present below, and will allow conversion across measures of D and β in multidimensional spaces.

4. Discussion

4.1. Mathematical Relationships between Ds and βs

Our results show that Voss [5] was correct regarding Equation (5)'s extension into n-dimensional measures of D with the limitations described therein. However, the way that β is commonly measured in images, $\beta_{(Surface)}$, is not that which Voss [5] described. Voss's [5] equation (Equation (5)) applies for the measure we call $\beta_{(Mountain\ Edge)}$. However, vision researchers typically use $\beta_{(Surface)}$. Whereas the difference between these two spectral decay rates is nonexistent for white noise, where $\beta = 0$, these measures are substantially different in the range over which these noises are fractal. Before commenting further on the different measures of β, we will first summarize the relationships for the fractal images discussed in this paper.

For the mountain profile fractal ($E = 1$), the Voss relationship of Equation (5) becomes:

$$D_{(Mountain\ Edge)} = 1 + (3 - \beta_{(Mountain\ Edge)})/2 \tag{6}$$

We have also shown in Section 3.3 that the Fourier spectral decay rates measured in 1- and 2-dimensional space are approximately related by:

$$\beta_{(Mountain\ Edge)} = \beta_{(Surface)} - 1 \tag{7}$$

over the range $1 < \beta_{(Mountain\ Edge)} < 3$ and $2 < \beta_{(Surface)} < 4$. Combining Equations (6) and (7) gives:

$$D_{(Mountain\ Edge)} = 1 + (4 - \beta_{(Surface)})/2 \qquad (8)$$

The relationship between β and $D_{(Surface)}$ can then be obtained using:

$$D_{(Surface)} = D_{(Mountain\ Edge)} + 1 = D_{(Coastal\ Edge)} + 1 \qquad (9)$$

We have not measured $\beta_{(Coastal\ Edge)}$ in our investigations. However, we expect that, if a coastal edge was unraveled by the process described by Zahn & Roskies [48], its β value will equal $\beta_{(Mountain\ Edge)}$ because $D_{(Coastal\ Edge)}$ is equivalent to $D_{(Mountain\ Edge)}$ and $E = 1$ applies to both the mountain and coastal edges.

4.2. Distinguishing βs

Our results provide the ranges of β over which the images are fractal. As Voss [5] noted, for D mountain ($1 < D_{(Mountain\ Edge)} < 2$), we have $1 < \beta_{(Mountain\ Edge)} < 3$. However, we have shown that β measured in a single variable-space (i.e., along a straight line path as $\beta_{(Mountain\ Edge)}$) diverges from β measured in a two-variable space (i.e., across a plane as $\beta_{(Surface)}$) to an extent that is characterized by Equation (7) for the range over which 2-dimensional noise is fractal. For D surface ($2 < D_{(Surface)} < 3$), we have $2 < \beta_{(Surface)} < 4$ and $1 < \beta_{(Mountain\ Edge)} < 3$. The fact that the β values measured by 1- and 2-dimensional Fourier transforms differ for fractal noises holds crucial consequences. The fractal structure of a terrain is quantified by $\beta_{(Mountain\ Edge)}$. Visual inspection of Figure 13 makes it immediately apparent that its value is significantly smaller than $\beta_{(Surface)}$ for fractals of topological dimension $E = 2$. Given that $\beta_{(Input)}$ matches $\beta_{(Surface)}$ rather than $\beta_{(Mountain\ Edge)}$, it is likely that many vision researchers have been misjudging the fractal content of their fractal terrains, or adapting them by an intuitive sense of the image's roughness. Equation (7) provides a formal justification for adjusting the β of 2-dimensional fractals.

The basis for this conversion lies in the difference in generating 1- vs. 2-dimensional noise. A pair of vectors can specify the phases and amplitudes of a 1-dimensional fractal noise pattern because they have only one phase at each frequency (for illustration, see the visualization of the amplitude vectors corresponding to three different input Betas (β_is) shown in Figure 6a–c and phase matrix shown in Figure 6d). In contrast, a 2-dimensional fractal pattern is generated from a matrix of amplitudes and a matrix of phases (for illustration, see the visualization of the amplitude matrices corresponding to three different input Betas (β_is) shown in Figure 7a–c and phase matrix shown in Figure 7d).

For 2- and higher-dimensional fractal noises, there are an increasingly greater number of inputs at increasingly high spatial frequencies (for illustration, see Figure 15, where the lowest frequency components have been centered). The number of inputs increases at a rate that is related to the distance from the lowest frequency (i.e., the radial distance in a low-spatial frequency-centered representation of Fourier space). Changing from a 1- to 2-variable space, weighting the input function $S_V(f)$ by f to increase the embedding dimension by 1 (from 1 to 2) requires a subtraction of 1 from β, as denoted by the following equation:

$$S_V(f) \times f = (f^{-\beta_i}) \times f = 1/f^{(\beta_i - 1)} \qquad (10)$$

4.3. A Generalized Equation to Relate Ds and βs

We postulate that the relationship between D and β continues to change with higher dimensional Fourier decomposition (for 3- and higher dimensional Fourier decomposition), such that the relationship between D and β can be described by the equation,

$$D = E + (F + 2 - \beta)/2 \qquad (11)$$

where F is the dimensional space of the Fourier transform (the number of variables with which the Fourier transform is performed), where $F \geqslant 1$, and $F < \beta < F + 2$ (as examples, $F = 1$ for $\beta_{(Mountain\ Edge)}$

and $F = 2$ for $\beta_{(Surface)}$). This new equation (Equation (11)) allows for conversion from D to both of the Fourier measurement techniques that can describe static images, and provides an extension of Mandelbrot's [1,4], Voss's [5], and Knill et al.'s [14] relationships that can describe spectral decay in dynamic fractal Brownian stimuli generated with Fourier, midpoint displacement, and other equivalent methods. Equation (11) extends Voss's [5] equation (Equation (5)) by generalizing the term for β from $\beta_{(Mountain\ Edge)}$.

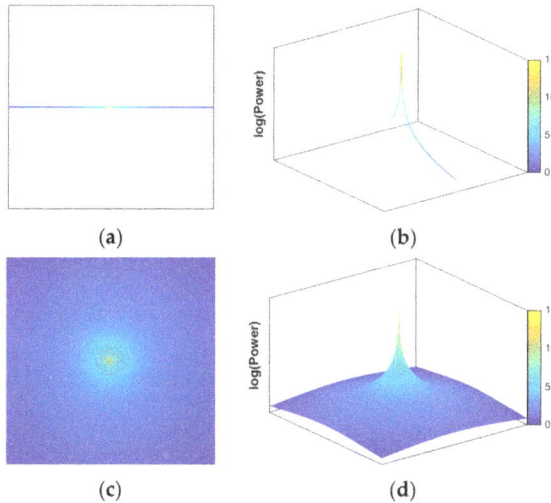

Figure 15. Real and imaginary frequency components of 1- and 2-dimensional fractal Fourier noise plotted in 2- and 3-dimensional spaces with color changing with frequency, such that higher frequency components are shown in cooler colors. (**a,b**) Amplitude-frequency plots of a 1-dimensional noise with low frequency components centered such that the amplitude of the higher frequency components fall at the edges of the plot; (**c,d**) Amplitude-frequency plots of 2-dimensional noise with low frequency components centered such that larger concentric circles indicate higher frequency components.

4.4. Importance of the Relationship between D and β for Current and Future Research

In addition to allowing for easy translation across the parameters D and β in aesthetics research, Equation (11) provides scaffolding for extension of basic vision research into questions related to visual sensitivity and the perception of fractal motion, and has far-reaching applicability to applied topics, including stress reduction and navigation.

To clarify the need for this new equation to allow for such forward progress, consider a hypothetical case of therapeutic intervention using fractal movies. From Equation (5) and previous research that suggests that low-to-moderate fractional dimensions ($1.3 \leqslant D \leqslant 1.5$) are optimal for stress reduction [49], a therapist might generate what are intended to be soothing movies of fractal noise with $\beta = 2.2$, thinking that β does not differ according to the number of variables with which the Fourier transform is performed. Meanwhile, the results of our analyses imply that such a series would be effectively space filling if $\beta_{(Volume)} = 2.2$. This is because Equation (11) implies the optimal range of values of $\beta_{(Volume)}$ for such an application would be $4 < \beta_{(Volume)} < 4.4$, because $E = 3$ and $F = 3$, where fractal noises are in the range $3 < \beta_{(Volume)} < 5$.

More generally, time represents a third dimension—yet to be explored—in the perception of fractal processes. An example would be a fractal pattern that undergoes fractal change over time. Responses to dynamic stimuli have a long history of consideration in vision research that continues today [50,51], though few have focused on perception of fractal motion [52,53]. Equation (11) provides the scaffolding to extend perceptual research into the study of dynamic fractals.

While Equation (11) supports the development of new lines of work into dynamic fractals, it also holds value in drawing conclusions across recent research using 2-dimensional fractal patterns in studies that have implications for aesthetics. Whereas Rainville and Kingdom [54] provide βs that are apparently in terms of $\beta_{(Mountain\ Edge)}$, they cite Knill et al. [14], who provided the relationship between D and β for surfaces. This highlights the difficulty associated with discerning the optimal range of β in aesthetics and vision research. More problematic is that because of the relative convenience of the respective algorithms' implementation, others report a combination of $D_{(Mountain\ Edge)}$ and $\beta_{(Surface)}$ values [23], for which there is no clear conversion provided in the published literature.

Finally, Equation (11) serves as a useful tool for converting between 2- and 3-dimensional representations of space, the problem we solve whenever we use a map to navigate. The recent work of Juliani et al. [28] asks individuals to navigate fractal environments. Under conditions such as these, the map typically has complexity in the range $1 < D_{(Coastal\ Edge)} < 2$, whereas the navigated environment has complexity in the range $2 < D_{(Surface)} < 3$, and the visually perceived scene has a spectral decay that likely falls off at a rate in the range $2 < \beta_{(Surface)} < 4$. While it is mathematically no less appropriate to describe all of these in terms of $\beta_{(Mountain\ Edge)}$, it is easier to interpret results described in units that reflect the experienced dimensional space precisely and explicitly. There is convenience to be gained by using this more general equation (Equation (11)) and its variables' boundary conditions rather than more specialized equations, such as those which have been put forth previously [5,14,21]. Equation (11) stems from a recognition that β varies with the number of variables with which the Fourier transform is applied. As such, it is important that we define which β is being used ($\beta_{(Line)}$, $\beta_{(Surface)}$, $\beta_{(Volume)}$, etc.) for easier interpretation of results and to facilitate the communication of future endeavors in interdisciplinary fractals research.

Acknowledgments: We thank Scott B. Stevenson (University of Houston College of Optometry) for useful discussions about the generation of noise images for stimulus presentation.

Author Contributions: All authors conceived and designed the experiments; Alexander J. Bies and Cooper R. Boydston contributed stimulus generation and analysis tools; and Alexander J. Bies performed the experiments, analyzed the data, and wrote the paper. All authors contributed to the review and final form of the manuscript.

Conflicts of Interest: The authors declare no conflict of interest.

Abbreviations

The following abbreviations are used in this manuscript:

β: Spectral slope
D: Fractal dimension
E: Euclidian dimension
F: dimensional space of the Fourier transform

References

1. Mandelbrot, B.B. *Fractals: Form, Chance, and Dimension*; Freeman: San Francisco, CA, USA, 1977.
2. Fournier, A.; Fussel, D.; Carpenter, L. Computer rendering of stochastic models. *Commun. ACM* **1982**, *25*, 371–384. [CrossRef]
3. Saupe, D. Algorithms for random fractals. In *The Science of Fractal Images*; Peitgen, H., Saupe, D., Eds.; Springer-Verlag: New York, NY, USA, 1982; pp. 71–136.
4. Mandelbrot, B.B. *The Fractal Geometry of Nature*; Freeman: San Francisco, CA, USA, 1983.
5. Voss, R.F. Characterization and measurement of random fractals. *Phys. Scripta* **1986**, *13*, 27–32. [CrossRef]
6. Fairbanks, M.S.; Taylor, R.P. Scaling analysis of spatial and temporal patterns: From the human eye to the foraging albatross. In *Non-Linear Dynamical Analysis for the Behavioral Sciences Using Real Data*; Taylor & Francis Group: Boca Raton, FL, USA, 2011.
7. Avnir, D.; Biham, O.; Lidar, D.; Malci, O. Is the geometry of nature fractal? *Science* **1998**, *279*, 39–40. [CrossRef]
8. Mandelbrot, B.B. Is nature fractal? *Science* **1998**, *279*, 738. [CrossRef]
9. Jones-Smith, K.; Mathur, H. Fractal analysis: Revisiting Pollock's drip paintings. *Nature* **2006**, *444*, E9–E10. [CrossRef] [PubMed]

10. Taylor, R.P.; Micolich, A.P.; Jonas, D. Fractal analysis: Revisiting Pollock's drip paintings (Reply). *Nature* **2006**, *444*, E10–E11. [CrossRef]

11. Markovic, D.; Gros, C. Power laws and self-organized criticality in theory and nature. *Phys. Rep.* **2014**, *536*, 41–74. [CrossRef]

12. Burton, G.J.; Moorehead, I.R. Color and spatial structure in natural scenes. *Appl. Opt.* **1987**, *26*, 157–170. [CrossRef] [PubMed]

13. Field, D.J. Relations between the statistics of natural images and the response properties of cortical cells. *J. Opt. Soc. Am. A* **1987**, *4*, 2379. [CrossRef] [PubMed]

14. Knill, D.C.; Field, D.; Kersten, D. Human discrimination of fractal images. *J. Opt. Soc. Am. A* **1990**, *7*, 1113–1123. [CrossRef] [PubMed]

15. van Hateren, J.H. Theoretical predictions of spatiotemporal receptive fields of fly LMCs, and experimental validation. *J. Comp. Physiol. A* **1992**, *171*, 157–170. [CrossRef]

16. Tolhurst, D.J.; Tadmor, Y.; Chao, T. Amplitude spectra of natural images. *Ophthalmic Physiol. Opt.* **1992**, *12*, 229–232. [CrossRef] [PubMed]

17. Field, D.J. Scale-invariance and self-similar wavelet transforms: An analysis of natural scenes and mammalian visual systems. In *Wavelets, Fractals, and Fourier Transforms*; Farge, M., Hunt, J.C.R., Vassilicos, J.C., Eds.; Clarendon Press: Oxford, UK, 1993; pp. 151–193.

18. Ruderman, D.L.; Bialek, W. Statistics of natural images: Scaling in the woods. *Phys. Rev. Lett.* **1994**, *73*, 814–817. [CrossRef] [PubMed]

19. Ruderman, D.L. Origins of scaling in natural images. *Vis. Res.* **1996**, *37*, 3385–3398. [CrossRef]

20. van der Schaaf, A.; van Haternen, J.H. Modeling the power spectra of natural images: Statistics and information. *Vis. Res.* **1996**, *36*, 2759–2770. [CrossRef]

21. Graham, D.J.; Field, D.J. Statistical regularities of art images and natural scenes: Spectra, sparseness, and nonlinearities. *Spat. Vis.* **2007**, *21*, 149–164. [CrossRef] [PubMed]

22. Hagerhall, C.M.; Purcell, T.; Taylor, R. Fractal dimension of landscape silhouette outlines as a predictor of landscape preference. *J. Environ. Psychol.* **2004**, *24*, 247–255. [CrossRef]

23. Spehar, B.; Taylor, R.P. Fractals in art and nature: Why do we like them? In Proceedings of the SPIE 8651, Human Vision and Electronic Imaging XVIII, 865118, Burlingame, CA, USA, 3 February 2013.

24. Spehar, B.; Wong, S.; van de Klundert, S.; Lui, J.; Clifford, C.W.G.; Taylor, R.P. Beauty and the beholder: The role of visual sensitivity in visual preference. *Front. Hum. Neurosci.* **2015**, *9*, 514. [CrossRef] [PubMed]

25. Bies, A.J.; Blanc-Goldhammer, D.R.; Boydston, C.R.; Taylor, R.P.; Sereno, M.E. Aesthetic responses to exact fractals driven by physical complexity. *Front. Hum. Neurosci.* **2016**, *10*, 210. [CrossRef] [PubMed]

26. Street, N.; Forsythe, A.M.; Reilly, R.; Taylor, R.; Helmy, M.S. A complex story: Universal preference vs. individual differences shaping aesthetic response to fractals patterns. *Front. Hum. Neurosci.* **2016**, *10*, 213. [CrossRef] [PubMed]

27. Spehar, B.; Walker, N.; Taylor, R.P. Taxonomy of individual variations in aesthetic responses to fractal patterns. *Front. Hum. Neurosci.* **2016**, *10*, 350. [CrossRef]

28. Juliani, A.W.; Bies, A.J.; Boydston, C.R.; Taylor, R.P.; Sereno, M.E. Navigation performace in virtual environments varies with the fractal dimension of the landscape. *J. Environ. Psychol.* **2016**, *47*, 155–165. [CrossRef] [PubMed]

29. Bies, A.J.; Kikumoto, A.; Boydston, C.R.; Greenfield, A.; Chauvin, K.A.; Taylor, R.P.; Sereno, M.E. Percepts from noise patterns: The role of fractal dimension in object pareidolia. In *Vision Sciences Society Meeting Planner*; Vision Sciences Society: St. Pete Beach, FL, USA, 2016.

30. Field, D.; Vilankar, K. Finding a face on Mars: A study on the priors for illusory objects. In *Vision Sciences Society Meeting Planner*; Vision Sciences Society: St. Pete Beach, FL, USA, 2016.

31. Hagerhall, C.M.; Laike, T.; Kuller, M.; Marcheschi, E.; Boydston, C.; Taylor, R.P. Human physiological benefits of viewing nature: EEG responses to exact and statistical fractal patterns. *Nonlinear Dyn. Psychol. Life Sci.* **2015**, *19*, 1–12.

32. Isherwood, Z.J.; Schira, M.M.; Spehar, B. The BOLD and the Beautiful: Neural responses to natural scene statistics in early visual cortex. *i-Perception* **2014**, *5*, 345.

33. Bies, A.J.; Wekselblatt, J.; Boydston, C.R.; Taylor, R.P.; Sereno, M.E. The effects of visual scene complexity on human visual cortex. In *Society for Neuroscience*, Proceedings of the 2015 Neuroscience Meeting Planner, Chicago, IL, USA, 21 October 2015.

34. Sprott, J.C. Automatic generation of strange attractors. *Comput. Graph.* **1993**, *17*, 325–332. [CrossRef]
35. Aks, D.J.; Sprott, J.C. Quantifying aesthetic preference for chaotic patterns. *Empir. Stud. Arts* **1996**, *14*, 1–16. [CrossRef]
36. Spehar, B.; Clifford, C.W.; Newell, B.R.; Taylor, R.P. Universal aesthetic of fractals. *Comput. Graph.* **2003**, *27*, 813–820. [CrossRef]
37. Taylor, R.P.; Spehar, B.; Van Donkelaar, P.; Hagerhall, C. Perceptual and physiological responses to Jackson Pollock's fractals. *Front. Hum. Neurosci.* **2011**, *5*, 60. [CrossRef] [PubMed]
38. Mureika, J.R.; Dyer, C.C.; Cupchik, G.C. Multifractal structure in nonrepresentational art. *Phys. Rev. E* **2005**, *72*, 046101. [CrossRef] [PubMed]
39. Forsythe, A.; Nadal, M.; Sheehy, N.; Cela-Conde, C.J.; Sawey, M. Predicting beauty: Fractal dimension and visual complexity in art. *Br. J. Psychol.* **2011**, *102*, 49–70. [CrossRef] [PubMed]
40. Hagerhall, C.M.; Laike, T.; Taylor, R.P.; Kuller, M.; Kuller, R.; Martin, T.P. Investigations of human EEG response to viewing fractal patterns. *Perception* **2008**, *37*, 1488–1494. [CrossRef] [PubMed]
41. Graham, D.J.; Redies, C. Statistical regularities in art: Relations with visual coding and perception. *Vis. Res.* **2010**, *50*, 1503–1509. [CrossRef] [PubMed]
42. Koch, M.; Denzler, J.; Redies, C. 1/f 2 characteristics and isotropy in the fourier power spectra of visual art, cartoons, comics, mangas, and different categories of photographs. *PLoS ONE* **2010**, *5*, e12268. [CrossRef] [PubMed]
43. Melmer, T.; Amirshahi, S.A.; Koch, M.; Denzler, J.; Redies, C. From regular text to artistic writing and artworks: Fourier statistics of images with low and high aesthetic appeal. *Front. Hum. Neurosci.* **2013**, *7*, 106. [CrossRef] [PubMed]
44. Dyakova, O.; Lee, Y.; Longden, K.D.; Kiselev, V.G.; Nordstrom, K. A higher order visual neuron tuned to the spatial amplitude spectra of natural scenes. *Nat. Commun.* **2015**, *6*, 8522. [CrossRef] [PubMed]
45. Menzel, C.; Hayn-Leichsenring, G.U.; Langner, O.; Wiese, H.; Redies, C. Fourier power spectrum characteristics of face photographs: Attractiveness perception depends on low-level image properties. *PLoS ONE* **2015**, *10*, e0122801.
46. Braun, J.; Amirshahi, S.A.; Denzler, J.; Redies, C. Statistical image properties of print advertisements, visual artworks, and images of architecture. *Front. Psychol.* **2013**, *4*, 808. [CrossRef] [PubMed]
47. Cutting, J.E.; Garvin, J.J. Fractal curves and complexity. *Percept. Psychophys.* **1987**, *42*, 365–370. [CrossRef] [PubMed]
48. Zahn, C.T.; Roskies, R.Z. Fourier descriptors for plane closed curves. *IEEE Trans. Comput.* **1972**, *3*, 269–281. [CrossRef]
49. Taylor, R.P. Reduction of physiological stress using fractal art and architecture. *Leonardo* **2006**, *39*, 245–251. [CrossRef]
50. Derrington, A.M.; Allen, H.A.; Delicato, L.S. Visual mechanisms of motion analysis and motion perception. *Ann. Rev. Psychol.* **2004**, *55*, 181–205. [CrossRef] [PubMed]
51. Silies, M.; Gohl, D.M.; Clandinin, T.R. Motion-detecting circuits in flies: Coming into view. *Ann. Rev. Neurosci.* **2014**, *37*, 307–327. [CrossRef] [PubMed]
52. Benton, C.P.; O'Brien, J.M.; Curran, W. Fractal rotation isolates mechanisms for form-dependent motion in human vision. *Biol. Lett.* **2007**, *3*, 306–308. [CrossRef] [PubMed]
53. Lagacé-Nadon, S.; Allard, R.; Faubert, J. Exploring the spatiotemporal properties of fractal rotation perception. *J. Vis.* **2009**, *9*. [CrossRef] [PubMed]
54. Rainville, S.J.; Kingdom, F.A.A. Spatial scale contribution to the detection of symmetry in fractal noise. *JOSA A* **1999**, *16*, 2112–2123. [CrossRef] [PubMed]

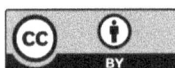

Part 2:
Symmetry in Human vision: Grouping and Preference

symmetry

MDPI

Article

Redundant Symmetry Influences Perceptual Grouping (as Measured by Rotational Linkage)

Barbara Gillam

School of Psychology, The University of New South Wales, Sydney 2052, Australia; b.gillam@unsw.edu.au;
Tel.: +61-2-9385-3522

Academic Editor: Marco Bertamini
Received: 8 February 2017; Accepted: 2 May 2017; Published: 9 May 2017

Abstract: Symmetry *detection* has long been a major focus of perception research. However, although symmetry is often cited as a "grouping principle", the effect of symmetry on grouping, an important form of perceptual organization, has been little measured. In past research, we found little spatio-temporal grouping for oblique lines symmetric around a horizontal axis during ambiguous rotary motion in depth. Grouping was measured by the degree to which the ambiguous motion direction was resolved for two elements in common (rotational linkage). We hypothesized that symmetry-based grouping would be stronger if symmetry was redundant i.e., carried by elements of greater complexity. Using the rotational linkage measure, we compared grouping for horizontally symmetric simple oblique lines and for lines composed of multiple conjoined orientations and found greater grouping for the more complex symmetric lines. A control experiment ruled out possible confounding factors and also showed a grouping effect of vertically aligned endpoints. We attribute the stronger grouping effect of redundant symmetry to the fact that it has a lower probability than does simple symmetry of arising from an accidental environmental arrangement.

Keywords: symmetry; grouping; redundancy; complexity; rotary motion in depth

---

1. Introduction

Symmetry is one of the defining characteristics of Gestalt "good figure" [1]. This implies that symmetric organizations will be preferred to asymmetric ones and that isolated elements will cohere into groups more readily if those elements are symmetric. More recently, Treder and Van der Helm [2] conclude that symmetry is a cue for the presence of one object, which also implies grouping. However, overwhelmingly, symmetry research explores its detection and saliency rather than its influence on perceptual organization, e.g., Barlow and Reeves [3]; Royer [4]; Wenderoth [5]; Tyler [6]; Wagemans [7]; Gurnsey, Herbert and Kenemy [8]. Although Locher and Wagemans [9] investigated the effect of grouping patterns and Bertamini, Friedenberg and Kubovy [10] the effect of contour organization on symmetry detection; the reverse influence has been little explored. Pomerantz and Kubovy [11] argued that it does not follow that because a property such as symmetry has salience, it plays a significant role in the process of organization. However, it has been known since the early work of Bahnsen [12], a student of Rubin [13], that a symmetric shape is more likely to be seen as a figure than an asymmetric one in a figure-ground task. This has been confirmed more recently by Peterson and Gibson [14] and Mojika and Peterson [15], who also showed that the effect of symmetry on figure-ground resolution was enhanced when several alternating symmetric regions were added to the display. Kanizsa and Gerbino [16] reported that convexity overrides symmetry in eliciting perception of figure, leading Pomerantz and Kubovy [11] to argue that since it is so easily overridden, symmetry probably plays little role in organization and only becomes available after elements are organized into units on other grounds. The Mojika and Peterson's [15] study showed, however, that with appropriate controls, symmetry is as effective as convexity.

Machilsen, Pauwels and Wagemans [17], stated that generally there has been "no certain benefit of symmetry on perceptual grouping" (p. 3), but they did show a small influence of vertical symmetry on the segregation of a pattern from a noisy background. It is well established that vertical symmetry is more salient than horizontal symmetry, a fact that is usually attributed to the ubiquitous vertical symmetry of biological structures. In a rare study extending these salience findings to perceptual organization, Gillam and McGrath [18] showed that two oblique lines arranged with vertical symmetry are grouped more than when arranged with horizontal symmetry and that the operative symmetry axis was retinal not environmental. The grouping criterion that these authors used was "rotational linkage" also used in the present experiments and described below.

The only other research we are aware of which measured the effect of symmetry on perceptual grouping is by Feldman [19] who measured the degree of grouping of two separate straight lines in various arrangements (See Figure 1) among which one pair (Figure 1E) had horizontal symmetry. His grouping criterion was the degree to which a given line pair showed an "object benefit". This is said to be present when comparisons of visual features are faster within a single object than between objects. Feldman found greatest object benefit for the symmetric figure (Figure 1E). However, Gillam [20], who studied the grouping of pairs of lines using the "rotational linkage" criterion, found that an almost identical figure to Feldman's Figure 1E (see Figure 2A) produced little grouping despite its symmetry. In accounting for the difference between the Feldman [19] and Gillam [20] results, it could be argued that the rotational linkage criterion is a more direct measure of grouping than object benefit, which measures a consequence of object formation rather than its determinants. The essence of rotational linkage (a term coined by Eby, Loomis and Solomon, [21]) is to present two or more lines (or objects) rotating in depth in *parallel projection*, which renders direction of motion (clockwise or counterclockwise) ambiguous (Wallach and O'Connell, [22]). The proportion of total exposure time during which the ambiguous rotation directions are resolved in common for several lines or objects is measured. Observers are asked to hold down a switch whenever individual elements appear to be rotating in opposite directions. Gillam [20] calls this "fragmentation time". Rotational linkage is measured as the total time minus the fragmentation time for a given number of rotations and provides a quantitative measure of grouping.

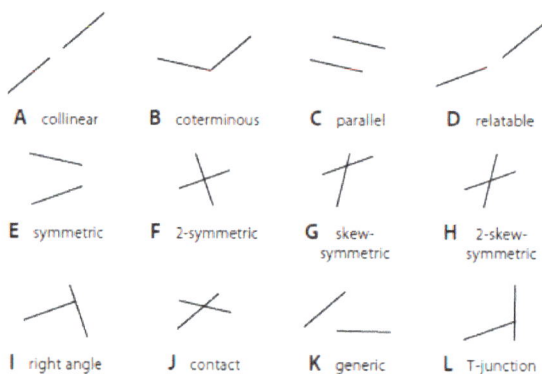

Figure 1. The stimulus figures used by Feldman [19]. See text.

Using the rotational linkage criterion, Gillam and colleagues have shown that the grouping of two lines is influenced by a number of stimulus factors including: (a) relative line orientation (Gillam, [20]); (b) line separation relative to length (Gillam, [23]; Gillam and Grant Jr., [24]); (c) axis of rotation

(Gillam and McGrath, [18]); and (d) common vanishing point with a surrounding frame (Gillam and Broughton, [25]). A general discussion of this approach to grouping can be found in Gillam [26].

The goal of the present research was to use the rotational linkage criterion to see whether the poor grouping (high rate of fragmentation) that we have generally found for the horizontally symmetric figure (Figure 2A) could be improved by increasing symmetry redundancy, which can be achieved by making the reflected lines more complex. Figure 2A has only two symmetrically arranged oblique straight lines. We compared fragmentation for this figure and for figures in which the horizontally symmetric straight oblique lines are replaced by similarly reflected lines made up of adjoined multiple orientations but with the same average orientation and separation as the lines of Figure 2A. These figures are shown in Figure 2B,C.

Our reason for using *horizontal* symmetry to investigate the effects of redundancy was that an earlier study (Gillam and McGrath, [18]) showed that Figure 2A turned 90 degrees to create *vertical* symmetry demonstrated strong rotational linkage leaving little scope for any additional effects of redundancy.

Greater grouping with more redundant symmetry is predictable on the grounds that symmetry in more complex figures is less likely than in simple figures to result from an accidental arrangement of two unrelated elements and is therefore more likely to be seen as a structural property. This outcome would be predicted by Rock's [27] view that perceptual resolutions avoid "coincidence". A similar outcome would follow from a Bayesian analysis (Barlow, [28]) in that more redundantly symmetric figures would have a higher probability of resulting from a distally symmetric arrangement. Symmetry *detection* on the other hand has been considered by van der Helm [2] to have a holographic structure in which the number of elements is irrelevant. Supporting evidence for this proposition, using blob stimuli, was reported by Csatho, van der Vloed and van der Helm [29]. Additionally, Baylis and Driver [30], using line stimuli more like those in the present study, found that the speed of symmetry detection for the two sides of a single object is not influenced by the complexity of the reflected contour. Finally, in a comprehensive visual evoked response study, Makin et al. [31] confirmed many aspects of the holographic model, including the fact that complexity has little effect on symmetry detection. Our hypothesis that redundant symmetry will facilitate grouping thus seems to be somewhat at odds with the general finding for symmetry detection. However, grouping based on symmetry will not necessarily be determined by the same factors as symmetry detection, which must occur prior to grouping.

2. Experiment 1

2.1. Method

The three figures used are shown drawn to scale at a quarter actual size in Figure 2. The axis of rotation is indicated by a dotted line. Observers sat at a distance of 140 cm from the screen with their eyes at the level of the midpoint of the object on the screen. The separation of the lines of Figure 2A along the axis of rotation was 2.5 cm (one degree). The average line orientation (15 degrees from the horizontal) and average separation were the same in all three figures. To achieve smooth motion, figures were presented on a computer-controlled Hewlett-Packard oscilloscope with a fast phosphor. A red filter placed over the screen eliminated faint ghosts caused by persistence. Each figure was presented for 10 rotations at a speed of 12 s per rotation. This slow smooth rotation has been found in the past to elicit ample opportunities for apparent change from fragmentation (opposite rotation) to rotational linkage. Although strict fixation was not required, a dot to guide location of looking was placed midway between the upper and lower sets of lines on the axis of rotation (which was not shown).

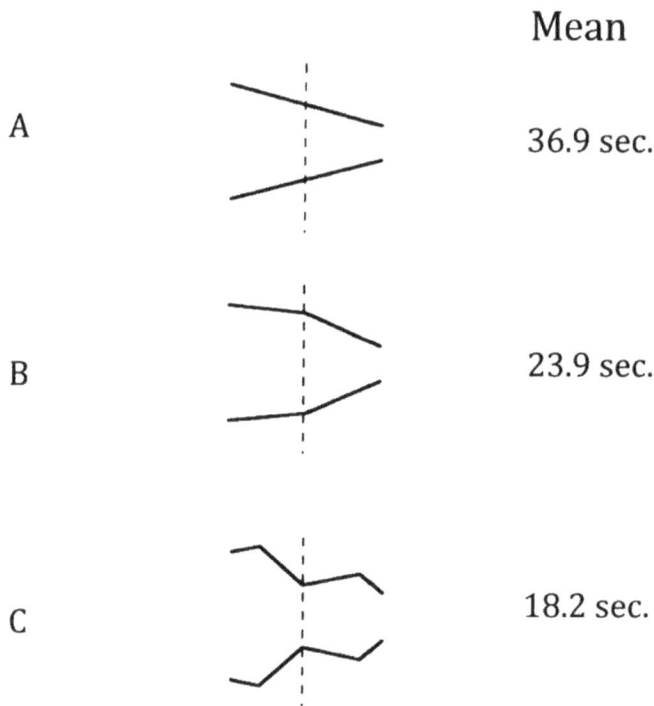

Figure 2. The figures used in Experiment 1 (drawn to one-quarter scale). The mean fragmentation time in seconds is shown next to each figure.

2.2. Observers

Participants in both experiments were volunteers from the State University of New York, State College of Optometry. For experiment 1, twelve students, ignorant of the rationale of the experiment, were used. Each observer was shown Figure 2A (known to readily fragment) and asked what he/she saw. As in all our grouping experiments, only those observers who spontaneously reported seeing fragmentation for Figure 2A in a pretest were used in the main Experiment. This ensured that they were clear about what they were supposed to respond to. Two of the twelve observers only reported fragmentation after it was suggested to them and were not used in the main experiment. The figures were presented for each observer in a different random order.

2.3. Results

The mean fragmentation time is shown next to each figure in Figure 2. An analysis of variance (ANOVA) showed a significant effect of figure (F = 7.29, df 2, 18 $p < 0.005$). Post-hoc Newman-Keuls tests showed that the mean for Figure 2A was significantly higher than the means for Figure 2B,C, (5.3 $p < 0.01$; 3.7 $p < 0.05$ respectively). Although Figure 2C had a lower mean fragmentation time (more grouping) than Figure 2B as predicted, these two means did not differ significantly from each other on a Newman-Keuls test.

The results support the hypothesis that symmetry carried by more complex elements (made up of multiple line orientations) results in greater grouping than symmetry carried by simple single line elements. It is possible that another difference between the simple and more complex stimuli is responsible rather than symmetry redundancy per se. It is unlikely however that the effect of complex symmetry arose from a fortuitous effect of the particular figures used, since Figure 2B,C differ considerably from each other. For example, Figure 2B is convex whereas Figure 2C is both convex and concave yet both enhanced grouping relative to Figure 2A. Experiment 2 explores these issues further.

3. Experiment 2

In this experiment, we attempted to replicate the basic finding of Experiment 1 with respect to complexity and to compare the effects of concave and convex symmetry. We also compared fragmentation time for symmetric figures and for similarly complex elements (lines with a mid-line orientation change) but not arranged symmetrically. Finally, in Experiment 2, we investigated the effect on grouping of offsetting the upper element horizontally from the lower element. This destroyed any reflective symmetry present while maintaining the same upper and lower elements as in the symmetric figures. This manipulation also explored vertical alignment of contour end points as a grouping factor.

3.1. Method

The figures used in Experiment 2 are shown drawn in Figure 3 at one-third actual size. There were four basic figures, each composed of an upper and lower element with endpoints vertically aligned and the same four figures with the upper and lower elements offset. The four basic figures were Figure 3A (Figure 2A from Experiment 1), Figure 3B (Figure 2B from Experiment 1, which was symmetric about a central horizontal axis and convex), Figure 3C (A concave figure symmetric about a central horizontal axis, which consisted of two lines per element that had the same average orientation and spacing as Figure 3A,B) and Figure 3D (A composite figure consisting of one line from Figure 3B and one from Figure 3C). Figure 3D provided a baseline non-symmetric figure against which to compare the symmetric Figure 3B,C from which its components were drawn. Finally, Figure 3E–H were the offset versions of the four basic Figure 3A–D respectively. These have the same components as the equivalent non-offset figures but lack symmetry.

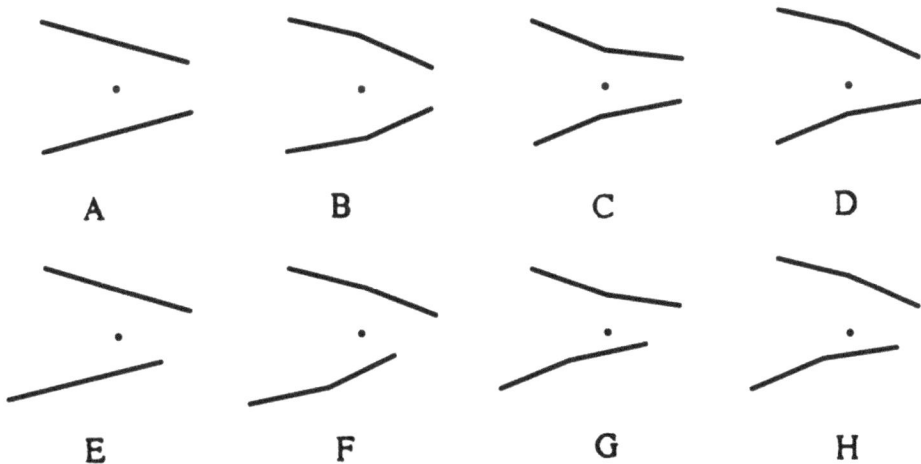

Figure 3. The figures used in Experiment 2 (drawn to one-third scale).

The method and observation distance were the same as in Experiment 1. All eight figures were presented rotating around a central vertical axis in parallel projection. There were initially 18 observers from a similar population as those used in Experiment 1 and ignorant concerning the rationale of the experiment. Three observers were rejected because they did not spontaneously report fragmentation in the pretest with the basic two-line Figure 2A. Thus 15 observers completed the experiment.

Stimuli were presented in a different random order for each observer. All figures were also presented for a second time to each observer in a different random order. The mean of the two presentations for each condition for each observer was used in the analysis.

3.2. Results

The means and standard errors of the fragmentation times for each condition are shown in Figure 4. Planned contrasts were carried out on the non-offset Figure 3A–D to test for an effect of complex symmetry. The mean fragmentation time for the more complex (redundant) symmetric Figure 3B,C were found to be significantly lower than for the simple symmetric Figure 3A and the asymmetric Figure 3D (F = 8.83, df 1, $p < 0.005$). A second planned contrast was carried out to examine the effect of offset. Offset was found to have a significant effect (F = 8.1, df 1, $p < 0.005$). The interaction between figure and offset was not significant.

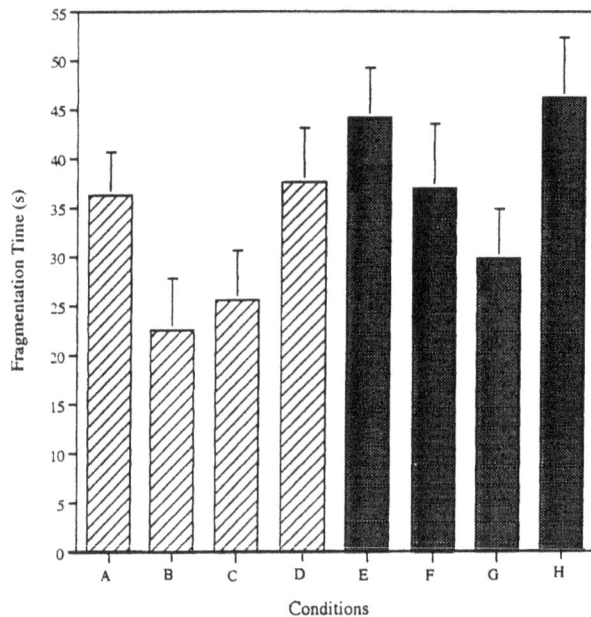

Figure 4. Means and standard errors for each figure used in Experiment 2.

3.3. Discussion

The hypothesis was again supported that horizontal symmetry supports grouping more effectively as it becomes more redundant. We also found a very general breakdown of grouping with horizontal offset of the elements. It is an ecological fact that the prevalence of vertically aligned contour edges is ubiquitous in the carpentered world. Our data suggest that it is also a grouping principle.

The data support the view that redundant symmetry is stronger evidence for structure than non-redundant symmetry. The more complex the symmetry, the greater the coincidence it would be for the symmetric layout to arise from a chance arrangement than from intrinsic structure. The visual system could have such contingencies built in to its responses either by evolution or learning. This argument could be made more strongly if in Experiment 1, symmetric (reflected) lines composed of four orientations (Figure 2C) had produced significantly more grouping than those composed of two lines (Figure 2B). Although there was a difference, the fact that it was not significant suggests that the grouping process may have a low ceiling with respect to symmetry redundancy.

Symmetry **2017**, *9*, 67

As mentioned in the introduction, the explanation we have proposed could also be couched in Bayesian terms.

4. Conclusions

Our past research showed that horizontal symmetry for a simple stimulus was ineffective in producing contour grouping. It appears from the present research that unlike vertical symmetry, horizontal symmetry requires a more complex line to be reflected to produce strong grouping. Barlow and Reeves [3] pointed out that symmetry could produce considerable processing advantages to an organism by allowing subsequent processes to deal with larger units. Gillam [20] pointed out the processing advantages of grouping in the processing of depth and motion. However, until the present studies, there is no direct evidence that symmetry produces grouping outside of figure-ground studies. The present data, however, provide evidence that symmetry results in spatio-temporal grouping if the elements reflected are sufficiently complex. This represents processing consequences of symmetry such as were foreshadowed by Barlow and Reeves [3] and shown for other stimulus factors by Gillam and colleagues (op. cit.). It does not seem likely that the grouping found for complex symmetry was occurring on other grounds.

Acknowledgments: This research was carried out when the author was on the Faculty of The State College of Optometry, SUNY, New York, NY, USA. It was supported by a grant from the U.S. National Institute of Mental Health (R01-MH30840). The author wishes to thank Tarryn Balsdon for help with the figures.

Conflicts of Interest: The author has no conflicts of interest with respect to this paper.

References

1. Koffka, K. *Principles of Gestalt Psychology*; Harcourt, Brace & World: New York, NY, USA, 1935.
2. Treder, M.S.; van der Helm, P.A. Symmetry versus repetition in cyclopean vision: A microgenetic analysis. *Vis. Res.* **2007**, *47*, 2956–2967. [CrossRef] [PubMed]
3. Barlow, H.B.; Reeves, B.C. The versatility and absolute efficiency of detecting mirror symmetry in random dot displays. *Vis. Res.* **1979**, *19*, 783–793. [CrossRef]
4. Royer, F. Detection of symmetry. *J. Exp. Psychol. Hum. Percept. Perform.* **1981**, *7*, 1186–1210. [CrossRef] [PubMed]
5. Wenderoth, P. The salience of vertical symmetry. *Perception* **1984**, *23*, 221–236. [CrossRef] [PubMed]
6. Tyler, C.W. Empirical aspects of symmetry perception. *Spat. Vis.* **1995**, *9*, 1–7. [CrossRef] [PubMed]
7. Wagemans, J. Characteristics and models of human symmetry detection. *Trends Cogn. Sci.* **1995**, *9*, 9–32. [CrossRef]
8. Gurnsey, R.; Herbert, A.M.; Kenemy, J. Bilateral symmetry embedded in noise is detected only at fixation. *Vis. Res.* **1998**, *38*, 3795–3803. [CrossRef]
9. Locher, P.J.; Wagemans, J. Effect of element type and spatial grouping on symmetry detection. *Perception* **1993**, *22*, 565–587. [CrossRef] [PubMed]
10. Bertamini, M.; Friedenberg, J.D.; Kubovy, M. Detection of symmetry and perceptual organization: The way a lock and key process works. *Acta Psychol.* **1997**, *95*, 119–140. [CrossRef]
11. Pomerantz, J.R.; Kubovy, M. Chapter 36 Theoretical Approaches to Perceptual Organization: Simplicity and Likelihood Principles. In *Handbook of Perception and Performance*; Boff, K.R., Kaufman, L., Thomas, J.P., Eds.; Wiley: New York, NY, USA, 1986; Volume 2.
12. Bahnsen, P. Eine Untersuchung über Symmetrie und Asymmetrie bei visuellen Wahrnehmungen. *Z. für Psychol.* **1928**, *108*, 129–154.
13. Rubin, E. *Synsoplevede Figurer*; Gyldendal: Copenhagen, Denmark, 1915.
14. Peterson, M.A.; Gibson, B.S. Must figure-ground organization precede object recognition? *Psychol. Sci.* **1994**, *5*, 253–259. [CrossRef]
15. Mojica, A.J.; Peterson, M.A. Display-wide influences on figure-ground perception: The case of symmetry. *Attn. Percept. Psychopys.* **2014**, *76*, 1069–1084. [CrossRef] [PubMed]
16. Kanizsa, G.; Gerbino, W. Convexity and Symmetry in Figure-Ground Organization. In *Vision and Artifact*; Henle, M., Ed.; Springer: New York, NY, USA, 1976; pp. 25–32.

17. Machilsen, B.; Pauwels, M.; Wagemans, J. The role of vertical mirror symmetry in visual shape detection. *J. Vis.* **2009**, *9*, 1–11. [CrossRef] [PubMed]
18. Gillam, B.; McGrath, D. Orientation relative to the retina determines perceptual organization. *Percept. Psychophys.* **1979**, *26*, 177–181. [CrossRef]
19. Feldman, J. Formation of visual "objects" in the early computation of spatial relations. *Percept. Psychophys.* **2007**, *69*, 816–827. [CrossRef] [PubMed]
20. Gillam, B. Perceived common rotary motion of ambiguous stimuli as a criterion of perceptual grouping. *Percept. Psychophys.* **1972**, *11*, 99–101. [CrossRef]
21. Eby, D.W.; Loomis, J.M.; Solomon, E.M. Perceptual linkage of multiple objects rotating in depth. *Perception.* **1989**, *18*, 427–444. [CrossRef] [PubMed]
22. Wallach, H.; O'Connell, D.N. The kinetic depth effect. *J. Exp. Psychol.* **1953**, *65*, 205–217. [CrossRef]
23. Gillam, B. Separation relative to length determines the organization of two lines into a unit. *J. Exp. Psychol. Hum. Percept. Perform.* **1981**, *7*, 884–889. [CrossRef] [PubMed]
24. Gillam, B.; Grant, T., Jr. Aggregation and unit formation in the perception of moving collinear lines. *Perception* **1984**, *13*, 659–664. [CrossRef] [PubMed]
25. Gillam, B.; Broughton, R. Motion capture by a frame: Global or local processing. *Percept. Psychophys.* **1991**, *49*, 547–550. [CrossRef] [PubMed]
26. Gillam, B. Observations on associative grouping: In honor of Jacob Beck. *Spat. Vis.* **2005**, *18*, 147–157. [CrossRef] [PubMed]
27. Rock, I. *The Logic of Perception*; MIT Press: Cambridge, MA, USA, 1993.
28. Barlow, H. Redundancy reduction revisited. *Netw. Comput. Neural Syst.* **2001**, *12*, 241–253. [CrossRef]
29. Csatho, A.; van der Vloed, G.; van der Helm, P.A. Blobs strengthen repetition but weaken symmetry. *Vis. Res.* **2003**, *43*, 993–1007. [CrossRef]
30. Baylis, G.C.; Driver, J. Perception of symmetry and repetition within and across visual shapes: Part-descriptions and object based attention. *Vis. Cogn.* **2001**, *8*, 163–196. [CrossRef]
31. Makin, A.D.J.; Wright, D.; Rampon, G.; Palumbo, L.; Guest, M.; Sheehan, R.; Cleaver, H.; Bertamini, M. An electrophysiological index of perceptual goodness. *Cereb. Cortex* **2016**, *26*, 4416–4434. [CrossRef] [PubMed]

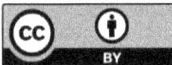

symmetry

MDPI

Article

Binocular 3D Object Recovery Using a Symmetry Prior

Aaron Michaux [1],*, Vikrant Kumar [2], Vijai Jayadevan [1], Edward Delp [1] and Zygmunt Pizlo [2]

[1]   School of Electrical and Computer Engineering, Purdue University, 465 Northwestern Avenue,
     West Lafayette, IN 47907, USA; vthottat@purdue.edu (V.J.); ace@ecn.purdue.edu (E.D.)
[2]   Department of Psychological Sciences, Purdue University, 703 3rd Street, West Lafayette, IN 47907, USA;
     vikrant1998@gmail.com (V.K.); zpizlo@purdue.edu (Z.P.)
*   Correspondence: amichaux@purdue.edu

Academic Editor: Marco Bertamini
Received: 16 January 2017; Accepted: 24 April 2017; Published: 28 April 2017

Abstract: We present a new algorithm for 3D shape reconstruction from stereo image pairs that uses mirror symmetry as a biologically inspired prior. 3D reconstruction requires some form of prior because it is an ill-posed inverse problem. Psychophysical research shows that mirror-symmetry is a key prior for 3D shape perception in humans, suggesting that a general purpose solution to this problem will have many applications. An approach is developed for finding objects that fit a given shape definition. The algorithm is developed for shapes with two orthogonal planes of symmetry, thus allowing for straightforward recovery of occluded portions of the objects. Two simulations were run to test: (1) the accuracy of 3D recovery, and (2) the ability of the algorithm to find the object in the presence of noise. We then tested the algorithm on the *Children's Furniture Corpus*, a corpus of stereo image pairs of mirror symmetric furniture objects. Runtimes and 3D reconstruction errors are reported and failure modes described.

Keywords: symmetry prior; symmetry detection; stereo; two-view geometry; 3D recovery

---

1. Introduction

The central importance of symmetry is well established in diverse fields such as physics, chemistry, mathematics, and art; however, it has received comparatively little attention in computer vision. Early computer vision researchers were interested in 3D recovery (for examples, see: [1–4]), and, as will be discussed later in this paper, symmetry is a powerful regularity that allows for 3D reconstruction. However, perhaps owing to the difficulty of the problem, interest in 3D recovery has been supplanted by machine learning approaches that almost always rely on purely 2D image features. (In the case of deep learning, instead of merely learning from 2D features, the 2D features themselves are learned from the training data [5].) Despite this trend in computer vision, it is widely recognized that human vision does perform 3D recovery [6], and, to this day, 3D recovery continues to be an important topic in computer vision.

Camera image formation is the forward problem of vision, and it is well-posed and well understood. Indeed, we know how to produce realistic looking images from 3D models [7]. However, there are an infinity of possible 3D models that can produce any given camera image, and that makes the inverse problem, 3D recovery from camera images, ill-posed [8]. In a classic 1985 paper, Poggio et al. [9] introduced the notion of computational vision, which uses regularization to solve early vision problems, such as 3D recovery. In essence, this means that all solutions to 3D recovery must involve a priori assumptions that constrain the possible recoveries. If we adopt a computational model of human cognition [10], as was done by David Marr [4], then the existence of innate a priori constraints also applies to human vision [11,12]. Considering that humans have definite ideas about the 3D shapes of objects that they perceive—Shepard and Metzler [13] proved as much with their classic experiment on the mental rotation of objects—it makes sense to investigate and understand what priors the human vision system uses in 3D shape perception.

Recent advances in human perception have shown that symmetry, and mirror symmetry in particular, is the most important prior in 3D shape perception [12,14,15]. Li et al. [16] argued further that an object's shape is defined by its symmetries. That is, an object has as much shape as it has symmetry or regularity. We consider it natural, therefore, to investigate mirror symmetry as an informative prior for 3D shape recovery in the spirit of Poggio et al.'s paradigm of computational vision.

In this paper, we present a new algorithm for performing 3D recovery for mirror symmetric objects from a pair of stereo images. There has been a small amount of persistent interest in using mirror symmetry to perform 3D recovery; however, almost no attempts use both mirror symmetry and two-view geometry at the same time. However, there is psychophysical evidence that the human visual system does precisely this: using both mirror symmetry and two-view geometry to aid 3D shape perception [17]. The advantage of combining mirror symmetry with two-view geometry is that each problem disambiguates the other, making it simpler to solve both simultaneously. (This is developed in Sections 3.2 and 3.3). For the sake of computational efficiency, we added the additional constraint that objects stand on a flat surface, or floor. This is easily arranged when capturing images in controlled conditions; however, most real world objects do stand on a flat surface [12], and there is psychophysical evidence that the human vision system takes advantage of this prior [18].

2. Related Works

As early as 1978, Marr and Nishihara [19] emphasized the importance of 3D representations in computer vision. In particular, Marr and Nishihara advocated for symmetric parts based on Binford's generalized cones [20]. However, this work did not address the mathematical problem of recovering 3D symmetric shapes from camera images. Kanade, 1981, did provide details for 3D reconstruction [3], but only for skew-symmetry (i.e., orthographic projections of planar symmetric figures). It was not until 1990 that Gordon first published details for 3D reconstruction from the perspective images of mirror symmetric objects [21], although Gordon credits the Oxford University engineer Guy Scott with the idea of calculating depth information from symmetry.

Since then, the field has grown immensely richer. A key observation was that mirror symmetry is a variant of two-view geometry [22]. That is, the image of a symmetric object allows for computing a second view of the same object. This is true except for degenerate cases and can be generalized to other types of symmetry. For example, the left and right side of the face are roughly identical, and thus the image of a face can be thought of as two aligned views of a single half. This provides a variety of mathematical invariants that form a theoretical basis for identifying symmetry, and for performing 3D reconstruction [23–25]—a field which could perhaps be called *structure from symmetry* [26].

The key practical problem in solving structure from symmetry is identifying which pairs of image points "go together". Returning to the example of the face, a point on the tip of the left ear goes with a specific point on the tip of the right ear: no other point will do. Registering these points in the 2D camera image is called the *symmetry correspondence problem*, and once done, the positions of the 2D points can be corrected at the subpixel level [27]. However, a general solution to the symmetry correspondence problem is currently beyond the state of the art. Few invariants exist for the general case problem, and any pair of imaged 2D curves is consistent with some 3D mirror symmetric interpretation [28].

It is natural to try to restrict the problem (following in the footsteps of Kanade) to orthographic images of planar symmetric figures, such as symmetric designs on walls and patterns on carpets. In this case, correspondences can be found using local 2D features that are robust, or invariant, to local affine distortions [29–32].

Despite challenges, solving symmetry correspondence for more general symmetric figures has been a topic of ongoing interest. One approach noted that mirror symmetry extends to the surface normals of a shape, providing a useful invariant for performing dense reconstruction using shape from shading [33]. Dense reconstruction has also been performed on mirror symmetric scenes by matching texture patches under smoothness constraints [34]. For scenes characterized by translational symmetry, dense reconstruction was performed using a graph-cut, with an energy function that incorporates symmetrical repetition [35].

More typically, researchers solve symmetry correspondences on edge maps by trying to register pairs of smooth contours. One early approach identified polygons in the 2D image that obey invariants for some form of 3D symmetry. These polygons are then registered with each other, allowing for 3D reconstruction [36]. Alternatively, it is possible to match line features directly in a loop that validates the match geometry for some form of 3D symmetry [37]. Instead of matching line features, one can attempt to trace pairs of contours, matching key features along the way, such as turning angle. Two studies follow this approach, using sets of human generated contours as input [38,39]. Öztireli et al. [40] extracted feature points and contours from rasterized images; however, human intervention is required to select points in order to facilitate curve matching. Sinha et al. [41] put forward an interesting dynamic programming approach that simultaneously extracts and matches contours; however, it can only work when the viewing angle of the 3D mirror symmetric object is restricted.

The algorithm presented in this paper solves symmetry correspondences on rasterized edge maps, and without human intervention, by using the two-view geometry of stereo image pairs to disambiguate possible correspondences. It is possible to perform 3D reconstruction from pairs of stereo images alone [22]; however, the results are usually noisy due to image pixelation. This paper presents an alternative point of view for using symmetry and two-view geometry together: symmetry can be used to improve the quality of 3D reconstructions, in effect performing subpixel accurate correspondence. This approach was pursued to clean up the 3D point clouds generated from the application of structure from motion [42,43].

Symmetry, however, does more than just provide subpixel correction, or accurate 3D reconstruction. Symmetry is a global property, and thus it can be used to perform *figure/ground organization*: localizing individual objects in a scene, and separating them from the background. In previous work, we investigated using mirror symmetry with two-view geometry to perform figure/ground organization [44]. However, as far back as 1997, Zabrodsky and Weinshall [45] observed that mirror symmetry and two-view geometry can be used together. They developed a graph based method for matching corresponding points, and tested it mainly on synthetic images. However, they also ran two tests using, respectively, three and five camera views of a 3D symmetric object and reported the average 3D reconstruction error on sparse sets of manually selected interest points. This can be taken as part of the inspiration for the algorithm presented in this paper.

3. Proposed Algorithm

We present an algorithm that performs 3D reconstruction of mirror symmetric objects from a pair of stereo images, where the symmetry is evident in the contours of the object. In many ways, the algorithm is a successor to the algorithm presented in [44]; however, it has been repurposed to perform 3D object reconstruction. Comparisons with [44] are detailed in Sections 4.3.1 and 4.3.3. While it is possible that this algorithm may have practical uses, it is a proof of concept for a family of methods that perform 3D object recovery using symmetries. The specific types of objects recovered depend on how the object's shape is defined. For this proof of concept, we use Definition 1 for the shape of an object.

Definition 1. *An object's shape is a set of 3D points that are mirror symmetric about two orthogonal planes of symmetry.*

This definition covers a variety of manufactured objects, including some pieces of furniture. One advantage of this definition is that the two planes of symmetry can be used to reconstruct the backs of objects. This is made clear in Sections 3.6 and 4.3.2. The reasons for restricting the algorithm to objects with definite edges, and the formulation of the 3D recovery as an optimization problem is developed in the rest of this section.

3.1. Notation

We use lowercase and uppercase bold symbols for points in $\mathbb{R}^2$ and $\mathbb{R}^3$, respectively. Therefore, for example, $x \in \mathbb{R}^2$, and $X \in \mathbb{R}^3$. Furthermore, we add a superscript asterisk for points in the respective projective spaces. Thus, $x^* \in \mathbb{P}^2$ and $X^* \in \mathbb{P}^3$. The exception is unit vectors in $\mathbb{R}^3$, which are written $\tilde{n}$ (lowercase because they have only two degrees of freedom). Subscripts refer to a particular camera, if relevant. For example, x_1^*, and x_2^* refer to point x^* in camera 1 and camera 2. The function $E(x^*)$ is used to convert homogeneous coordinates into equivalent Cartesian points. Thus, $\|E(x^*)\|$ refers to the L^2 norm of the Cartesian equivalent to the homogeneous coordinate x^*.

In this paper, we use a pinhole camera model and only consider calibrated cameras. We use K for the intrinsic camera matrix, and $P = K[R \,|\, t]$ for the camera matrix. R and t are the extrinsic camera parameters: R a rotation matrix, and $t = -RC$, where C is the coordinates of the camera center. Again, we use subscripts if a particular camera is indicated. Thus, $x_1^* = P_1 X^*$ gives the projection of point X^* in camera 1. All intrinsic parameters are assumed to be known, as is the relative rotation and translation between the camera pair, and thus we use a calibrated stereo system.

Sometimes, we need to refer to the reprojection error of an image point relative to some estimate of a 3D point. For example, point X^* may be imaged in camera 1 as point x^*, but with some errors. In this case, the reprojection error is expressed as: $d(x^*, P_1 X^*) = \|E(x^*) - E(P_1 X^*)\|$. For those unfamiliar with homogeneous coordinates, camera matrices, and projective spaces, please refer to Hartley and Zisserman [22].

3.2. 3D Mirror Symmetry and Projective Geometry

An object is mirror symmetric in 3D if the object is invariant (unchanged) when reflected through a single plane of symmetry, $\pi = \begin{bmatrix} \tilde{n}^\top & d \end{bmatrix}^\top$. Thus, Equation (1) holds true for any point on the object S:

$$\forall U \in S, \quad \exists V \in S \quad s.t. \quad V = U - 2(\tilde{n}^\top U + d)\tilde{n}. \tag{1}$$

In this formulation of the plane equation, $\pi = \begin{bmatrix} \tilde{n}^\top & d \end{bmatrix}^\top$, the point plane distance is given by $\tilde{n}^\top U + d$, and $\tilde{n}$ (a unit vector) gives the normal to the symmetry plane, which will henceforth be referred to as the *direction of symmetry*. A mirror symmetric object is shown in Figure 1.

Object Definition 1 refers to two orthogonal planes of symmetry. In this case, Equation (1) is true for each plane of symmetry, and furthermore, the planes of symmetry are orthogonal to each other. Planes π_1 and π_2 are orthogonal to each other if, and only if, the respective directions of symmetry are orthogonal to each other.

We use a pinhole camera model for a calibrated camera with intrinsic matrix K, and with neither radial nor skew distortion. Let P be the camera matrix, and let U^* and V^* be mirror symmetric points obeying the relationship given in Equation (1) (i.e., when expressed as Cartesian points in $\mathbb{R}^3$). Thus $u^* = PU^*$ and $v^* = PV^*$ are the points imaged by the camera.

The 3D line joining U and V has direction $\tilde{n}$. Imagine starting at point U and traveling toward and through point V and continuing an infinite distance: to a point on π_∞, the plane at infinity in $\mathbb{P}^3$. This creates a new point $N^* = \begin{bmatrix} \tilde{n}^\top & 0 \end{bmatrix}^\top$, which has no Cartesian equivalent in $\mathbb{R}^3$. Then $n^* = PN^*$ is the *vanishing point* associated with the plane of symmetry. It is a rule of projective geometry that points on lines in $\mathbb{P}^3$ are imaged to points on lines in $\mathbb{P}^2$ (see [22]), and because U^*, V^*, and N^* are all co-linear, then so are u^*, v^*, and n^*. We call u^* and v^* *corresponding points*, since they are related to each other by the mirror symmetry of U^* and V^*. All corresponding points for the image of a mirror-symmetric object are co-linear with the vanishing point.

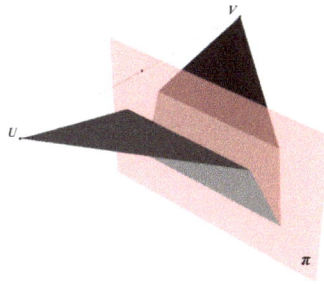

Figure 1. The figure is mirror symmetric about the plane $\pi = \begin{bmatrix} \tilde{n}^\top & d \end{bmatrix}^\top$. This means that every point U is related to some point $V = U - 2(\tilde{n}^\top U + d)\tilde{n}$—for example, the wing-tips, as shown above. The line joining U to V is parallel to the direction of symmetry, $\tilde{n}$, the normal of the symmetry plane.

This brings us to the mathematical relationship for reconstructing 3D points U and V up to scale from their imaged points u and v, given that the vanishing point, n, is known. First, write $U = \|U\|\tilde{u} + C$, and $V = \|V\|\tilde{v} + C$, where C is the camera center, and $\tilde{u}$ and $\tilde{v}$ are unit vectors. Let KR be the left-most 3×3 block of the camera matrix $P = K[R \mid t]$. This makes $\tilde{u} = (KR)^{-1}u^* / \|(KR)^{-1}u^*\|$, and $\tilde{v} = (KR)^{-1}v^* / \|(KR)^{-1}v^*\|$. Let $\tilde{n} = (KR)^{-1}n^* / \|(KR)^{-1}n^*\|$ be the direction vector in $\mathbb{R}^3$ derived from the vanishing point. Note that $\tilde{n}$ is the direction of symmetry set by the symmetry plane normal. Now, consider the angles between $\tilde{n}$, and $\tilde{u}$ and $\tilde{v}$. Specifically, let $\theta = \cos^{-1}(\tilde{u}^\top \tilde{n})$ and $\phi = \cos^{-1}(\tilde{v}^\top \tilde{n})$. The angles θ and ϕ are illustrated in Figure 2.

Referring again to Figure 2, the line joining U and V is, by definition, parallel to the line extending from the camera center, C, down the direction of symmetry $\tilde{n}$. Let U' be the point on the ray through $\tilde{n}$ such that $CU'U$ makes a right angle triangle, and let $\lambda = \|U - U'\|$ be the distance between U and U'. Then, by construction, $\sin\theta = \lambda / \|U\|$. Similarly, if V' is the point on the ray through $\tilde{n}$ such that $CV'V$ makes a right angle triangle, then $\sin\phi = \lambda / \|V\|$. The relationship $\lambda = \|U - U'\| = \|V - V'\|$ holds because the four points $\{U, V, U', V'\}$ form a rectangle. This gives Equation (2), which relates the length $\|V\|$ relative to $\|U\|$, with the angle formed by their direction vectors with the direction of symmetry. This relationship is shown in Figure 2:

$$\frac{\sin\theta}{\sin\phi} = \frac{\|V\|}{\|U\|}. \tag{2}$$

To solve for U and V, note that their midpoint lies on the symmetry plane $\pi = \begin{bmatrix} \tilde{n}^\top & d \end{bmatrix}^\top$. That is: $\frac{1}{2}(U + V)^\top \tilde{n} + d = 0$. Thus, $(U + V)^\top \tilde{n} = \left(\|U\|\tilde{u} + C + \frac{\sin\theta}{\sin\phi}\|U\|\tilde{v} + C\right)^\top \tilde{n} = -2d$, giving Equation (3):

$$\|U\| = \frac{-2(d + C^\top \tilde{n})}{\tilde{u}^\top \tilde{n} + \frac{\sin\theta}{\sin\phi}\tilde{v}^\top \tilde{n}}. \tag{3}$$

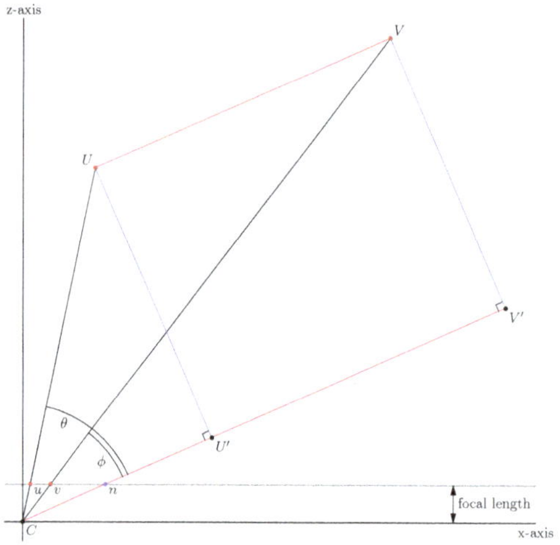

Figure 2. Diagram that shows the relationship expressed in Equation (2). Specifically because the points $\{U, V, U', V'\}$ form a rectangle, the length $\lambda = \|U - U'\| = \|V - V'\|$. Then, we have the ratio $\sin\theta / \sin\phi = \|V\|/\|U\|$. The diagram is patterned after [44]. An interactive 3D version of this diagram is available in the supplementary materials.

Substitute from Equation (3) into Equation (2) to calculate the length $\|V\|$. Note that this formula requires a calibrated camera with a finite focal length because, otherwise, the angles θ and ϕ cannot be determined. Furthermore, the image points u and v must be distinct. There is a degenerate case when the plane of symmetry goes through the camera center, in which case both the numerator and denominator of Equation (3) become zero. (i.e., $d + C^\top\tilde{n} = 0$, and the denominator can be rearranged to show that $\tan\theta + \tan\phi = 0$.) Except for this degenerate case, a set of 3D mirror symmetric points can be recovered up to scale from a vanishing point, and a set of corresponding points in the image. The scale of the recovered object is set by d, the distance between the symmetry plane and the origin. For further discussion, see [44]. See [21,28,46] for alternative formulations.

3.3. Solving the Symmetry Correspondence Problem with Two-View Geometry

Solving the symmetry correspondence problem is all that is required to solve for the 3D shape of a mirror symmetric object. However, as described in Section 2, there is no known robust and general purpose method for solving symmetry correspondence, and it remains a topic of ongoing research. Indeed, so long as they are co-linear with the vanishing point, one can select arbitrary pairs of corresponding points and reconstruct a 3D object [12]. This applies in the continuous case as well, and any pair of 2D curves is consistent with some pair of 3D mirror symmetric curves [28]. One key issue is that a degenerate viewing angle can hide details in the images of one or both of the 3D curves, as is shown in Figure 3.

If we consider 3D mirror symmetry and two-view geometry together, the situation is simplified. For a two-view camera system, a single point in 3D is imaged in two different cameras. That is, point X^* is imaged in camera 1 as $x_1^* = P_1 X^*$ and in camera 2 as $x_2^* = P_2 X^*$. This pair of points, x_1^* and x_2^*, is also known as a *corresponding pair*, but for the binocular correspondence problem. (for complete coverage, see [22].)

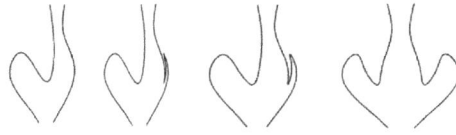

Figure 3. These four images are generated from the same pair of 3D mirror symmetric curves but seen from different vantage points. On the far left, the viewing angle is such that the curve images do not suggest 3D symmetry. Nonetheless, the relationship is there, and it becomes clear as the view is rotated, especially in the two right-most images. These images were published in [28].

Consider shape S as a set of points in $\mathbb{R}^3$. Each camera gives a unique image of the points in S, and thus a prospective pair of 3D symmetric curves are imaged uniquely in each camera. This observation underlies Equation (4), which states that when the points $X \in S$ are projected using camera matrix P_i, the reprojection error (defined in Section 3.1) to a point in the relevant binary edge map $\texttt{EdgeMap}_i$ is less than some threshold ϵ. (A binary edge map is a binary image where each pixel indicates the presence or absence of an edge.). For two-view geometry, we have $i \in \{1, 2\}$:

$$\forall X^* \in S \quad \exists x_i^* \in \texttt{EdgeMap}_i, \quad s.t. \quad d(x_i^*, P_i X^*) < \epsilon. \tag{4}$$

Taken together, Equations (1) and (4) specify a 3D mirror symmetric shape that is consistent with evidence in two (or perhaps more) camera images. Only two visible edge points are required for each image. Figure 4 illustrates what is gained by combining mirror symmetry with two-view geometry. Let U and V be 3D points that are mirror symmetric about a symmetry plane π with direction of symmetry $\tilde{n}$. Let u_1 and u_2 be the images of U in cameras 1 and 2, and likewise, let v_1 and v_2 by the images of V in cameras 1 and 2. The points u_1 and v_1 are symmetric corresponding points, and must be co-linear with n_1, the image of $\tilde{n}$ on the plane at infinity (as described in Section 3.2). Likewise, u_2 and v_2 are co-linear with n_2 in the second camera image. Note also that u_1 and u_2 correspond in the binocular sense, and so do v_1 and v_2. Each individual point participates in two different epipolar geometries, and thus the entire system is over-constrained, with the locations of each of the four points constrained by both the direction of symmetry, $\tilde{n}$, and *Fundamental matrix* [22], which constrains the locations of binocularly corresponding points according to the relative rotation and translation between the two cameras. Thus, Equations (1) and (4) together specify 3D points that are consistent with this over-constrained geometry and provide an avenue to solve both the binocular and the symmetry correspondence problem at the same time. In effect, the symmetry correspondence problem disambiguates the binocular correspondence problem, and vice versa. This restricts the algorithm to those objects whose mirror symmetry is evident in the binary edge maps of both images. When one or both projected points are missing (for example, they are occluded, or not picked up by edge detection), then that pair of 3D points are omitted in shape S.

The proposed algorithm requires an efficient method for validating if a given shape S satisfies the image evidence. We first calculate binary edge maps for each image using the Canny operator with an adaptive filter [47]. The edge points are loaded into an R-tree [48], thus creating a spatial index for the edge points in each image. Then, for each point $X^* \in S$, the spatial index is used to query the closest point to $E(P_i X^*)$ in camera i. The reprojection error is given by the L^2 distance between the queried point and the projected point, and this error must be less than ϵ. This procedure has average time complexity $O(mnk)$, where m is the number of cameras, $n = |S|$ is the number of 3D points in shape S, and k is the expected time complexity for looking up single points from the spatial index.

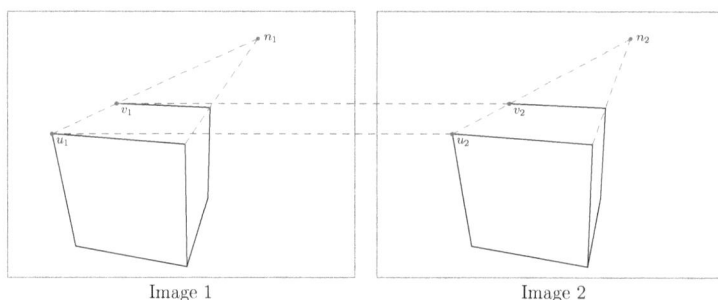

Figure 4. Points u_1 and u_2 are the images of some point $U \in \mathbb{R}^3$, and points v_1 and v_2 are the images of some point $V \in \mathbb{R}^3$. Let $\tilde{n}$ be the direction vector between U and V, and N^* the intersection of $\tilde{n}$ with the plane at infinity (see Section 3.2). Let n_1 and n_1 be the images of N^* in camera 1 and 2. Then, as described in Section 3.2, u_1, v_1, and n_1 are co-linear, and likewise u_2, v_2, and n_2 are co-linear. Furthermore, u_1 and u_2 are co-linear with the binocular epipole, a point in $\mathbb{P}^2$ calculated from the relative rotation and translation between the two cameras. See [22] for a full treatment. Likewise, v_1 and v_2 are also co-linear with the binocular epipole. This creates an over-constrained system, where the image points u_1, v_1, u_2, and v_2 are restricted by the direction vector between the two 3D points that generated them (i.e., U and V), and the relative rotation and translation between the two cameras.

3.4. Using a Floor Prior

Most objects stand on a floor, or flat surface, and there is psychophysical evidence that the human visual system uses some sort of floor prior [12,18]. Using a floor prior is similar to the "Manhattan World" assumption [49], where a scene is assumed to have three global vanishing points related to an orthogonal basis in $\mathbb{R}^3$. In this case, the normal to the floor plane corresponds to the "up direction" in a Manhattan World. However, the floor prior by itself is more flexible, admitting objects with a single plane of symmetry (thus two vanishing points in total), or perhaps other symmetries. Furthermore, floor plane estimation is robust and stable under two-view geometry when many floor points are visible—a typical scenario when a particular application allows for the control of camera viewing angles.

We assume that objects stand (or lie) on the floor, and that their symmetry planes are orthogonal to the floor plane. This restricts the object's direction of symmetry to the one-dimensional subspace orthogonal to the floor plane normal. The projection of this subspace is called the *horizon line*, and is the intersection of the image plane with the plane parallel to the floor that also contains the camera center.

The floor prior is found using a procedure developed by Li et al. [46]. First, a disparity map is calculated using OpenCV's StereoBM algorithm [50], which matches patches of texture between a pair of rectified stereo gray-scale images. Triangulation [22] is then applied to the disparity map to generate a 3D point cloud. Finally, *Random sample consensus* (RANSAC [51]) is used to find the equation of the plane that contains the most 3D points within a specified error threshold. This method works well when the floor is visible and is robust to the noise typical of 3D reconstructions from stereo image pairs.

3.5. Finding Symmetry Planes

As pointed out in Section 3.2, finding vanishing points is equivalent to finding the direction of symmetry for a symmetry plane. The proposed algorithm extends existing feature based approaches to vanishing point detection by taking advantage of both 3D symmetry and two-view geometry. Equation (3) shows that the vanishing point alone would be enough to recover the 3D object up to scale; however, scale is important in two-view geometry and is required for Equation (4). Thus, we must estimate both the direction of symmetry and d, the distance between the symmetry plane and the origin.

We use the Harris operator [52] with parameters set to over detect corner features. Corner features are then registered with each other across both input images using the disparity map previously calculated when finding the floor prior. Let $\eta = \begin{bmatrix} \tilde{g}^\top & d_\eta \end{bmatrix}^\top$ be the equation for the floor, where $\tilde{g}$ is suggestive of the direction of gravity. Let x_i^* be an image point in camera i. Equation (5) is the ray-plane intersection that denotes the point on the floor plane that images to x_i^*. This situation is illustrated in Figure 5:

$$F(x_i^*, i) = C_i - \frac{\tilde{g}^\top C_i + d_\eta}{\tilde{g}^\top (KR)_i^{-1} x_i^*} (KR)_i^{-1} x_i^*. \tag{5}$$

If we assume that u_i^* and v_i^* are a corresponding pair of points, then the direction of symmetry, $\tilde{n}$, can be estimated in camera i by finding the unit vector between $F(u_i^*, i)$ and $F(v_i^*, i)$. Equation (6) gives the estimate for $\tilde{n}$ by averaging across both cameras:

$$\tilde{n} = \frac{1}{2} \sum_{i=1}^{2} \frac{F(u_i^*, i) - F(v_i^*, i)}{\|F(u_i^*, i) - F(v_i^*, i)\|}. \tag{6}$$

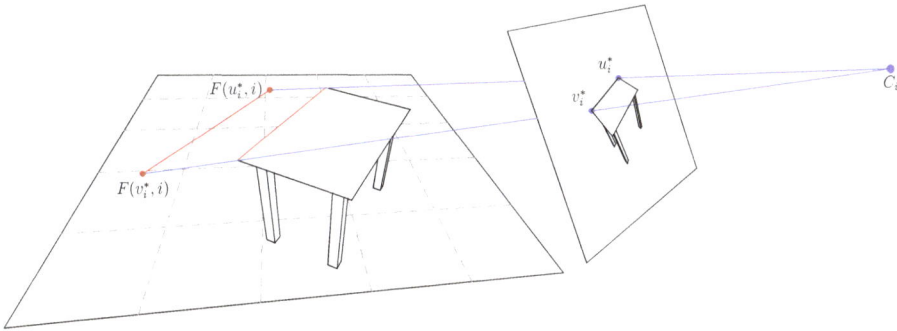

Figure 5. Method for estimating the direction of symmetry $\tilde{n}$ from assumed corresponding points u_i^* and v_i^*. Equation (5) is used to find $F(u_i^*, i)$, and $F(v_i^*, i)$, the points on the floor plane that image to u_i^* and v_i^*. The vector $F(u_i^*, i) - F(v_i^*, i)$ is an estimate for the direction of symmetry, but for a single pair of points in a single camera. Equation (6) estimates $\tilde{n}$ by averaging the normalized estimates across all cameras.

To estimate d, note that if U and V are symmetric about π, then the midpoint $M = \frac{1}{2}(U + V)$ must lie on the symmetry plane. That is, $M^\top \tilde{n} = d$. To find M, we first select an arbitrary d, say $d' = 1$. Then, using Equations (2) and (3), we recover U_i and V_i to scale, but for each camera image. Then, $\hat{m}_i = \frac{1}{2}(KR)_i^{-1}(U_i + V_i)$ is the back projection from camera center C_i that images to point m_i^* in camera image i. That is, $m_i^* = P_i(\hat{m}_i + C_i)$. We then use triangulation [22] in Equation (7) to estimate d by first finding M:

$$d = \texttt{triangulate}(P_1(\hat{m}_1 + C_1),\ P_2(\hat{m}_2 + C_2))^\top \tilde{n}. \tag{7}$$

Symmetry planes are recovered for all pairs of detected corners; however, many solutions can be discarded immediately. The equations above are over-determined, and while every solution is guaranteed to be orthogonal to the floor, the resulting reprojection error may be large for 3D points recovered using Equations (2) and (3). Thus, we only keep those solutions that have reprojection errors for all corner features less than a threshold ϵ, as specified in Equation (8):

$$\Pi = \{\pi : (U_i, V_i) = \xi(\pi, P_i, u_i^*, v_i^*),\quad d(u_i^*, P_i U_i), d(v_i^*, P_i V_i) < \epsilon,\quad i \in \{1, 2\}\}, \tag{8}$$

where u_i^*, v_i^* is every pair of corner features registered across both images by the disparity map calculated in Section 3.4, π is the resulting symmetry plane found by solving Equations (6) and (7), and $(U_i, V_i) = \xi(\pi, P_i, u_i^*, v_i^*)$ gives the two solutions for Equations (2) and (3) in camera image i. This operation has worst time complexity $O(n^2)$ in the number of corner features detected, since we are testing all unique sets of two corner features chosen from the set of all detected corner features.

3.6. Two Orthogonal Symmetry Planes

To find orthogonal symmetry planes, we consider all pairs of hypotheses in Π specified in Equation (8). The worst case time complexity is $O(n^4)$, since, in theory, we could be testing all unique sets of four corner features from the set of all detected corner features. In practice, however, most pairs of corners are already discarded by using Equation (8) when generating the set Π. We specify the reprojection error of a pair of planes as the maximum reprojection error of one of the points in one of the cameras that was involved in generating one of the symmetry plane hypotheses. This is specified by Equation (9), where u_{ij}^* and v_{ij}^* are the pair of image points that originally generated symmetry plane hypothesis j in image i, and U_{ij} and V_{ij} are calculated using symmetry plane hypothesis j in image i:

$$\texttt{error}(\pi_1, \pi_2) = max\left(d(u_{ij}^*, P_i U_{ij}), d(v_{ij}^*, P_i V_{ij})\right) \quad i, j \in \{1, 2\}. \tag{9}$$

Every pair of symmetry plane hypotheses in Π is considered, and Nelder–Mead [53] is applied to minimize the error specified in Equation (9) after forcing the symmetry planes to be orthogonal. The set Π' is then the set of all the hypothesis pairs whose optimized error is less than some threshold ϵ.

Note that using two planes of symmetry allows for reconstructing the backs of objects, which are normally occluded in the camera images. Because all the points in object S obey Equation (1) for every symmetry plane, then every point $X \in S$ can be reflected in one or both symmetry planes, relating it to three other points in S. This means that points on the visible front of the object are related to occluded points on the back of the object, and thus that back of the object can be recovered. This is not possible when objects have only a single plane of symmetry; however, even in this case, the backs of objects can be recovered using additional assumptions, such as planarity [12].

This observation requires that we modify Equation (4) so that we do not attempt to try to find image evidence for points that we expect to be occluded. To do this, we take each set of four points that are related through the two symmetry planes, and we remove the point that is furthest from the camera center. We then combine these sets of three points to make $S' \subset S$, and apply Equation (4) to the points in S'.

3.7. Recovering Objects with Short Curves

A 3D shape, defined by Definition 1, can be recovered for every symmetry-plane-pair in Π', by using Equations (2) and (3) on all pairs of edge points in a single image. According to Equation (4), the recovered 3D points must project to an edge point within a set threshold, ϵ, for all camera images. In a method similar to RANSAC [51], the final recovered 3D shape is simply that with the largest number of 3D points that are consistent with Equation (4).

In theory, this has worst case time complexity $O(n^2)$ in the number of edge points, since we could be considering all unique sets of two edge points from the set of all detected edge points. However, as outlined in Section 3.2, the images of symmetric points must be co-linear with the vanishing point derived from the relevant symmetry plane. Therefore, the proposed algorithm sorts all edge points by the angle subtended with the vanishing point, and then a local search is performed about each point to find co-linear points that solve for 3D points that obey the threshold specified in Equation (4). The expected time complexity is $O(n \log n + nm)$, where $O(n \log n)$ is the time complexity for sorting edge points, and nm is the expected number of comparisons made across all m camera images in the local search for co-linear points.

In practice, incidental arrangements of edge points lead to some false positive 3D points that are not filtered out by applying Equation (4). Almost all of these incidental points can be removed by considering short continuous runs of edge points, which we call contours. Instead of finding "best" or "meaningful" contours—an expensive operation that may introduce instabilities—we split the runs of edge points at approximately equally spaced intervals. We then select several points on each contour, and solve for the 3D points as before; however, in addition to filtering the results by Equation (4), we also add the additional constraint that the corresponding edge points must lie within a set distance along some contour. Not only does this procedure reduce the number of false positive points in the recovered shape, it also dramatically improves the speed of the computation by reducing the number of edge points being considered with each recovery.

3.8. Overview of Algorithm

Figure 6 gives a flow chart, and dependency graph, for the algorithm. Many steps can be executed in parallel, and individual steps can also make good use of parallelism. In particular, estimating the floor (Section 3.4), finding symmetry hypotheses (Sections 3.5 and 3.6), and calculating solutions (Section 3.7) can each have their time complexities divided by the available parallelism.

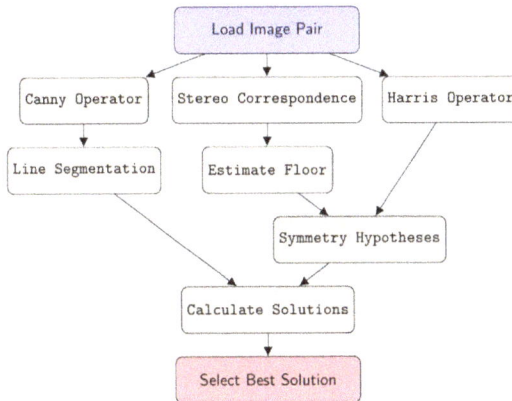

Figure 6. Flow chart of proposed 3D recovery algorithm.

Table 1 lists the algorithm parameters, which are chosen with reference to the properties of the relevant equations. Increasing the reprojection thresholds results in more false positives in the recovered 3D shape. The algorithm is robust to changes in the other parameters, including contour length.

Table 1. Algorithm parameters. For details on the *random sample consensus* algorithm (RANSAC), see: [51].

Parameter	Reference	Value
RANSAC iterations for floor estimation	Section 3.4	500 iterations
RANSAC threshold for floor estimation	Section 3.4	0.1 m
Harris block size	Section 3.5	3
Harris k	Section 3.5	0.01
Object point reprojection threshold	Equation (4)	$\epsilon = 1.5$ pixels
Symmetry plane reprojection threshold	Equation (8) and Section 3.6	$\epsilon = 1.5$ pixels
Contour length	Section 3.7	15 pixels

4. Results

We have presented an algorithm for performing 3D object recovery for mirror symmetric objects from pairs of images. We ran two simulations to test aspects of this algorithm. In simulation 1, Section 4.1, we compared Triangulation [22]—the standard 3D recovery algorithm for two-view geometry—to the formula derived in Section 3.2, which performs 3D recovery using mirror symmetry. In simulation 2, Section 4.2, we generated synthetic images of random mirror symmetric shapes with one versus two planes of symmetry, and with random noise features, in order to examine how well the algorithm solves the correspondence problem. In Section 4.3, we present results for the algorithm on a corpus of real image pairs. Since the algorithm is a repurposed refinement of previous work on figure/ground organization [44], we compare the new algorithm to this previous work.

4.1. Simulation 1

The algorithm presented in this paper addresses, in part, two different problems: the correspondence problem and the 3D recovery problem. The correspondence problem involves selecting sets of corresponding image points that share some geometric property. For example, consider Figure 4. The points u_1 and u_2 are corresponding points for the binocular correspondence problem, and u_1 and v_1 are corresponding points for the symmetry correspondence problem. Furthermore, all four points, u_1, v_1, u_2, and v_2, are corresponding points for both the symmetry and binocular correspondence problems together. Solving a given correspondence problem involves identifying a set of image points.

The 3D recovery problem involves calculating points in 3D from sets of corresponding points and is usually performed with a mathematical formula. By contrast, solving a correspondence problem usually involves some type of search. Triangulation [22] is the standard method for performing 3D recovery from a pair of binocular corresponding points. In Section 3.2, we developed an equation for 3D recovery from a pair of corresponding points for the symmetry correspondence problem. The reader may guess that this 3D recovery should be more accurate, on average, than any 3D reconstruction performed on corresponding points for the binocular correspondence problem, including Triangulation, because the latter is inherently sensitive to noise [22].

The supplementary materials include animations of a figure recovered from real image pairs (described fully in Section 4.3), using either Triangulation, or Equations (2) and (3) from Section 3.2. In all cases, the correspondence problem was solved using the symmetry based algorithm presented in this paper; only the last step—3D recovery—is different. The 3D figure recovered using Triangulation features peculiar "planar" clustering, which is caused by pixelation in the camera images. The recovered 3D points jump from plane to plane as the difference between the corresponding points changes by one pixel. This is a well known problem and can only be ameliorated by subpixel correction before Triangulation is performed. The animation files show qualitatively that recovery based on symmetry is unquestionably better than Triangulation. The pixel-related artifacts of binocular recovery are almost never symmetrical with respect to the common symmetry plane of the object, and so, these artifacts are corrected by adding the symmetry constraint. However, as we show below, Triangulation is more sensitive to noise even when controlling for pixelation.

In this simulation, we compare 3D recovery using Triangulation, versus using Equations (2) and (3) for pairs of points, as opposed to whole objects. We generated one random pair of 3D points at a time. The points were uniformly distributed over a $4 \times 4 \times 4$ m^3 box centered 3 m directly in front of the simulated camera. A single pair of points is obviously mirror symmetrical with respect to the plane that bisects them. This plane was computed and used for the recovery based on Equations (2) and (3). These two 3D points were projected, as continuous variables, to a pair of simulated images using a calibrated stereo camera with a 12-cm baseline, a 66-deg horizontal field of view. After the two image points (in $\mathbb{R}^2$) were calculated, a variable amount of Gaussian white noise was added. The standard deviation of the Gaussian white noise was specified in pixels, which is relative to the assumed 800×600 image format. The simulated image points were never rounded (to the nearest pixel) so that the simulation is a valid approximation for other image resolutions. Thus, the noise in our experiment simulates other natural processes, other than pixelation, that affect image formation. Either Triangulation or Symmetry (Equations (2) and (3)) were used to perform 3D recovery from a pair of image points. Figure 7 shows the error in recovery (in meters) as a function of the standard deviation of the added Gaussian white noise (in pixels). Each data point in the graph is the average error from 1 million replications. In each replication, one pair of random 3D points was generated and recovered. Note that the use of the true symmetry plane in this simulation when a single pair of points was recovered represents the fact that the estimated symmetry plane of an object consisting of hundreds of points is very stable precisely because many pairs of points are used to estimate that plane. This is the unique advantage of incorporating a spatially global constraint.

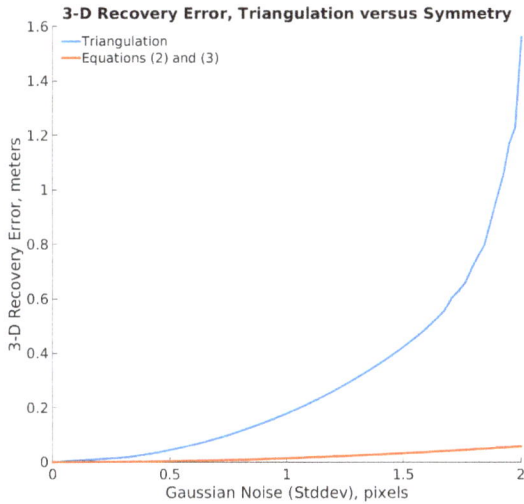

Figure 7. Top curve: error in 3D recovery using Triangulation [22] as a function of image noise. Bottom curve: error in 3D recovery using symmetry (Equations (2) and (3)) as a function of image noise.

Figure 7 clearly shows that 3D recovery using Triangulation is more sensitive to noise, which could come from image pixelation, or other aspects of camera system, such as uncorrected lens distortion. Recovery using Equations (2) and (3) was more than an order of magnitude more accurate at all levels of noise, except zero noise, when recovery was identical for both methods.

4.2. Simulation 2

In this simulation, we used random synthetic figures to assess how well the present algorithm solves the correspondence problem for shapes with one or two planes of symmetry, and in the presence of noise. We followed [17] to generate random synthetic shapes with a single plane of symmetry. These shapes are bilaterally symmetric, have planar surfaces, a flat base, and are made out of three rectangular boxes joined to each other. The same procedure was used for shapes with two planes of symmetry; however, the shape was flatted across the top, with the height chosen to keep the total volume unchanged. The shapes averaged $35 \times 47 \times 34$ cm^3. Please refer to [17] for precise details on how these shapes are generated.

To generate random noise, we sampled 3D points uniformly in a $2 \times 2 \times 2$ m^3 box centered at a point 2.5 m in front of the camera center. Each 3D point became the point of intersection for two 3D lines, each 10-cm long, and sitting on a plane with a random orientation. The orientation of the plane was generated by sampling from a uniform distribution for the orientation vector's inclination and azimuth.

The random shape and noise features were then projected to a pair of 800×600 simulated images using a calibrated stereo camera with a 12-cm baseline, and a 66-deg horizontal field of view. A random shape with two planes of symmetry and 250 noise features is shown in Figure 8a,b. The crossed noise features were specifically chosen to generate lots of corner detections, since these are used to find symmetry planes, as described in Section 3.5. Furthermore, the lines were made long enough so that most of the projected lines would not be easily filtered out when finding correspondences, as described in Section 3.7.

The proposed algorithm then attempted 3D recovery on the composited image pairs. The image pairs contained no texture information with which to estimate the floor plane, so the orientation of the floor—a plane orthogonal to the shapes one or two symmetry planes—was given to the algorithm. Correct correspondence (true positives), incorrect correspondences (false positives), and missed correspondences (false negatives) were then counted, and used to generate a *precision* and *recall* score for each image pair. Figure 8c,d shows the recovered 3D shape as seen from the two camera views.

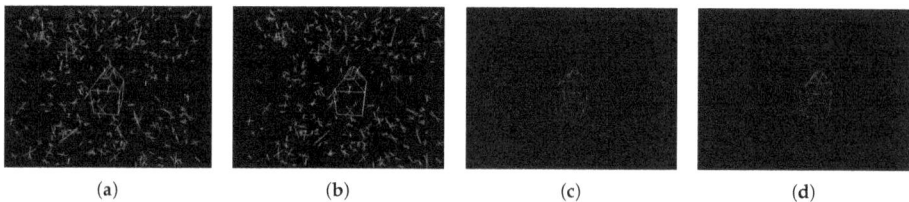

(a)   (b)   (c)   (d)

Figure 8. Input shape with two planes of symmetry, and random noise. (**a**,**b**) show the right and left camera image, respectively. The shape was recovered by the proposed algorithm, and (**c**,**d**) show the recovered 3D shape as seen by the left and right camera, respectively. An animation of the recovered shape is included in the supplementary materials.

Figure 9a shows precision and recall scores as a function of the percentage of noise features in the images, for shapes with one or two planes of symmetry. Ten random scenes were generated for each level of noise, and in each condition. (i.e., one or two planes of symmetry.) The percentage noise is calculated as 1 minus the number of visible corners in the synthetic shape (a maximum of 16) divided by the number noise features (each cross is a single noise feature). This data was generated using $\epsilon = 1.5$, the default "object point reprojection threshold" listed in Table 1, which is the ϵ used in Equation (4). We expected that as this threshold was loosened, recall would rise, and precision would fall. This is indeed the case, as shown in Figure 9b, which gives the same results but for $\epsilon = 5$.

We conclude that the method for solving the correspondence problem is robust to incidental noise. Furthermore, adding a second plane of symmetry does improve the robustness of the algorithm: precision is better, and recall does not suffer, or is better as in Figure 9b.

4.3. Experiment

To assess the algorithm on real images, we needed a corpus of stereo image pairs of objects, with two orthogonal planes of symmetry, standing on a clearly visible floor. The authors of [46] kindly made available the *Children's Furniture Corpus*, which is now available in the supplementary materials. This corpus consists of eighty-nine 800×600 grayscale image pairs of 11 exemplars, nine of which have two orthogonal planes of symmetry, and two with single planes of symmetry. Images were captured under typical indoor lighting conditions using a Point Grey Bumblebee2® stereo camera (Point Grey, Richmond, BC, Canada), with a 12-cm baseline, and a 66-deg horizontal field of view. Each exemplar averaged 1.87 m from the camera, sitting in the middle of the frame on flat blue carpet, and was captured from roughly equally spaced orientations.

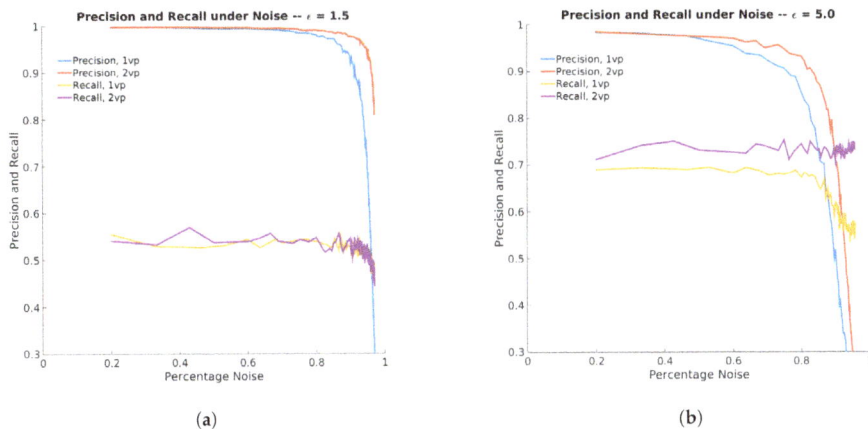

Figure 9. Precision and recall scores as a function of the percentage of noise features in the input images, for randomly generated shapes with one or two symmetry planes (vanishing points). (**a**) shows precision and recall for the algorithm's default parameters, listed in Table 1. We see that recall is similar for both types of shapes; however, precision is better for shapes with two symmetry planes. Furthermore, precision is more robust to noise for shapes with two symmetry planes; (**b**) shows precision and recall when $\epsilon = 5$. This is the ϵ in Equation (4). Loosening this threshold increases recall at the cost of lowered precision. Both precision and recall are better for two symmetry planes, indicating that the extra symmetry plane improves the algorithms performance due to the additional constraints that it provides.

The physical exemplars (pieces of furniture) were measured by hand with a tape measure, and Autodesk® Maya® (Maya 2016, Autodesk Inc., San Rafael, CA, USA) was used to create 3D models. Custom made software was then used to annotate each corpus image. Annotations consisted of extrinsic and intrinsic camera parameters, and the hand made Autodesk® Maya® model file (a triangle mesh) along with rotation, translation, and scale parameters. This is sufficient to place the mesh in 3D space, and project it to each camera image.

To measure the accuracy of the 3D recovery of shape S, we summed the average minimum distances between each point $X \in S$ and some point on triangle Δ in the hand-made 3D ground truth mesh, Ξ, with the average of the minimum distance between each vertex $V \in \Xi$ and some point $X \in S$. This is specified by Equation (10):

$$\text{error}(S, \Xi) = \left(\frac{1}{|S|} \sum_{X \in S} \underset{\Delta \in \Xi}{arg\,min}\, d(X, \Delta) \right) + \left(\frac{1}{|\Xi|} \sum_{V \in \Xi} \underset{X \in S}{arg\,min}\, d(V, S) \right). \tag{10}$$

Recovery was then performed on four 16 core Intel® Xeon® E7-8800v3 processors (Intel, Santa Clara, CA, USA), running Ubuntu® 14.04 (Canonical, London, UK). The algorithm produced output for all but two pairs of input images. Failure modes are discussed in Section 4.3.2. The average runtime was 2.41 s, and the average error, according to Equation (10), was 2.79 cm, or just over 1 inch. This error is the approximate thickness of the furniture surfaces, and, in part, contains errors in the hand made models. The results are summarized in Table 2, which shows the average speed and error for each exemplar. Table 3 shows sample 3D reconstructions.

4.3.1. Baseline for Comparison

This study is unique in that it reports the error in 3D object recovery over a corpus of images, when using projective geometry, and a mirror symmetry prior. To the authors knowledge, there is no comparable study, with either qualitative results being presented [25,30,34,37,41,54], errors only being reported on a few keypoints for only one or two images [45,55,56], or the approach is otherwise incomparable [29,31–33,35,42,43], or too restricted to be able to produce 3D recoveries from raster images such as those found in the Children's Furniture Corpus [3,21,26,38–40,57]. The authors suggest that more quantitative studies on corpora of camera images are needed, and have made the *Children's Furniture Corpus* available in the supplementary materials of this paper.

Michaux et al. [44] utilizes a similar method for disambiguating the symmetry and binocular correspondence problems, described in Section 3.3, and also uses a floor prior. Although this work aims to localize multiple objects in a scene at once, it can be adapted to perform 3D object recovery. The algorithm in this paper is an elaboration of [44], and thus we chose [44] as a baseline for comparison. The nature of those elaborations, and their effect on the speed and accuracy of 3D recovery, is discussed in Section 4.3.3.

Table 2. Experimental results were collected for the *Children's Furniture Corpus*, and a modified version of Michaux et al. [44] was used as a baseline for comparison. The second column denotes the number of image pairs for the given exemplar. Errors were calculated using Equation (10) and are reported in centimeters, along with a 95% confidence interval. Runtimes are reported in seconds, also with a 95% confidence interval. The algorithm failed to generate results for two image pairs of the Rubbish Bin, as discussed in Section 4.3.2.

Exemplar	#	Proposed Method	Michaux et al. [44]
Curved Stand	8	1.90 ± 1.69 cm 1.97 ± 0.41 s	3.42 ± 1.49 cm 8.96 ± 4.28 s
Short Stand	7	2.16 ± 0.27 cm 1.56 ± 1.47 s	4.94 ± 4.44 cm 3.52 ± 1.65 s
Bookshelf	8	2.13 ± 2.59 cm 2.30 ± 0.50 s	2.81 ± 2.86 cm 9.75 ± 3.25 s
Short Dense Stand	5	3.04 ± 1.17 cm 2.89 ± 3.90 s	6.21 ± 2.67 cm 4.14 ± 4.08 s
Mid Dense Stand	6	3.38 ± 2.48 cm 3.37 ± 4.14 s	4.74 ± 3.06 cm 8.25 ± 6.71 s
Tall Dense Stand	7	3.46 ± 5.76 cm 5.69 ± 7.34 s	5.20 ± 1.64 cm 18.17 ± 17.46 s
Short Table	8	2.96 ± 3.19 cm 1.45 ± 1.09 s	5.39 ± 5.36 cm 4.03 ± 1.53 s
Long Table	7	2.61 ± 4.08 cm 1.51 ± 1.25 s	5.52 ± 7.61 cm 5.68 ± 2.40 s
Rubbish Bin	6	2.54 ± 1.64 cm 0.89 ± 1.85 s	9.67 ± 8.43 cm 6.40 ± 5.56 s
Total/Average	63	2.66 ± 3.50 cm 2.41 ± 4.00 s	5.13 ± 5.65 cm 7.86 ± 10.71 s

Table 3. 3D reconstructions. The left two columns show the pair of the input images. The right two columns show 3D reconstructions, where the view has been rotated. The displayed objects are, from top to bottom: Curved Stand, Short Stand, Bookshelf, Short Dense Stand, Mid Dense Stand, and Long Table. Animation files are available in the supplementary materials. The recovered objects have two symmetry planes, and are thus naturally divided into four quadrants.

Input (Left Image)	Input (Right Image)	120-deg Rotation	240-deg Rotation

4.3.2. Discussion

The algorithm produced 3D reconstructions for all input image pairs, except for two image pairs of the Rubbish Bin. 3D reconstructions were, in general, excellent, with most recovered 3D points close to edges or surfaces on the annotated ground truth 3D meshes. The backs of objects were recovered, even though they were occluded, because the occluded points were related to points on the front of the object by reflections through one or both symmetry planes, as described in Section 3.6.

This contributes to the structure of the objects being clearly visible and identifiable to human viewers, who, presumably also recover the backs of the objects. Despite these successes, several failure modes were identified, as were opportunities for improvement.

Reducing the object point reprojection threshold, ϵ (see Table 1), resulted in significantly cleaner looking objects; however, recoveries were also sparser without affecting errors calculated by Equation (10). This is caused by the algorithm finding all the correspondences for edge points that are less than ϵ. Most edge points participate in multiple correspondence pairs, including erroneous correspondences that are "close enough", according to Equation (4). Solving this problem is not as simple as limiting edge points to single correspondences, since pixelated images require multiple correspondences for single edge points. This happens when the pair of mirror-symmetric curves are not equidistant to the camera, and thus image to 2D contours of different lengths. The pixels on the shorter contour must then participate in multiple correspondences in order to recover all of the points on the longer contour. This particular problem deserves consideration, and is important for generating more accurate and aesthetically pleasing 3D recoveries; however, it does not affect the basic structure of the recovery.

3D reconstruction depends on corner detection producing the required two pairs of corners that characterize the symmetry planes of the object, as shown in Figure 10a. Furthermore, these corners must appear in both images, and be registered with each other successfully. If no such set of four corners is found, then the algorithm fails. This happened for two images pairs of the Rubbish bin, one shown in Figure 10b. Corner detection worked well for the other corpus images; however, it does represent a potential algorithmic instability.

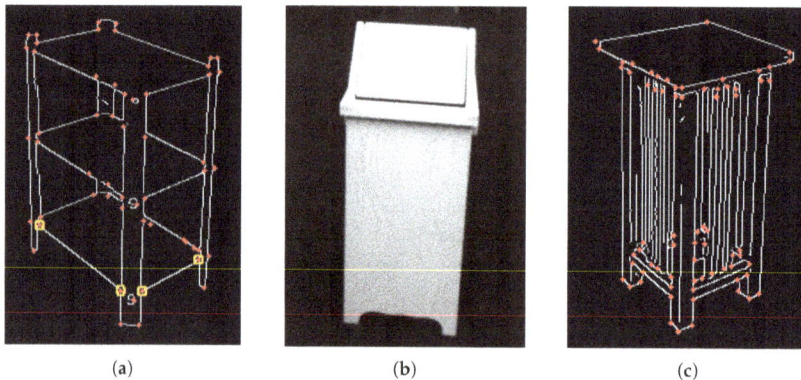

(a) (b) (c)

Figure 10. The importance of corner detection. (**a**) 3D recovery fails unless at least two pairs of corner features appear that reveal the required symmetry planes. In this edge map of an image of the Bookshelf, detected corners are marked in red, and a sufficient set of four corners is marked by yellow circles; (**b**) degenerate view of the Rubbish Bin. Recovery fails because the back of the object is not visible, and corner detection cannot be used to determine one of the planes of symmetry; and (**c**) runtime suffers when corner detection produces many corner pairs that generate symmetry hypotheses orthogonal to the floor, as is the case in this image of the Tall Dense Stand. These hypotheses are not filtered out by Equation (8), and runtime tends towards $O(n^4)$ in the number of detected corners. Runtime for this image was 11.48 s.

As described in Section 3.6, the worst case runtime is $O(n^4)$ in the number of detected corners. (The worst runtime was 11.48 s, for an image pair of the Tall Dense Stand shown in Figure 10c.) The algorithm can be modified to use any method for detecting symmetry planes, and there are many fast methods for finding vanishing points that can be used to calculate directions of symmetry for prospective symmetry planes.

Some 3D recoveries were poor even when symmetry planes were detected correctly. This was due to instabilities caused by degenerate cases inherent in the geometrical foundations of the algorithm. Consider the image of the Bookshelf shown in Figure 11a. The image itself is almost mirror symmetric in 2D, indicating that the symmetry plane contains (or runs close to) the center of perspective projection. As discussed in Section 3.2, this degenerate case prevents recovering 3D depth information from symmetry. As such, 3D recovery must rely on two-view geometry, which, in general, is noisy due to pixelation in the image [22]. However, two-view geometry also has a degenerate case. The Bumblebee2® camera (Point Grey, Richmond, BC, Canada) produces pairs of rectified images [22], which confounds solving binocular correspondence for points on horizontal lines. This means that Equation (4) is not particularly useful in disambiguating symmetry correspondences. Nonetheless, the algorithm produced recognizable output even in this pathological case, as shown in Figure 11b,c.

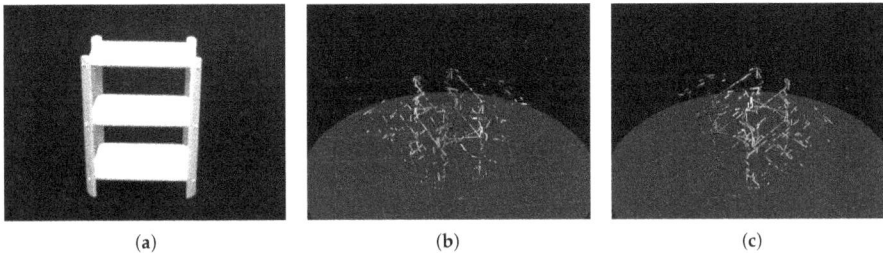

| (a) | (b) | (c) |

Figure 11. Degenerate views. (**a**) 3D recovery is poor even though symmetry planes can be estimated via corner detection. The image of the object is almost symmetrical in 2D, which means that the symmetry plane contains (or runs close to) the camera center. This makes 3D recovery numerically unstable, as described in Section 3.2. Furthermore, many of the lines are almost horizontal, a degenerate case when solving binocular correspondence for two-view geometry with rectified cameras [22], which is the case here. (**b,c**) show 3D recoveries with the view rotated by 120-deg and 240-deg. An animation file is available in the supplementary materials.

4.3.3. Comparison to Baseline

As shown in Table 2, the proposed method is both faster and more accurate than the baseline for comparison, [44]. The reasons for this lie in the differences between the two algorithms. We believe that the main reason for the more consistent and accurate results of the proposed algorithm lies in how vanishing points were detected. Firstly, Equation (9) uses the L^∞ norm, while [44] utilizes an equation similar to Equation (8), but based on the L^2 norm. Our analysis found that the L^∞ was much better suited to filtering out erroneous correspondences and should always be preferred to the L^2 norm.

Secondly, the baseline utilizes Equation (4) over the entire edge map of both input images, while the proposed algorithm also utilizes short pieces of curves. Using short pieces of curves proved to be an important innovation, because, as noted in Section 3.7, many incidental arrangements of edge points will still satisfy Equation (4). By utilizing short curves, we ensure that Equation (4) applies to contiguous sets of points—a powerful restriction. Our analysis showed that it was sufficient to work on the end points of the curve segments, and simply ensure that they are connected. This vastly improved the stability and performance of the algorithm.

Thirdly, the baseline identifies symmetry planes using RANSAC, while the proposed algorithm, searched across sets of four automatically detected corner features, and uses a closed form expression to make initial estimates of symmetry planes (Equations (5)–(7)). This means that the proposed algorithm depends on corner detection, as described in Section 4.3.2; however, we found that, in general, the symmetry plane detection was much better than the baseline.

Finally, the most obvious difference is that the baseline uses a shape definition based on just a single plane of symmetry, as opposed to two planes of symmetry. The choice of two planes of symmetry provides additional constraints on recovered points, as specified by Equation (9), and also provides a simple mechanism for recovering occluded surfaces. This results in more accurate estimates of the vanishing points (more points are involved when optimizing Equation (9)), as well as more complete figures. However, note that the backs of most exemplars are not completely occluded in the corpus images, and when [44] performed well, it was almost as accurate as the proposed algorithm, even though it utilized just one plane of symmetry. The exception was the Rubbish Bin, an object whose rear facing contours are always occluded. In this case, the baseline's performance compared least favorably to the proposed algorithm. In brief, the refined method presented in this paper is faster and more robust than the baseline.

5. Conclusions

The results suggest that mirror symmetry—a biologically motivated prior—is useful in performing 3D recovery from pairs of stereo images. However, the algorithm was designed and tested on a specific class of symmetrical objects, namely, those with two orthogonal planes of symmetry. Although this presented potential performance issues, discussed in Section 3.6, it also allowed for straightforward recovery of the backs of objects. The formulation relied on the 3D mirror symmetry of the objects being evident in edge maps of input image pairs. Practically speaking, this limits the application of the algorithm to objects with clearly visible contours—a typical restriction for solving the symmetry correspondence problem.

The failure modes discussed in Section 4.3.2 suggest that the algorithm could benefit from numerous small improvements, such as better or faster vanishing point detection. Furthermore, the algorithm has good precision (it rarely recovers false points); however, recall is limited (it tends to miss parts of objects). It is reasonable, therefore, to use the algorithms output as a starting point for completing the entire figure, perhaps using a smoothness constraint to do contour completion.

Larger improvements are also possible. First, there is no reason why the algorithm cannot be reformulated for an object definition for shapes with single planes of symmetry, while still recovering the backs of objects. This involves adding extra constraints to the object; however, these constraints may be useful in other ways. For example, as pointed out in [12], combining mirror symmetry with planarity is sufficient to recover occluded surfaces under common conditions. Many objects have planar surfaces, and psychophysical evidence suggests that humans use a planarity prior when recovering the shape of mirror symmetric curves [58].

Relaxing the use of the floor prior raises interesting questions as well. The algorithm can be modified to do this by simply letting Π (from Equation (8)) be generated from all pairs of corner features, and Π' from all pairs of symmetry hypotheses in Π. Although the runtime would suffer, the algorithm would still recover 3D shapes, including objects floating through the air. One caveat is that part of the accuracy of the symmetry hypotheses in Π (and thus Π') comes from the floor prior. This is because direct 3D recovery from stereo image pairs tends to be noisy, and the direction of symmetry would have to be calculated from those noisy recoveries. One way around this is to use pairs of hypotheses (from Π') as the initialization point for some optimization procedure that modifies the symmetry plane parameters in order to maximize the number of recovered 3D points that obey Equation (4). This could potentially mean orders of magnitude more evaluations of Equation (4). These computational problems would be alleviated by finding better methods for estimating the vanishing points of objects, or perhaps other innovations with how Equation (4) is handled.

Another interesting problem is to consider solving the symmetry correspondence problem for single uncalibrated images. Solving this problem will have many immediate applications because the Internet is full of uncalibrated images of symmetric objects. The focal length of an uncalibrated image can be estimated from two orthogonal directions, if we assume that the principal point is the center of the image [59]—usually close enough if the image has not been cropped. Therefore, in theory, camera calibration could be performed from images of symmetrical objects. This may be related to how the human vision system calibrates itself [60].

The authors believe that advances in computer vision lie in a deep understanding of the priors used by the human visual system. There is a straightforward logical argument for why this is so: if we assume a computational model of human cognition, then the powerful capabilities of the human vision system are founded in the innate priors that it uses. We have used two-view geometry as a crutch to explore possible ways for solving symmetry correspondence and pointed out several small and large problems that remain to be solved. A robust and general purpose solution for the symmetry correspondence problem would significantly advance the state of the art and also have immediate applications.

Supplementary Materials: The following are available online at www.mdpi.com/2073-8994/9/5/64/s1: The *Children's Furniture Corpus*. Animation files for reconstructions shown in Table 3, and Figures 8 and 11 can be found at https://osf.io/qdzz6/. This url also contains an animation of the curved stand with 3D recovery performed using Triangulation, as described in Section 4.1. An interactive 3D version of Figure 2 is available at http://www.pageofswords.net/symmetry-equation/.

Acknowledgments: This research was supported by the National Eye Institute of the National Institutes of Health under award number 1R01EY024666-01. The content of this paper is solely the responsibility of the authors and does not necessarily represent the official views of the National Institutes of Health.

Author Contributions: Aaron Michaux designed and implemented the proposed algorithm, and co-wrote the paper. Vikrant Kumar handcrafted the 3D models, annotated the data set, and assisted in writing. Zygmunt Pizlo, Vijai Jayadevan and Edward Delp participated in theoretical discussions that laid the basis for the paper's algorithm, reviewed the math, and co-wrote the paper.

Conflicts of Interest: The authors declare no conflict of interest.

References

1. Horn, B. Understanding image intensities. *Artif. Intell.* **1977**, *8*, 201–231.
2. Witkin, A. Recovering surface shape and orientation from texture. *Artif. Intell.* **1981**, *17*, 17–45.
3. Kanade, T. Recovery of the three-dimensional shape of an object from a single view. *Artif. Intell.* **1981**, *17*, 409–460.
4. Marr, D. *Vision: A Computational Investigation into the Human Representation and Processing of Visual Information*; Henry Holt and Co., Inc.: New York, NY, USA, 1982.
5. Hinton, G. Learning multiple layers of representation. *Trends Cogn. Sci.* **2007**, *11*, 428–434.
6. Dickinson, S. Challenge of image abstraction. In *Object Categorization: Computer and Human Vision Perspectives*; Cambridge University Press: New York, NY, USA, 2009.
7. Chalmers, A.; Reinhard, E.; Davis, T. *Practical Parallel Rendering*; CRC Press: Boca Raton, FL, USA, 2002.
8. Tikhonov, A.N.; Arsenin, V.Y. *Solutions of Ill-Posed Problems*; Winston: Washington, DC, USA, 1977.
9. Poggio, T.; Torre, V.; Koch, C. Computational vision and regularization theory. *Nature* **1985**, *317*, 314–319.
10. Pinker, S. *How the Mind Works*; W. W. Norton & Company: New York, NY, USA, 1997.
11. Tsotsos, J.K. *A Computational Perspective on Visual Attention*; MIT Press: Cambridge, MA, USA, 2011.
12. Pizlo, Z.; Li, Y.; Sawada, T.; Steinman, R. *Making a Machine That Sees Like Us*; Oxford University Press: Oxford, UK, 2014.
13. Shepard, S.; Metzler, D. Mental rotation: Effects of dimensionality of objects and type of task. *J. Exp. Psychol. Hum. Percept. Perform.* **1988**, *14*, 3–11.
14. Vetter, T.; Poggio, T.; Bülthoff, H. The importance of symmetry and virtual views in three-dimensional object recognition. *Curr. Biol.* **1994**, *4*, 18–23.
15. Sawada, T.; Li, Y.; Pizlo, Z. Shape Perception. In *The Oxford Handbook of Computational and Mathematical Psychology*; Oxford University Press: Oxford, UK, 2015; p. 255.
16. Li, Y.; Sawada, T.; Shi, Y.; Steinman, R.; Pizlo, Z. Symmetry Is the sine qua non of Shape. In *Shape Perception in Human and Computer Vision*; Springer: London, UK, 2013; pp. 21–40.
17. Li, Y.; Sawada, T.; Shi, Y.; Kwon, T.; Pizlo, Z. A Bayesian model of binocular perception of 3D mirror symmetrical polyhedra. *J. Vis.* **2011**, *11*, 11.
18. Palmer, E.; Michaux, A.; Pizlo, Z. Using virtual environments to evaluate assumptions of the human visual system. In Proceedings of the 2016 IEEE Virtual Reality (VR), Greenville, SC, USA, 19–23 March 2016; pp. 257–258.

19. Marr, D.; Nishihara, H. Representation and Recognition of the Spatial Organization of Three-Dimensional Shapes. *Proc. R. Soc. Lond. B Biol. Sci.* **1978**, *200*, 269–294.

20. Binford, T. Visual perception by computer. In Proceedings of the IEEE Conference on Systems and Control, Miami, FL, USA, 15–17 December 1971; Volume 261, p. 262.

21. Gordon, G. Shape from symmetry. In Proceedings of the Intelligent Robots and Computer Vision VIII: Algorithms and Techniques, Philadelphia, PA, USA, 1 March 1990; Volume 1192, pp. 297–308.

22. Hartley, R.; Zisserman, A. *Multiple View Geometry in Computer Vision*; Cambridge University Press: Cambridge, UK, 2003.

23. Rothwell, C.; Forsyth, D.; Zisserman, A.; Mundy, J. Extracting projective structure from single perspective views of 3D point sets. In Proceedings of the Fourth IEEE International Conference on Computer Vision, Berlin, Germany, 11–14 May 1993; pp. 573–582.

24. Carlsson, S. *European Conference on Computer Vision*; Springer: Berlin/Heidelberg, Germany, 1998; pp. 249–263.

25. Van Gool, L.; Moons, T.; Proesmans, M. Mirror and Point Symmetry under Perspective Skewing. In Proceedings of the Computer Vision and Pattern Recognition, San Francisco, CA, USA, 18–20 June 1998; pp. 285–292.

26. Hong, W.; Yang, A.; Huang, K.; Ma, Y. On symmetry and multiple-view geometry: Structure, pose, and calibration from a single image. *Int. J. Comput. Vis.* **2004**, *60*, 241–265.

27. Penne, R. Mirror symmetry in perspective. In *International Conference on Advanced Concepts for Intelligent Vision Systems*; Springer: Berlin/Heidelberg, German, 2005; pp. 634–642.

28. Sawada, T.; Li, Y.; Pizlo, Z. Any pair of 2D curves is consistent with a 3D symmetric interpretation. *Symmetry* **2011**, *3*, 365–388.

29. Cham, T.; Cipolla, R. Symmetry detection through local skewed symmetries. *Image Vis. Comput.* **1995**, *13*, 439–450.

30. Cham, T.; Cipolla, R. Geometric saliency of curve correspondences and grouping of symmetric contours. In *European Conference on Computer Vision*; Springer: Berlin/Heidelberg, Germany, 1996; pp. 385–398.

31. Cornelius, H.; Loy, G. Detecting bilateral symmetry in perspective. In Proceedings of the IEEE Computer Vision and Pattern Recognition Workshop, New York, NY, USA, 17–22 June 2006; p. 191.

32. Cornelius, H.; Perd'och, M.; Matas, J.; Loy, G. Efficient symmetry detection using local affine frames. In *Scandinavian Conference on Image Analysis*; Springer: Berlin/Heidelberg, Germany, 2007; pp. 152–161.

33. Shimshoni, I.; Moses, Y.; Lindenbaum, M. Shape reconstruction of 3D bilaterally symmetric surfaces. *Int. J. Comput. Vis.* **2000**, *39*, 97–110.

34. Köser, K.; Zach, C.; Pollefeys, M. Dense 3D reconstruction of symmetric scenes from a single image. In *Joint Pattern Recognition Symposium*; Springer: Berlin/Heidelberg, Germany, 2011; pp. 266–275.

35. Wu, C.; Frahm, J.; Pollefeys, M. Repetition-based dense single-view reconstruction. In Proceedings of the IEEE Computer Vision and Pattern Recognition, Colorado Springs, CO, USA, 20–25 June 2011; pp. 3113–3120.

36. Yang, A.; Huang, K.; Rao, S.; Hong, W.; Ma, Y. Symmetry-based 3D reconstruction from perspective images. *Comput. Vis. Image Underst.* **2005**, *99*, 210–240.

37. Bokeloh, M.; Berner, A.; Wand, M.; Seidel, H.; Schilling, A. Symmetry detection using feature lines. *Comput. Graph. Forum* **2009**, *28*, 697–706.

38. Cordier, F.; Seo, H.; Park, J.; Noh, J. Sketching of mirror-symmetric shapes. *IEEE Trans. Vis. Comput. Graph.* **2011**, *17*, 1650–1662.

39. Cordier, F.; Seo, H.; Melkemi, M.; Sapidis, N. Inferring mirror symmetric 3D shapes from sketches. *Comput.-Aided Des.* **2013**, *45*, 301–311.

40. Öztireli, A.; Uyumaz, U.; Popa, T.; Sheffer, A.; Gross, M. 3D modeling with a symmetric sketch. In Proceedings of the Eighth Eurographics Symposium on Sketch-Based Interfaces and Modeling, Vancouver, BC, Canada, 5–7 August 2011; pp. 23–30.

41. Sinha, S.; Ramnath, K.; Szeliski, R. Detecting and Reconstructing 3D Mirror Symmetric Objects. In *European Conference on Computer Vision*; Springer: Berlin/Heidelberg, Germany, 2012; pp. 586–600.

42. Gao, Y.; Yuille, A. Symmetric bon-rigid structure from motion for category-specific object structure estimation. In *European Conference on Computer Vision*; Springer: Berlin/Heidelberg, Germany, 2016; pp. 408–424.

43. Cohen, A.; Zach, C.; Sinha, S.; Pollefeys, M. Discovering and exploiting 3D symmetries in structure from motion. In Proceedings of the IEEE Computer Vision and Pattern Recognition, Providence, RI, USA, 16–21 June 2012; pp. 1514–1521.

44. Michaux, A.; Jayadevan, V.; Delp, E.; Pizlo, Z. Figure-ground organization based on three-dimensional symmetry. *J. Electron. Imaging* **2016**, *25*, 061606.

45. Zabrodsky, H.; Weinshall, D. Using bilateral symmetry to improve 3D reconstruction from image sequences. *Comput. Vis. Image Underst.* **1997**, *67*, 48–57.

46. Li, Y.; Sawada, T.; Latecki, L.; Steinman, R.; Pizlo, Z. A tutorial explaining a machine vision model that emulates human performance when it recovers natural 3D scenes from 2D images. *J. Math. Psychol.* **2012**, *56*, 217–231.

47. Canny, J. A computational approach to edge detection. *IEEE Trans. Pattern Anal. Mach. Intell.* **1986**, *6*, 679–698.

48. Beckmann, N.; Kriegel, H.; Schneider, R.; Seeger, B. The R*-tree: An efficient and robust access method for points and rectangles. *ACM Sigmod Rec.* **1990**, *19*, 322–331.

49. Coughlan, J.; Yuille, A. Manhattan world: Orientation and outlier detection by bayesian inference. *Neural Comput.* **2003**, *15*, 1063–1088.

50. Bradski, G. The OpenCV Library. Avaiable online: http://www.drdobbs.com/open-source/the-opencv-library/184404319 (accessed on 16 January 2017).

51. Fischler, M.; Bolles, R. Random sample consensus: a paradigm for model fitting with applications to image analysis and automated cartography. *Commun. ACM* **1981**, *24*, 381–395.

52. Harris, C.; Stephens, M. A combined corner and edge detector. In Proceedings of the Fourth Alvey Vision Conference, Manchester, UK, 31 August–2 September 1988; pp. 147–151.

53. Olsson, D.; Nelson, L. The Nelder–Mead simplex procedure for function minimization. *Technometrics* **1975**, *17*, 45–51.

54. François, A.; Medioni, G.; Waupotitsch, R. Reconstructing mirror symmetric scenes from a single view using 2-view stereo geometry. In Proceedings of the IEEE International Conference on Pattern Recognition, Quebec, QC, Canada, 11–15 August 2002; Volume 4, pp. 12–16.

55. Fawcett, R.; Zisserman, A.; Brady, M. Extracting structure from an affine view of a 3D point set with one or two bilateral symmetries. *Image Vis. Comput.* **1994**, *12*, 615–622.

56. Mitsumoto, H.; Tamura, S.; Okazaki, K.; Kajimi, N.; Fukui, Y. 3D reconstruction using mirror images based on a plane symmetry recovering method. *IEEE Trans. Pattern Anal. Mach. Intell.* **1992**, *14*, 941–946.

57. Huynh, D. Affine reconstruction from monocular vision in the presence of a symmetry plane. In Proceedings of the Seventh IEEE International Conference on Computer Vision, Kerkyra, Greece, 20–27 September 1999; Volume 1, pp. 476–482.

58. Sawada, T.; Li, Y.; Pizlo, Z. Detecting 3D mirror symmetry in a 2D camera image for 3D shape recovery. *Proc. IEEE* **2014**, *102*, 1588–1606.

59. Li, B.; Peng, K.; Ying, X.; Zha, H. Simultaneous vanishing point detection and camera calibration from single images. In *International Symposium on Visual Computing*; Springer: Berlin/Heidelberg, Germany, 2010; pp. 151–160.

60. Pirenne, M. *Optics, Painting & Photography*; JSTOR; Cambridge University Press: Cambridge, UK, 1970.

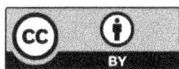

symmetry

MDPI

Article

Matching Visual and Acoustic Mirror Forms

Ivana Bianchi [1,*], Roberto Burro [2], Roberta Pezzola [3] and Ugo Savardi [2]

[1] Department of Humanities, University of Macerata, Macerata 62100, Italy
[2] Department of Human Sciences, University of Verona, Verona 37129, Italy; roberto.burro@univr.it (R.B.); ugo.savardi@univr.it (U.S.)
[3] Guitar Maestro, Fermo 63900, Italy; r.pezzola@libero.it
* Correspondence: ivana.bianchi@unimc.it; Tel.: +39-0733-258-4320

Academic Editor: Marco Bertamini
Received: 24 January 2017; Accepted: 2 March 2017; Published: 10 March 2017

Abstract: This paper presents a comparative analysis of the ability to recognize three mirror forms in visual and acoustic tasks: inversion (reflection on a horizontal axis), retrograde (reflection on a vertical axis) and retrograde inversion (reflection on both horizontal and vertical axes). Dynamic patterns consisting of five tones in succession in the acoustic condition and five square dots in succession in the visual condition were presented to 180 non-musically expert participants. In a yes/no task, they were asked to ascertain whether a comparison stimulus represented the "target" transformation (i.e., inversion, retrograde or retrograde inversion). Three main results emerged. Firstly, the fact that symmetry pertaining to a vertical axis is the most easily perceived does not only apply to static visual configurations (as found in previous literature) but also applies to dynamic visual configurations and acoustic stimuli where it is in fact even more marked. Secondly, however, differences emerged between the facility with which the three mirror forms were recognized in the acoustic and visual tasks. Thirdly, when the five elements in the stimulus were not of the same duration and therefore a rhythmic structure emerged, performance improved not only in the acoustic but also (even more significantly) in the visual task.

Keywords: visual symmetry; acoustic symmetry; mirror form detection; inversion; retrograde; retrograde inversion; dynamic stimuli

---

1. Introduction

Over the years psychologists have devoted a lot of attention to the perception of visual symmetry ([1]; for a review, see [2,3]). Extensive experimental research has demonstrated convincingly that mirror symmetry on a vertical axis is easier to identify than mirror symmetry on a horizontal or oblique axis [4–16], even at very short exposure times [4,9,17–21]. There is also evidence that infants are already able at the age of 4 months to distinguish symmetry on a vertical axis from other forms of visual symmetry [22–27]. This has led scholars to theorize that a hardwired mechanism underlies the human perception of mirror reflections, in particular on a vertical axis.

In contrast, only a few studies, carried out some time ago, have investigated the recognition of acoustic symmetry (known as "mirror forms") in non-expert listeners [28–33]. Furthermore, to the best of our knowledge, there is no previous study on whether it is possible to create a systematic parallel between the ability to recognize the same mirror forms in two sense modalities, in this case visual and acoustic. The experiment described in the present paper addresses this issue and to this end the participants carried out both an acoustic recognition task and a visual recognition task. In the acoustic task, short melodies consisting of a sequence of five notes were presented to the participants, immediately followed by another melody which was one of the three possible mirror transformations of the initial melody (Figure 1a): retrograde (i.e., the notes are played in reversed order) which correspond to a reflection around a vertical axis; inversion (i.e., the initial melody is played with the intervals inverted, so that for example a rising minor third becomes a falling minor third) which corresponds to a reflection around a horizontal axis or retrograde inversion (i.e., the inverted notes are played in retrograde) which corresponds to a double reflection around both horizontal and vertical axes. Corresponding stimuli were presented in the visual tasks (see Appendix A). In this case, the initial stimulus consisted of a sequence of five dots, appearing one after the other, and the subsequent comparison stimulus consisted of another sequence of five dots which represented one of the three mirror transformations of the initial pattern (Figure 1b).

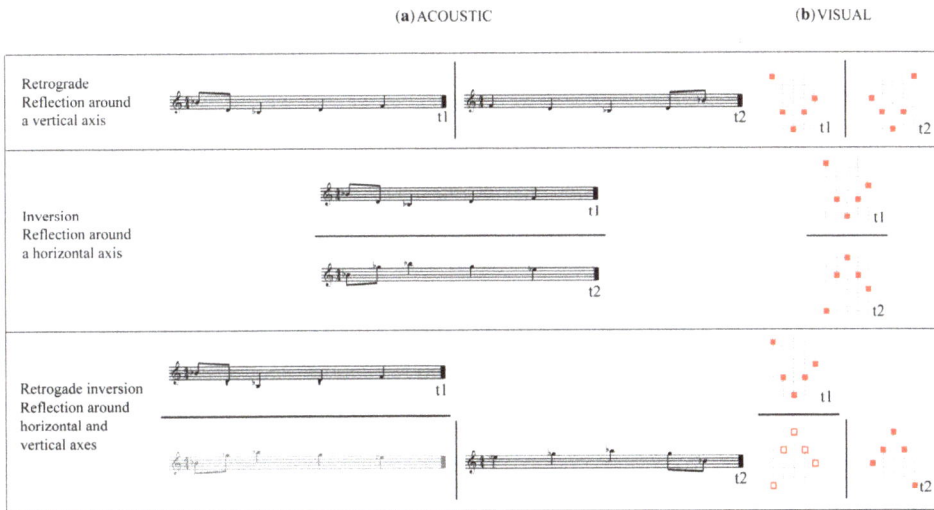

Figure 1. A representation of the three types of transformation (mirror forms) studied in: (**a**) acoustic task; and (**b**) visual task. The standard stimulus was presented first (t1), then the comparison stimulus (t2) followed after a 1 s Inter Stimulus Interval (ISI).

Visual and acoustic perception are two different sense modalities with different underlying physiological mechanisms and therefore differences in people's ability to detect the three symmetrical transformations in the two sense modalities are to be expected. However, cross modal correspondence is a well-known phenomenon in psychology [33–36]. It is implied in one of the traditional methods used in psychophysics, i.e., cross modal matching, in which people are asked to match the apparent intensity of various stimuli across two sensory modalities (e.g., adjusting the brightness of a light to match the loudness of a sound). Experimental tasks in which people are asked to identify an object which they have been shown by means of touch have also been used (for instance, in Sperry's famous split brain experiment [37]) as well as a shape-sound matching task which was first described in the "takete-maluma" study [38,39]. Over the years, cross modal correspondence has been consistently found with reference to a variety of sensory modalities but the phenomenon is very well documented for visual and acoustic modalities. The perception of an invariant relationship between audio and visual stimulation emerges at very precocious ages. At 4–5 months infants are able to detect synchrony between visual and acoustic stimuli [40,41], to make associations between sounds and changes in the direction of a movement [42,43], to match faces and voices (e.g., [44,45]) and to recognize similarities between the common rhythmic structures, tempo, and duration of auditory and visual events ([46–48]; see [49], for a review). Within this cross-modal context it is also well known that humans spontaneously describe auditory pitch spatially (e.g., [50–52]). The correspondence between symmetrical acoustic and visual patterns addressed in the present study is based precisely on this spatial correspondence:

the vertical distance between the dots in the visual stimuli corresponds to the distance between the notes in the acoustic stimuli which indicates the pitch (see Appendix A).

The three transformations studied in the present paper (retrograde transformation, inversion and retrograde inversion) were widely used in theories of compositional techniques originating in the 20th century which were known as dodecaphony. Dowling [30] was the first to investigate and experiment in order to discover whether listeners with no musical experience are able to recognize these three mirror forms. He used short melodies and a short-term recognition memory task in which the participants were presented with musical sequences consisting of five tones of equal duration followed by the corresponding mirror transformation (inversion, retrograde, and retrograde inversion). After being given information about the three kinds of mirror forms, listeners were asked to judge whether the two melodies presented corresponded to one of them. Blocks of trials were run separately for each of the three forms. Performance was above chance for all three forms, although the task turned out to be difficult. At presentation times similar to those used in the present study (i.e., at five tones presented in 2.5 s), the retrograde mirror form was easier to recognize than the inversion form, and both were more easily recognized than the retrograde inversion form. However, in a faster presentation condition (i.e., five tones per second, which means that the overall duration of the stimulus was 1 s), the inversion form turned out to be the easiest with the retrograde intermediate and the retrograde inversion forms proving the most difficult. There were no differences in the ease with which the three mirror forms were recognized in another study [31] with a different experimental task and longer melodies. Participants first listened to some extracts from the *Wind Quintet* (Op. 26) and the *String Quartet* (No. 4, Op. 37) by Arnold Schoenberg and became familiar with them. Probe stimuli were then presented, consisting either of the prime form or an inversion of the prime form (beginning on the same tone), the retrograde of the prime form (without transposition) and the retrograde inversion of the prime form (the non-transposed retrograde of the inversion). Participants in the experiment were asked to recognize whether the probe stimulus was a mirror form of the *Wind Quintet* or the *String Quartet* (respectively Melodies 1 and 2). Their accuracy was above a chance level performance, but no differences in their performance emerged between the three mirror forms and this was interpreted as an indication that the listeners found it equally easy to recognize the inversion, retrograde and retrograde inversion mirror forms. However, these findings can also be interpreted simply as showing that people have an ability to recognize a certain relatedness between the comparison stimulus and one of the two standard melodies, independently of whether or not they were able to recognize the specific mirror form. Individual differences were found, with accuracy correlated to the level to which the participants had previously studied music. We will go back to the differences in outcomes relating to the experimental conditions in the final discussion.

In one of the conditions studied by Dowling [30], before performing an acoustic task, the participants were presented with an analogous visual recognition task. The standard stimulus (a pattern consisting of five dots which was similar to the notational representations of the melodies in the acoustic experiment) appeared on the left-hand side of the page, while four comparison stimuli were presented on the other side of the page. One of these four configurations was the target mirror form which the participants were required to identify. Only 10 stimuli were used in this preliminary visual phase. Dowling predicted that doing the visual task first would lead to an improvement in performance in the acoustic task since it would provide more information relating to the structure of the configurations to be identified in the subsequent task. Contrary to his prediction, no significant improvements emerged in the condition including the preliminary visual task, and there was in effect only a slight tendency in that direction (i.e., 65% correct responses when there was a preliminary visual task vs. 59% in the acoustic task without the preliminary visual task). In the present study we go beyond the idea of a visual task as a preliminary training task and address a systematic direct comparison between the participants' performance with corresponding sets of visual and acoustic stimuli (using 96 stimuli for the visual condition and 96 stimuli for the acoustic condition). Moreover, our study provided a bi-directional perspective on the possible facilitator effect of performing the task across modalities as the two groups of participants performed the two tasks in a different order (i.e., first the visual task and then the acoustic task or vice versa).

There were four main specific aims in this research. The first was to verify whether naïve subjects (i.e., non-expert listeners) are able to recognize mirror forms in acoustic stimuli. The findings in previous literature regarding this issue are controversial. Secondly, we aimed to assess whether there was a difference in performance in the two sense modalities, a comparison made possible by the fact that the participants performed both the visual and acoustic task with corresponding stimuli. This represents the main innovation in the study. The third aim, related to the second, was to explore whether there are cross-modal facilitator effects influencing the ease with which mirror forms are recognized in one sense modality after doing the same task in another sense modality (i.e., when the visual task follows the acoustic task or vice-versa). This might provide insights regarding whether the detection of symmetry in the sequential conditions analyzed in this study are specific to each sensory domain or whether cross modal facilitation effects emerge. The fourth aim was to assess the role of Rhythm. There are contrasting results from previous studies regarding the role of the rhythm of a melody (determined by the varying duration of the notes) on the ability to recognize the three mirror forms. According to some (e.g., [32,53]), non-isochronism makes recognizing the mirror forms easier. In other studies [31,54], it has been found that it is more difficult to recognize melodic patterns with non-isochronous stimuli as compared to isochronous stimuli. It has to be noted, however, that in the latter studies, the isochronous and non-isochronous stimuli also differed in other ways related to their melodic structure and therefore there is no clear evidence that isochronism was the critical factor. All of the stimuli used in the present study were made up of five elements (five tones for the acoustic stimuli and five square dots for the visual stimuli) which appeared one after the other. In one condition (isochronism), all of the elements were of the same duration, i.e., 600 ms, while in another condition (non-isochronism), they were of two different durations, i.e., 400 ms and 800 ms. The study not only made it possible to test the effect of this characteristic (isochronism vs. non-isochronism) in the acoustic condition, but also provided first indications of whether it has a similar role in the recognition of visual symmetry in short dynamic sequences.

2. Materials and Methods

2.1. Participants

180 undergraduate students and adults with no musical expertise participated in the study. All had normal or corrected to normal vision and reported normal hearing. All participants performed both the visual (V) and acoustic task (A), and all responded to both the isochronous and non-isochronous stimuli. Order and Target mirror form were the only two variables which were studied between subjects. Ninety of participants performed the visual task before the acoustic task (order VA), while the other 90 were exposed to the two tasks in the opposite order (AV). The inversion mirror form was the target for 30 participants, the retrograde mirror form was the target for 30 other participants, and the retrograde inversion mirror form was the target for the remaining 30 participants. We opted for a single target detection task rather than asking the participants to classify each stimuli according to which of the three mirror forms it represented, due to the fact that in previous studies it had been found that this type of acoustic task is difficult for non-experts and that it is easier for people to recognize one single target.

The study was approved by the Ethics Committee of the University of Verona as the local ethics committee responsible and was conducted in accordance with the Declaration of Helsinki (revised 2008). All participants gave their written informed consent in accordance with the local ethics committee requirements.

2.2. Procedure

The experiment started with a training phase during which participants were familiarized with all of the three mirror forms (inversion, retrograde, retrograde inversion) by means of three visual representations and three acoustic examples such as those shown in Figure 1, one for each of the three mirror forms. The idea behind exposing the participants to all three forms was that this would help them to understand the mechanism by contrasting or differentiating between the various different forms. The participants were allowed to hear and see examples of each of the three mirror forms as many times as they wanted until they felt they were familiar with them. The instructions followed. They were shown on a computer screen and read out by the experimenter. In the instructions, participants were told that four series of 48 stimuli would be presented (192 stimuli in total) and that each stimulus would consist of a pair of short melodies or a pair of visual patterns which were related to each other in terms of one of the three mirror forms. One of these forms was randomly assigned to each participant as his/her "target" and it was explained to them that the task consisted of recognizing whether the pair of melodies or the pair of visual patterns in each stimulus were related in terms of their target mirror form (yes/no task). An interval of 1 s separated the presentation of the standard stimulus and the comparison stimulus. Participants had 3 s to respond (in a response sheet) before the next pair was presented.

Two of the four series of stimuli involved visual stimuli (V), one series of 48 isochronous stimuli and another series of 48 non-isochronous stimuli. The other two series involved the acoustic version of the same stimuli (A), one series of 48 isochronous stimuli and another series of 48 non-isochronous stimuli. Participants in the AV condition were first exposed to the two acoustic series and then to the two visual series; participants in the VA condition were exposed first to the visual series and then to the acoustic series. All of the participants responded to the four series of stimuli, with short pauses of four minutes between one series and the next. The overall duration of the experiment was 36 min.

A stand alone software (programming language: Actionscript 3 for Adobe AIR runtime environments) was used for the presentation of the visual and acoustic stimuli. A Dell P2210 56 cm (22 In.) screen (Dell, Round Rock, TX, USA) with a resolution of 1680 × 1050 pixels (475 × 300 mm, equivalent to approximately 43.2 × 28.1 degrees of visual angle at the recommended viewing distance 650 mm) and a refresh rate of 60 Hz was used for the experiment. The visual stimuli were made up of 1680 × 1050 pixels and thus filled the entire screen. The visual stimuli consisted of five small square red dots presented in succession, with each dot lasting 600 ms in the isochronous condition, and 400 ms or 800 ms in the non-isochronous condition, and disappearing when the next dot appeared on the screen (i.e., the inter-dot interval was null). Each stimulus started from left to right and was centered with respect to the screen. The acoustic stimuli were created using MakeMusic Finale 2011 (MakeMusic Corporate, Boulder, CO, USA) at a sampling rate of 44,100 Hz–32 bit (and presented with Creative Sound Blaster Audigy FX PCIe 5.1 (Creative Technology, Singapore, Asia) using high quality loudspeakers Audioengine A2+ (Audioengine, Austin, TX, USA). Auditory stimuli were equalized for overall sound pressure using Audition CC 2015 (Adobe Systems Software, San Jose, CA, USA). The stimuli consisted of five tones (Timbre: Guitar; attack: 10 ms; decay: 31 ms). Each tone had an overall duration of 600 ms in the isochronous condition, and 400 ms or 800 ms in the non-isochronous condition. The inter-tone spacing was null.

Both visual and acoustic stimuli lasted a total of 3 s in the isochronous condition (600 ms × 5 elements) and 3.2 s in the non-isochronous condition (800 ms × 3 elements + 400 ms × 2 elements).

2.3. Stimuli

The number of elements in each acoustic stimulus (i.e., five notes), the overall duration of the stimuli (3–3.2 s), and the duration of the interval between the standard stimulus and the comparison stimulus (i.e., 1 s) were defined based on the previous literature on the same subject (in particular [30]) for the purposes of comparison. Due to the fact that a general finding in previous studies was that it is not easy for untrained listeners to recognize acoustic mirror forms, we followed the criterion of choosing conditions—not only in terms of duration but also of the types of intervals and the range of tones (octaves)—which facilitated the recognition of the three mirror forms [29,30,32,53–55]. For instance, all of the acoustic stimuli were in a major or minor key, with each stimulus starting with an initial note (either E3 or E4) followed by other notes chosen from among the first, third and fifth notes of the key and an additional non-chord passage note from the same key (that is, either the second, fourth, sixth or seventh note). Moreover, in all of the stimuli used in the acoustic experiment, the five pitches which made up each stimulus varied within a range of one octave, which according to Pedersen [55] is associated with better performance in same/different tasks using melodic patterns. In the present study, it was also necessary to use a narrow range of tones in order to guarantee that the corresponding visual stimuli would be perceived as unified. In fact, according to the proximity law of grouping [56], if there was too great a distance between the five elements in each visual stimulus, then there would have been a risk that the participants would perceive two or more separate groups of elements and not one unified pattern. Lastly, we also controlled other features such as the contour and length of the final interval which, according to previous literature, could influence the ability to recognize acoustic melodies in mirror forms. The complete set of variables used in the creation of the stimuli was as follows:

(i) *Sense modality: acoustic (A), visual (V).* The stimuli consisted of a short sequence of five tones in the acoustic task and of five square dots appearing in sequence in the visual task. The latter "corresponded" to a visual representation of the acoustic stimuli (see Appendix A).

(ii) *Mirror Form: inversion (INV), retrograde (RET), retrograde inversion (RETINV).* Three comparison stimuli were obtained for each standard stimulus by means of applying one of the three mirror form transformations: inversion, retrograde or retrograde inversion.

(iii) *Rhythm: isochronous (ISO), non-isochronous (N-ISO).* The stimuli presented in the isochronous condition were the same as those presented in the non-isochronous condition in terms of the shape of the configuration. What varied was the duration of each of the five tones (A) or dots (V) in the configuration. The duration was fixed at 600 ms in the isochronous condition while in the non-isochronous condition, three elements had a duration of 800 ms (half-notes) and two elements had a duration of 400 ms (quarter-notes). In the non-isochronism condition a grouping effect emerged which meant that the participants perceived a kind of "rhythm" in the succession of the tones or dots. The overall duration of the stimulus (3–3.2 s) made the condition comparable to Dowling's best performance condition (2.5 s).

(iv) *Contour.* The shape of the contour was determined by the number of inversion points, as in [30,31], i.e., the points where increments in pitch height (for the acoustic stimuli) or spatial height (for the visual stimuli) are followed by a decrement; or, vice versa, decrements in pitch height (for the acoustic stimuli) or spatial height (for the visual stimuli) are followed by an increment. Given that each stimulus was formed of five notes (or dots), the maximum number of points where there could be an inversion was three, giving a maximum of 14 different possible contours (see Table 1). In order to contain the levels of this variable, we selected only eight out of the 14 contours (those which are not in parentheses in Table 1). The eight types of contour used in the experiment thus contained 0, 1, 2 or 3 inversion points. In the statistical analyses, contour was a random effect.

(v) *Final interval: long or short.* In [31], the length of the final interval impacted on the participants' ability to recognize the acoustic mirror forms. Despite the fact that in their experiment the stimuli used were different to those used in the present study as they were longer and characterized by wider octave extensions and a greater tonal and temporal complexity, a decision was made to take this variable into account in the creation of the stimuli with the result that there were two versions of the final interval for each of the eight contours: long (L), i.e., between seven and twelve semitones, and short (S), i.e., less than four semitones. This variable was considered as a random effect in our statistical analyses.

Table 1. Possible types of contour in the five element configurations, defined in terms of increment (+) or decrement (−) of each note/dot as compared to the previous note/dot in terms of pitch height (for the acoustic stimuli, i.e., notes) or spatial height (for the visual stimuli, i.e., dots).

Number of Points of Inversion	Contour
0	++++
0	− − − −
1	+++−
1	(− − −+)
1	(+− − −)
1	(−+++)
1	(++− −)
1	− −++
2	(−++−)
2	+− −+
2	(++−+)
2	− −+−
3	+−+−
3	−+−+

Note: The eight patterns used in the study are those which are not in parentheses.

In total, 192 pairs of stimuli were presented to each participant in the experiment (2 Sense modalities × 8 Contours × 2 Final intervals × 2 Rhythms × 3 Mirror forms).

The Target (inversion, retrograde or retrograde inversion mirror forms) and the Order of the two sense modalities (visual-acoustic; acoustic-visual) were studied between subjects. All the other variables—Sense modality (acoustic, visual), Rhythm (isochronism, non-isochronism), Contour (8 levels) and Final Interval (long, short)—varied within subjects.

2.4. Statistics and Data Analysis

Data were analyzed in terms of the Signal Detection Theory (SDT) [57,58]. Responses were classified as either Hit (H), Correct Rejection (CR), False Alarms (FA) or Missing (M). The a priori proportion of "signals" (target stimulus) and noise (non-target stimulus) was 1/3 since all the stimuli presented to participants consisted of three different mirror forms and each participant was requested to target only one of these, meaning that there was one "yes" response and two "no" responses. This was taken into account when calculating the Hit Rate, i.e., the probability of responding "yes" on signal/target trials, and False Alarm Rate, i.e., the probability of responding "yes" on noise/non-target trials. In SDT, the binary answers (i.e., yes/no) of a set of participants are modeled as being influenced by two distinct factors, a perceptual sensitivity component and a response bias. In other words, two people with similar perceptual sensitivity capabilities may have different inclinations to answer "yes" or "no", or they might modify their inclination (i.e., response bias) in relation to the costs/benefits associated with each of the responses. To calculate sensitivity and response bias, we used two non-parametric measures, i.e., A' and B'', respectively [59]. We used these non-parametric measures instead of the traditional measure of sensitivity d' (d-prime) since, according to SDT, d' is unaffected by response bias (i.e., it is a pure measure of sensitivity) only if two assumptions are satisfied regarding the decision variable: (1) the signal and noise distributions are both normal; and (2) the signal and noise distributions have the same standard deviation. Since these two assumptions cannot actually be tested in yes/no tasks, non-parametric measures of sensitivity were advisable in this case. Several non-parametric measures of sensitivity and response bias have been proposed (e.g., [60,61]) but the most popular are A' and B''. These were devised by Pollack and Norman [62]; a complete history is provided by [63]. The formulas for computing A' and B'' are:

If Hit (H) > False Alarm (FA):

$$A' = \frac{1}{2} + \frac{(H - FA) \times (1 + H - FA)}{4 \times H \times (1 - FA)} \tag{1}$$

If (FA) > (H):

$$A' = \frac{1}{2} - \frac{(FA - H) \times (1 + FA - H)}{4 \times FA \times (1 - H)} \tag{2}$$

and:

$$B'' = \frac{(1 - H) \times (1 - FA) - H \times FA}{(1 - H) \times (1 - FA) + H \times FA} \tag{3}$$

Our main focus was to test whether there were different degrees of sensitivity (A') to the three mirror forms in one or both of the sense modalities. When differences in sensitivity were found, we also studied whether there were differences in response bias (i.e., B''). If there was greater sensitivity relating to one of the mirror forms as compared to the others and if this correlated with a response bias in the same direction, this would mean that the participants found it easier to detect that specific mirror form and that this was associated with a tendency to be more conservative in their responses (i.e., they tended to respond "no" more frequently than "yes"). If greater sensitivity was associated with no difference in response bias, then this could be taken as an indication that the participants found it easier to detect that specific mirror form but without this being associated with a specific response bias. And if greater sensitivity was associated with a response bias in the opposite direction, this could be interpreted as an indication that the participants found it easier to detect that specific mirror form as compared to the other mirror forms, and that this coexisted with a more liberal response bias (i.e., a bias towards "yes"). The A' and B'' values for each individual participant were recalculated for every interaction between the fixed effects that we were interested in studying. A series of Generalized Mixed effect Models (GLMMs) were then performed on these A' and B'' values. Based on an initial exploration of the data (see Section 3.1), we decided not to collapse the data by Subject and always entered this variable in the GLMMs models as a random effect. In all the following GLMMs, Sense Modality, Mirror Forms and Rhythm were always studied as fixed effects, while Contour, Final Interval and Subjects always entered the models as random effects.

When the range of the dependent variable is between 0 and 1 (as in the case of A'), the most suitable type of GLMM is the binomial family and logit link function [64,65]. In order to use the same type of analysis for B'' (whose values ranged between -1 and 1, with positive numbers representing a conservative bias, i.e., a tendency to answer "no", while negative numbers representing a liberal bias, i.e., a tendency to answer "yes", and with 0 representing no bias), a linear transformation was preliminarily applied to the original B'' values in order to rescale them within the interval 0–1 $((B'' + 1)/2)$.

All analyses were carried our using the statistical software program R 3.3.1, with the "lme4" [66], "car" [67], "lsmeans" [68], and "effects" [69] packages. We performed Mixed Model ANOVA Tables (Type 3 tests) via likelihood ratio tests [70–72] implemented in the "afex" package [73]. Bonferroni corrections were applied to post-hoc comparisons.

3. Results

3.1. Ease of Recognition

The scatter plots of A' values in Figure 2 provide a first overview of the participants' average sensitivity. The degree of sensitivity was assessed according to the ease with which the participant recognized the target mirror forms in the acoustic (diagrams on the left) and visual (diagrams on the right) tasks. The A' values typically range from 0 to 1, with 0.5 indicating that the signal cannot be distinguished from noise, and 1 which corresponds to perfect performance. Values less than 0.5 may arise from sampling error or indicate that the participant was somewhat confused when responding.

We know from previous literature on the recognition of acoustic mirror forms that the task is difficult for non-expert subjects, whereas no former data are available concerning how easy/difficult it is to recognize corresponding dynamic visual configurations. A straightforward comparison between the A' values obtained in our study and previous findings is not possible since in previous literature the analysis was usually based on the frequency of correct responses and did not compare the two correct responses (H, CR) or the two types of error (M, FA) as Signal Detection Theory presupposes. What is usually reported is that the number of correct responses was significantly different from chance (0.50) but that the task turned out to be difficult [30].

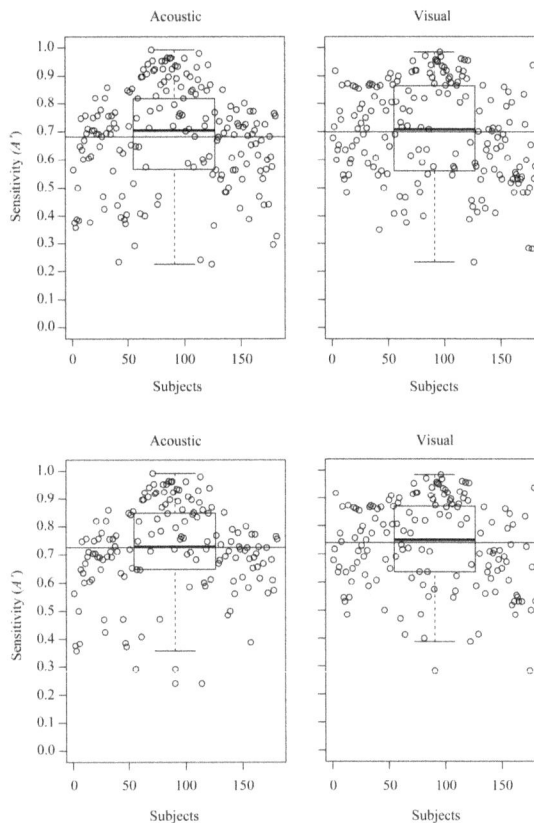

Figure 2. Scatter plots of the participants' average sensitivity (A') and corresponding box plots around the median in the Acoustic task and Visual task (the box is between the upper and lower quartile; whiskers represent the maximum and minimum values excluding outliers; the long thin horizontal line displayed within each plot represents the mean). The two top scatter plots refer to all of the sample data. The two bottom scatter plots refer to the sample data after elimination of participants with low sensitivity (i.e., $A' < 0.6$) in both tasks.

In the top two diagrams in Figure 2, the original sample of participants is displayed. They show that the average sensitivity (represented by the thin horizontal line) was $M_{A'} = 0.682$ (*Standard Deviation* (*SD*) = 0.177) in the Acoustic task and $M_{A'} = 0.699$ (*SD* = 0.172) in the Visual Task. The medians (displayed in the box plots) are slightly above these values. The scatter plots also reveal that while most of the participants performed overall better than chance ($A' > 0.6$: 71% in the acoustic task and 67% in the visual task), and that some of them performed very well ($A' > 0.8$: 27% in the acoustic task and 36% in the visual task), the task was in effect not very easy. Indeed a percentage of participants that is certainly not negligible had sensitivity values around 0.5 ($0.4 < A' < 0.6$: 20% in the acoustic task and 29% in the visual task), which indicates that they were not able to distinguish signal (i.e., the target mirror forms) from noise (i.e., the other two mirror forms). Moreover, 9% of participants in the acoustic task and 4% in the visual task had sensitivity values between 0.2 and 0.4. This suggests that they confused the target form which they were supposed to be looking for with one of the other two mirror forms. This is not as strange as it may seem given that the three mirror forms all consisted of a similar type of transformation in that they were all mirror reflections.

Participants with an overall sensitivity less than 0.6 in both tasks were eliminated from the dataset (i.e., around 16% of the initial 180 participants) before the subsequent statistical analyses were done (the new dataset is provided as Supplementary Material: file "database_sym"). Since the aim of the study was to test whether different sensitivity to the "same" mirror forms emerged in the two sense modalities, participants with a sensitivity >0.6 in *one* of the two tasks but not in the other were considered meaningful cases and for this reason were included in the dataset. The new values relating to average sensitivity in the two tasks (represented by the thin horizontal line in the two bottom diagrams in Figure 2) are $M_{A'} = 0.726$ ($SD = 0.154$) in the Acoustic task and $M_{A'} = 0.740$ ($SD = 0.153$) in the Visual Task.

3.2. Ease of Recognition of the Three Mirror Forms in the Two Sense Modalities

In order to study the participants' sensitivity to the three different Mirror Forms in the two Sense Modalities, we conducted a first GLMM on A' with Sense Modality and Mirror Forms as fixed effects. Both of these main effects turned out to be significant (Mirror Forms: ChiSq = 53.489, df = 2, $p < 0.0001$; Sense Modality: ChiSq = 91.212, df = 1, $p < 0.0001$), as was their interaction (ChiSq = 2202.414, df = 2, $p < 0.0001$). As shown in Figure 3 and as confirmed by post-hoc tests and the descriptive statistics for the raw data (i.e., Mean and *SD*—as reported in Table 2), the participants were more sensitive to the retrograde mirror form, i.e., a reflection on a vertical axis, in both the visual and acoustic tasks (RET_A vs. INV_A: EST = 0.261, SE = 0.027, z-ratio = 9.352, $p < 0.0001$; RET_A vs. RETINV_A: EST = 0.198, SE = 0.029, z-ratio = 6.680, $p < 0.0001$; RET_V vs. RETINV_V: EST = 0.228, SE = 0.029, z-ratio = 7.682, $p < 0.0001$; RET_V vs. INV_V: EST = 0.096, SE = 0.027, z-ratio = 3.451, $p = 0.008$).

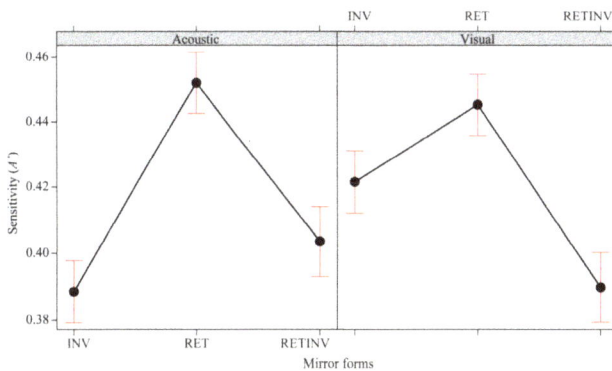

Figure 3. Effect plots of the interaction between Mirror form (Inversion (INV), Retrograde (RET), Retrograde Inversion (RETINV)) and Sense Modality (acoustic, vision) on participants' sensitivity (A'). Results are given on the logit scale used in the Generalized Mixed effect Models (GLMM) analysis. Error bars represent a 95% confidence interval.

Table 2. Mean sensitivity (A') and mean response bias (B'') relating to the three mirror forms (Inversion (INV), Retrograde (RET), Retrograde Inversion (RETINV)) in the two sense modalities, with corresponding standard deviations (*SD*).

MIRROR FORM_Sense Modality	A'	B''
RET_acoustic	$M = 0.833$ ($SD = 0.139$)	$M = 0.154$ ($SD = 0.464$)
INV_acoustic	$M = 0.645$ ($SD = 0.148$)	$M = 0.167$ ($SD = 0.288$)
RETINV_acoustic	$M = 0.681$ ($SD = 0.096$)	$M = 0.381$ ($SD = 0.286$)
RET_visual	$M = 0.811$ ($SD = 0.154$)	$M = -0.124$ ($SD = 0.454$)
INV_visual	$M = 0.736$ ($SD = 0.122$)	$M = 0.019$ ($SD = 0.311$)
RETINV_visual	$M = 0.646$ ($SD = 0.136$)	$M = 0.228$ ($SD = 0.356$)

An analyses of the response biases (see Table 2, B'') revealed that, in general, greater sensitivity in the detection of the retrograde transformation was also associated with a more conservative bias in the other two mirror forms (i.e., a tendency to respond "no"). This was found for all comparison, except one (B'': RET_V vs. RETINV_V: EST = -0.392, SE = 0.071, z-ratio = -5.457, $p < 0.0001$; RET_V vs. INV_V: EST = -0.210, SE = 0.067, z-ratio = -3.109, $p = 0.028$; RET_A vs. RETINV_A: EST = -0.230, SE = 0.071, z-ratio = -3.209, $p = 0.02$; RET_A vs. INV_A: EST = -0.064, SE = 0.067, z-ratio = -0.954, $p = 1.000$).

A comparison between the sensitivity relating to the visual task and that relating to the acoustic task revealed that participants were more sensitive to the inversion mirror form (i.e., a reflection on a horizontal axis) in the visual task than in the acoustic task (INV_V vs. INV_A: EST = 0.137, SE = 0.003, z-ratio = 44.424, $p < 0.0001$). In terms of the percentage of correct responses (Hit + Correct Rejection), participants correctly responded to 66% of the total number of inversion mirror forms presented in the visual task and to 60% of the total number of inversion mirror forms presented in the acoustic task. As the analysis of B'' revealed (Table 2), this difference in sensitivity was also associated with more conservative responses (i.e., with a bias towards responding "no") in the acoustic task as compared to the visual task (INV_V vs. INV_A: EST = -0.141, SE = 0.003, z-ratio = -42.347, $p < 0.0001$).

Sensitivity to the other two mirror forms also differed between the two sense modalities, with greater sensitivity to both the retrograde and the retrograde inversion mirror forms in the acoustic task (RET_A vs. RET_V: EST = 0.027, SE = 0.003, z-ratio = 9.558, $p < 0.0001$; RETINV_A vs. RETINV_V: EST = 0.057, SE = 0.003, z-ratio = 16.392, $p < 0.0001$). The percentage of correct responses (Hit + Correct Rejection) for the retrograde mirror form was 76% in the acoustic task and 73% in the visual task and for the retrograde inversion mirror form, the percentage of correct responses was 61% in the acoustic task and 58% in the visual task. The analyses revealed that participants were not only better at detecting these two mirror forms (i.e., retrograde and retrograde inversion) in the acoustic as compared to the visual task, but also that their responses for both mirror forms were more conservative (i.e., with a bias towards responding "no") in the visual task as compared to the acoustic task (B'': RET_V vs. RET_A: EST = 0.287, SE = 0.003, z-ratio = 84.057, $p < 0.0001$; RETINV_V vs. RETINV_A: EST = 0.125, SE = 0.003, z-ratio = 35.473; $p < 0.0001$).

3.3. Cross Modality Facilitation Effects

A second GLMM was conducted (with Order, Sense Modality and Mirror Forms as fixed effects) in order to test whether sensitivity increased as a consequence of the order in which the two tasks were performed, i.e., acoustic followed by visual or visual followed by acoustic. No main effect of Order emerged (ChiSq = 0.717; df = 1; $p = 0.396$) which indicates that sensitivity was not improved *in general* by presenting the visual and acoustic tasks in a specific order. However, as the significant interaction between Order, Sense Modality and Mirror form indicated (ChiSq = 1086.764; df = 2; $p < 0.0001$), and as post-hoc tests clarified, facilitation effects across modalities did emerge for one mirror form, i.e., the retrograde mirror form (Figure 4).

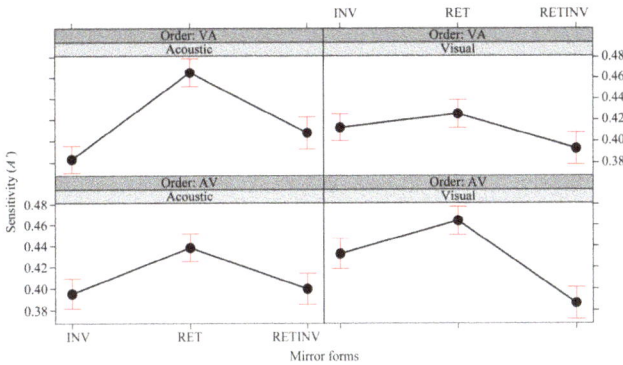

Figure 4. Effect plots of the interaction between Order (VA: Visual followed by Acoustic, AV: Acoustic followed by Visual), Sense Modality (Acoustic, Visual) and Mirror form (Inversion (INV), Retrograde (RET), Retrograde Inversion (RETINV)) on sensitivity (A'). Results are given on the logit scale used in the Generalized Mixed effect Models (GLMM) analysis. Error bars represent a 95% confidence interval.

Sensitivity to the retrograde mirror form in the visual task was increased after participants had carried out the acoustic task. In other words, the participants' sensitivity when they were asked to detect the retrograde pattern visually (i.e., a reflection around a vertical axis) increased when the visual task followed the acoustic task (AV) as compared to when the visual task was performed first (VA) (RET_V_AV: $M = 0.871$, $SD = 0.111$; RET_V_VA: $M = 0.752$, $SD = 0.168$; RET_V_AV vs. RET_V_VA: EST = 0.155, SE = 0.038, z-ratio = 4.006, $p = 0.004$). No difference due to the order of the visual and acoustic tasks in terms of the participants' sensitivity was found for the other two mirror forms. As the analysis of B'' revealed, the difference in sensitivity found for the retrograde transformation was also associated with a change in the response bias: participants' responses turned out to be more liberal (i.e., with a bias towards "yes") when the visual task was performed after the acoustic task, while there was a slightly more conservative bias (i.e., a bias towards "no") when the visual task was performed first (RET_V_AV: $M = -0.286$, $SD = 0.493$; RET_V_VA: $M = 0.039$, $SD = 0.341$; RET_V_AV vs. RET_V_VA: EST = -0.410, SE = 0.093, z-ratio = -4.394, $p < 0.0001$).

3.4. The Effects of the Isochronism versus Non-Isochronism (Rhythm)

A third GLMM with Sense Modality and Rhythm as fixed effects was conducted to test whether sensitivity to the three mirror forms varied when the elements forming the pattern had different (non-isochronism (N-ISO)) or identical (isochronism (ISO)) durations. A main effect of Rhythm emerged (ChiSq = 329.85, df = 1, $p < 0.0001$) and there was a significant interaction with Sense Modality (ChiSq = 168.97, df = 1, $p < 0.0001$). As shown in Figure 5 and confirmed by post-hoc tests (see also the mean values reported in Table 3), participants had greater sensitivity in the non-isochronous condition in both sense modalities (ISO_A vs. N-ISO_A: EST = -0.011, SE = 0.002, z-ratio = -4.213, $p < 0.001$; ISO_V vs. N-ISO_V: EST= -0.058, SE = 0.002, z-ratio = -22.161, $p < 0.0001$). However, the effect was stronger in the visual task. In the isochronous condition, participants were equally sensitive in both the visual and acoustic tasks (ISO_A vs. ISO_V: EST = 0.005, SE = 0.002, z-ratio = 2.007, $p = 0.268$), while in the non-isochronous condition, sensitivity was greater in the visual task (N-ISO_A vs. N-ISO_V: EST = -0.041, SE = 0.002, z-ratio = -16.745, $p < 0.0001$). The analysis of B'' revealed that in the acoustic task participants were in general more conservative in their responses than in the visual task (ISO_A vs. ISO_V: EST = 0.178, SE = 0.003, z-ratio = 55.752, $p < 0.0001$; N-ISO_A vs. N-ISO_V: EST = 0.205, SE = 0.003, z-ratio = 72.260, $p < 0.0001$). While in the acoustic task there was no difference in the response bias between the two rhythm conditions (ISO_A vs. N-ISO_A: EST = -0.007, SE = 0.003, z-ratio = -2.463, $p = 0.10$), a difference was found in the visual task where participants were more conservative in the isochronous condition (ISO_V vs. N-ISO_V: EST = 0.066, SE = 0.003, z-ratio = 19.849, $p < 0.0001$)—despite the fact that the mean values indicate a very small response bias.

Table 3. Mean sensitivity (A') and mean response bias (B''), with corresponding standard deviations, relating to the three mirror forms (inversion, retrograde, retrograde inversion) in the two sense modalities and in the isochronism versus non-isochronism conditions.

MIRROR FORM_Sense Modality	A'	B''
ISO_acoustic	M = 0.726 (SD = 0.165)	M= 0.213 (SD = 0.415)
N-ISO_acoustic	M = 0.722 (SD = 0.172)	M = 0.219 (SD = 0.421)
ISO_visual	M = 0.722 (SD = 0.171)	M = 0.010 (SD = 0.430)
N-ISO visual	M = 0.752 (SD = 0.168)	M = −0.026 (SD = 0.467)

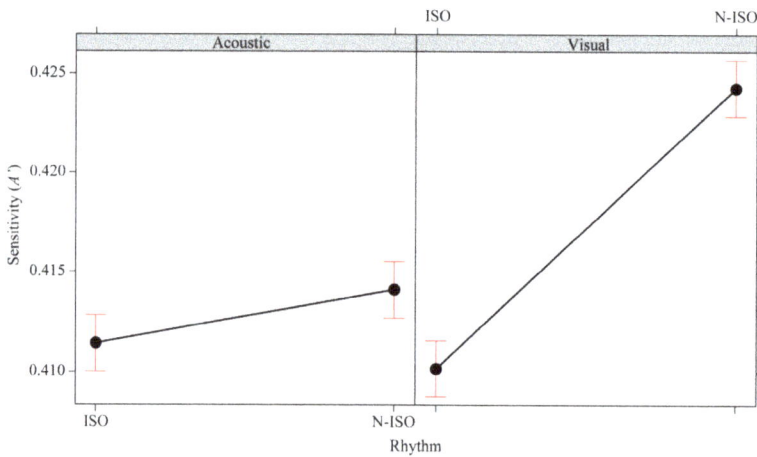

Figure 5. Effect plot of the interaction between Rhythm and Sense Modality (Acoustic, Visual) on sensitivity (A'). Results are given on the logit scale used in the Generalized Mixed effect Models (GLMM) analysis. Error bars represent a 95% confidence interval.

4. Discussion and Conclusions

One of the basic problems affecting the study of visual perception is to explain how the observer recognizes stimuli in his/her environment which undergo continuous and various transformations of shape and size (the constancy problem). In acoustic perception too the issue of whether people are able to perceive two melodies as being "the same" even if all the notes have been changed is an old problem dating back to von Ehrenfels [74] who used this example to establish his definition of Gestalt qualities. We know that melodies may be transposed, speeded up or slowed down (within certain limits) without compromising the listener's ability to recognize them as "the same" tune. The transformations considered in this paper (i.e., mirror forms) consist of "reflections" of the melodic pattern as a whole which may take the form of an upside down transformation (inversion), a back to front transformation (retrograde) or an upside down and back to front transformation (retrograde inversion). The ability to recognize these mirror forms has been addressed in this paper from a new perspective as both the visual and acoustic recognition of corresponding symmetrical patterns was studied for the purposes of comparison. Moreover, in addition to providing new information regarding the acoustic perception of the three mirror forms to be added to the few (discordant) findings in previous literature, the study also aimed to produce new data on the visual detection of mirror symmetry when sequential patterns and a sequential detection task are considered.

Studies on symmetry detection in dot patterns have confirmed that the visual system is efficient at detecting symmetry, even at very brief presentation times, i.e., stimulus presentations less than 160 ms (e.g., [17,18,21]), during which it is not possible to apply intentional pair-wise comparison strategies based on eye movement or shifts in spatial attention. Processes involving pair-wise comparisons and the intentional matching of corresponding dot-pairs have been hypothesized to support symmetry detection (e.g., [75]), especially when highly demanding tasks are involved, such as the discrimination of perfectly symmetrical versus nearly symmetrical patterns [76]. The type of stimuli and the task used in the study presented in this paper are different from those used in traditional visual symmetry detection tasks (in both static and dynamic conditions) in which the pattern elements are presented simultaneously (for a review and application of various types of methods see [77]). In our experiment, the elements forming each pattern (i.e., the five square dots) appeared in succession over approximately 3 s and not simultaneously. Moreover the two "halves" forming the symmetrical configuration were also presented in succession (i.e., one after the other) divided by a one second Inter Stimulus Interval (ISI). Many researchers have shown that symmetry is easier to detect than a simple repeated pattern when the symmetry is within an object, i.e., there is a "within-object relation", while repetition is easier to detect when the matching parts belong to different objects, i.e., there is a 'between-object relation' (e.g., [78–80]). In a sense, the conditions which were used in the present study can be considered to be more similar to a between-object matching than a within-object matching and as such it is very different from the automatic rapid symmetry detection conditions reported by most researchers. The task described in this paper likely involved pairwise comparison processes and stimulated matching strategies to compare the two series of elements, which made the task more demanding and difficult.

Three main findings emerged. Firstly, our results provide further evidence (in addition to the findings in previous literature regarding static and dynamic visual configurations—see the papers cited in the introduction) that symmetry around a vertical axis is particularly easy to recognize. Our findings show that this also applies to the case of sequential visual configurations and acoustic stimuli. The preference for this type of symmetry seems to be even more evident in the case of auditory perception than it is for visual perception as indicated by the following findings from the present study: (i) acoustic sensitivity to symmetry around a vertical axis (the retrograde mirror form) was significantly greater than sensitivity to the corresponding visual stimuli (see Figure 3); and (ii) recognizing the retrograde mirror form in the visual task was easier after the acoustic task but not vice versa (Figure 4). This suggests that even though the reflection around a vertical axis (the retrograde mirror form) was one of the two mirror forms which the participants found easier to detect visually, performing the acoustic task first increased their sensitivity to the visual equivalent, whereas performance in the acoustic task remained the same with or without prior visual "training".

Secondly, despite the fact that a preference for symmetry around a vertical axis (the retrograde mirror form) was common to both sense modalities, the participants did not in general display the same sensitivity in the two types of task. Differences between the two sense modalities emerged for all three mirror forms: reflections around a vertical axis (retrograde) and reflections around a vertical and horizontal axis (retrograde inversion) were more easily recognized in the acoustic task than in the visual task, while reflections around a horizontal axis (inversion) were more easily recognized in the visual task than in the acoustic task. These differences, in addition to the fact that we did not find a general training effect (i.e., a main effect) depending on the order in which the tasks were performed, suggests that the two tasks were relatively independent.

Thirdly, in the present study, performance in the acoustic task improved when the five elements in the stimuli were not of the same duration and a rhythmic structure therefore resulted. This outcome is in agreement with previous evidence on the role of rhythm in tasks involving the recognition of acoustic mirror forms [32,53] but it contrasts with other results indicating that better performances were associated with isochronous melodies (e.g., [31]—although in this case longer melodies and other melodic features also co-varied). The findings in our study demonstrate that non-isochronism facilitates not only the recognition of acoustic mirror forms, but also greatly enhances performance in the recognition of sequential visual patterns (Figure 5). This is an interesting new result concerning the visual perception of symmetry. The different duration of the five elements in the sequence creates grouping effects. We speculate that these local organizations, rather than the "global spatial structure" (which is three seconds long), might provide a useful hint. The spatial relationships perceived between these sub-units (which are simpler and shorter) offer anchor points for a pair-wise comparison strategy to be applied. In our experimental conditions, the overall duration of the event to be judged was around 7 s: the first pattern was presented over approximately three seconds followed by a one second ISI and then the other 3 s long pattern. Iconic memory has a much lower capacity than echoic memory (e.g., [81,82]). Therefore it is reasonable to suppose that the grouping effects provided by rhythm in the non-isochronous conditions offer simplification strategies for the pair-matching comparison which is particularly useful for visual memory.

Our main focus in this paper was to study the participants' sensitivity to the three mirror forms. However, whenever a significant difference in sensitivity emerged, the response bias was also analyzed. A constant finding in all the analyses of B'' carried out in the paper was that a lower degree of sensitivity was associated with a conservative response bias. This means that, in this study, when the participants found it difficult to identify the target (i.e., in the case of the mirror forms which they were less sensitive to), they tended to deny the presence of the target pattern.

One of the thought-provoking results emerging from this study regards the difficulty with which inversion mirror forms (i.e., reflections around a horizontal axis) were recognized in the acoustic task. This confirms the evidence found by Dowling [30] in similar presentation conditions (i.e., five tones in 2.5 s). When the results of the visual task were compared to those of the acoustic task, it became clear that it was more difficult to detect the inversion transformation as compared to the retrograde transformation in both sensory modalities but the participants' sensitivity to inversion was significantly greater in the visual task than in the acoustic task. In Dowling's [30] original study, the inverse transformation was more easily detected than the retrograde transformation in the faster condition (i.e., when the five tones were presented in 1 s). On the one hand, this finding indicates the sensitivity of the outcomes to the specific temporal condition considered but this is not dissimilar to the fact that in other dynamic conditions symmetry detection is easier with dynamic as compared to static presentations only at certain optimal frequencies (see [77]). On the other hand, it provides cues for speculation about the differences between the two conditions. In the faster condition studied by Dowling [30], the five tones forming each melody were not simultaneously presented but nearly so: all five tones were presented within 1 s. The overall acoustic event was quite long (the probe stimulus, 1 s, was followed by a 2 s ISI and then by the comparison stimulus, another 1 s), but the global spatial structure of the five tones could be grasped as a whole. Conversely, in the slower presentation condition (two tones/s) which was similar to that used in this study, the overall acoustic structure cannot be grasped unless it is sequential. In the latter condition, i.e., when the global structure is difficult to grasp as a whole, the identity of the elements forming the sequence is probably decisive as it permits the invariance between the two "halves" of the symmetrical configuration to be noticed. This identity is preserved in the retrograde transformation (if not transposed) but not in the inversion transformation. Indeed, in the retrograde transformation, the pitch of the notes in the initial stimuli and in the comparison stimuli remains unchanged: only the order in which they are played is reversed (i.e., the first tone in the comparison stimulus is the last in the initial stimulus; the second tone in the comparison stimulus is the fourth tone in the initial stimulus etc.—see Figure 1a). Conversely, in the inversion mirror form, only the first note remains unchanged in the standard and comparison stimuli. The other four tones change in pitch with respect to the initial tones (see Figure 1a). Evidence of the importance of identity of pitch in the retrograde transformation emerges from the studies showing that when the retrograde transformation is transposed (and therefore the pitch of the notes no longer corresponds to that of the initial melody), people's ability to detect symmetry severely deteriorates [33].

The finding that sensitivity to inversion was lower than sensitivity to the retrograde transformation in both sensory modalities is however in line with overall evidence that upside-down inversions in mirrors (and in general in perception) represent a more severe violation than left to right reversals (e.g., [83–87]).

Taken as a whole, the results of our experiment might contribute to the discussion on the role of global and local factors in the perception of symmetry in sequential versus simultaneous conditions when various sense modalities are considered (for a revision of how the importance of global factors as opposed to local elements have been incorporated into many different theoretical accounts or models of the visual detection of mirror symmetry, see [13]).

The long-standing debate on how many mechanisms underlie the detection of mirror symmetry (e.g., [7,19,20,75,79,88–90]) might also be revived by the addition of new hypotheses regarding cross-modal or modal-specific processes. The issue of the existence of independent or related processing paths underlying the perception of visual and acoustic symmetry is well worth investigating as is the question of whether there are independent or related processing paths underlying the perception of symmetry in dynamic and static visual configurations. This might be further extended to embodied experiences of mirror symmetry related to the proprioception of one's own body structure or of specific body movements as well as to haptic symmetry perception (e.g., [91–94]). We might also ask about the relationship between the proprioceptive and tactile perception of symmetry and the acoustic processing of symmetry in congenitally blind people whose visual experiences of symmetry are lacking [60,95–100]. When assessed in terms of brain processing, these topics would add to the list of open questions on the subject revised by Bertamini and Makin [101]. We know that the detection of visual and haptic symmetry appears to rely on common brain areas such as the lateral occipital complex in sighted individuals and that in both early blind and sighted (but blindfolded) control subjects, the detection of tactile symmetry is associated with a network implicating frontal and parietal cortical areas (i.e., the medial frontal and superior parietal cortices) [95]. However, in the case of early blind individuals, a significant activation in the retinotopic (i.e., primary visual cortex) and object-selective areas (i.e., lateral occipital and fusiform cortices) was also observed. The activation observed in blind subjects in the early visual cortex during tactile discrimination is in line with previous evidence of cross-modal cortical plasticity in cases of blindness [102]. We might ask how this relates to the cortical activation which occurs during the detection of acoustic symmetry.

Supplementary Materials: The following are available online at www.mdpi.com/2073-8994/9/3/39/s1, Table S1: database_sym.

Acknowledgments: This work was supported by funds of the Department of Human Sciences at the University of Verona under Grant (ex60%MIUR). We thank two anonymous reviewers whose observations have helped us to improve the quality of the paper.

Author Contributions: Ivana Bianchi, Roberta Pezzola and Ugo Savardi conceived and designed the experiment; Roberto Burro and Roberta Pezzola performed the experiment; Roberto Burro and Ivana Bianchi analyzed the data; Ivana Bianchi, Roberta Pezzola, Roberto Burro and Ugo Savardi wrote the paper and contributed to its revision.

Conflicts of Interest: The authors declare no conflict of interest. The founding sponsors had no role in the design of the study; in the collection, analyses, or interpretation of data; in the writing of the manuscript, and in the decision to publish the results.

Appendix A

The set of acoustic and corresponding visual standard stimuli used in the study are shown in Figure A1).

In Figure A1, the section headed A_IS and A_NIS shows the notes played in the isochronous acoustic condition (i.e A_IS, in which all sounds were of the same duration, in this case 600 ms) and the notes played in the non-isochronous acoustic condition (i.e., A_NIS, in which the sounds were of two different durations with the chromes lasting 400 ms and the quarter-notes lasting 800 ms). For readers who are not familiar with musical notation, please note that the flat and sharp alterations are only signaled at the first note (as by convention) but they hold until the end of the bar, which in our case means until the end of the stimulus.

The corresponding visual stimuli are shown in the section headed V: in the isochronous condition, each dot remained on the screen for 600 ms before disappearing; in the non-isochronous condition, some dots (i.e., those corresponding to the chromes in the acoustic stimuli) lasted 400 ms and the others lasted 800 ms. The grids in the background of the visual stimuli are shown here so that the correspondence between the spatial distance and the difference in pitch in the acoustic stimuli is clear, but these were not displayed in the actual stimuli shown to the participants.

Each of the 32 standard stimuli was presented in association with the three corresponding mirror transformations: retrograde, inversion and retrograde inversion. This means that 96 pairs of standard and comparison stimuli (32 × 3) were presented to the participants in the acoustic task and 96 corresponding pairs (32 × 3) were presented in the visual task.

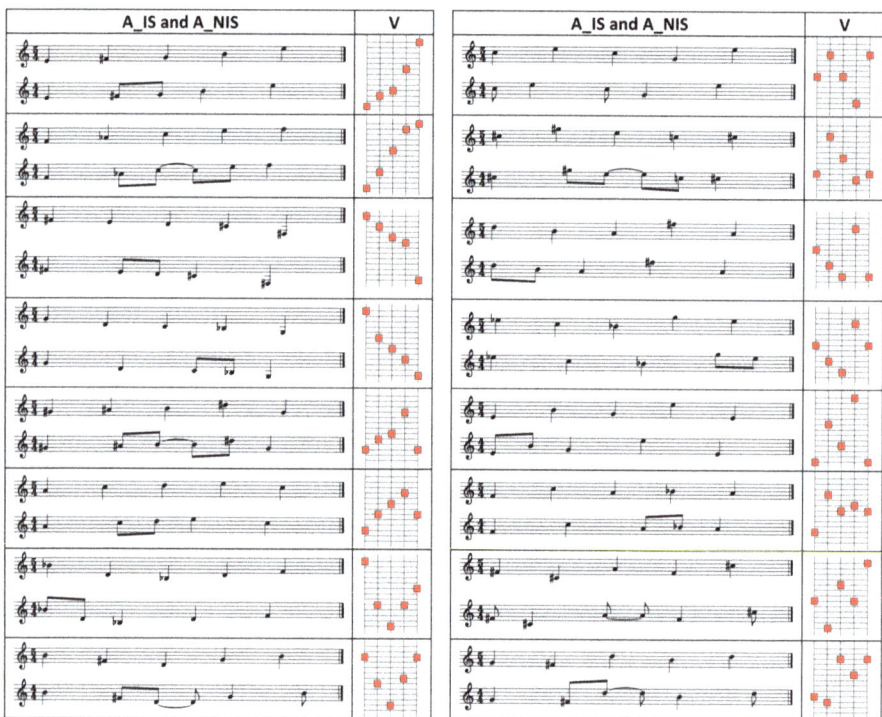

Figure A1. The standard stimuli used in the experiment. The figure shows the notes played in the isochronous acoustic condition and in the non-isochronous acoustic condition (A_IS and A_NIS), and the corresponding visual stimuli (V).

References

1. Van der Helm, P.A. Symmetry perception. In *The Oxford Handbook of Perceptual Organization*; Wagemans, J., Ed.; Oxford University Press: Oxford, UK, 2014; pp. 108–128.
2. Giannouli, V. Visual symmetry perception. *Encephalos* **2013**, *50*, 31–42.
3. Treder, M.S. Behind the looking-glass: A review on human symmetry perception. *Symmetry* **2010**, *2*, 1510–1543. [CrossRef]
4. Carmody, D.P.; Nodine, C.F.; Locher, P.J. Global detection of symmetry. *Percept. Mot. Skills* **1977**, *45*, 1267–1273. [CrossRef] [PubMed]

5. Corballis, B.; Beale, I. *The Psychology of Left and Right*; Lawrence Erlbaum Associates: Hillsdale, NJ, USA, 1976.

6. Goldmeier, E. Similarity in visually perceived forms. *Psychol. Issues* **1972**, *8*, 1–136. [PubMed]

7. Herbert, A.M.; Humphrey, G.K. Bilateral symmetry detection: Testing a 'callosal' hypothesis. *Perception* **1996**, *25*, 463–480. [CrossRef] [PubMed]

8. Wagemans, J. Detection of visual symmetries. *Spat. Vis.* **1995**, *9*, 9–32. [CrossRef] [PubMed]

9. Locher, P.; Nodine, C. The perceptual value of symmetry. *Comput. Math. Appl.* **1989**, *17*, 475–484. [CrossRef]

10. Locher, P.; Wagemans, J. The effects of element type and spatial grouping on symmetry detection. *Perception* **1990**, *22*, 565–587. [CrossRef] [PubMed]

11. Rock, I.; Leaman, R. An experimental analysis of visual symmetry. *Acta Psychol.* **1963**, *21*, 171–183. [CrossRef]

12. Royer, F.L. Detection of symmetry. *J. Exp. Psychol. Hum. Percept. Perform.* **1981**, *7*, 1186–1210. [CrossRef] [PubMed]

13. Wagemans, J. Characteristics and models of human symmetry detection. *Trends Cogn. Sci.* **1997**, *1*, 346–352. [CrossRef]

14. Wenderoth, P. The salience of vertical symmetry. *Perception* **1994**, *23*, 221–236. [CrossRef] [PubMed]

15. Wenderoth, P. The effects of dot pattern parameters and constraints on the relative salience of vertical bilateral symmetry. *Vis. Res.* **1996**, *36*, 2311–2320. [CrossRef]

16. Zimmer, A.C. Foundations for the measurement of phenomenal symmetry. *Gestalt Theory* **1984**, *6*, 118–157.

17. Barlow, H.B.; Reeves, B.C. The versatility and absolute efficiency of detecting mirror symmetry in random dot displays. *Vis. Res.* **1979**, *19*, 783–793. [CrossRef]

18. Julesz, B. Figure and ground perception in briefly presented isodipole textures. In *Perceptual organization*; Kubovy, M., Pomerantz, M., Eds.; Erlbaum: Hillsdale, NJ, USA, 1981; pp. 27–57.

19. Palmer, S.E.; Hemenway, K. Orientation and symmetry: Effects of multiple, rotational, and near symmetries. *J. Exp. Psychol. Hum. Percept. Perform.* **1978**, *4*, 691–692. [CrossRef] [PubMed]

20. Tyler, C.W.; Hardage, L.; Miller, R.T. Multiple mechanisms for the detection of mirror symmetry. *Spat. Vis.* **1995**, *9*, 79–100. [CrossRef] [PubMed]

21. Wagemans, J.; Van Gool, L.; Dydewalle, G. Detection of symmetry in tachistoscopically presented dot patterns: Effects of multiple axes and skewing. *Percept. Psychophys.* **1991**, *50*, 413–427. [CrossRef] [PubMed]

22. Baylis, G.C. Visual parsing and object-based attention: A developmental perspective. In *Cognitive Neuroscience of Attention*; Richards, J.E., Ed.; Lawrence Erlbaum Associates, Inc.: Mahwah, NJ, USA, 1998; pp. 251–286.

23. Bornstein, M.H.; Ferdinandsen, K.; Gross, C.G. Perception of symmetry in infancy. *Dev. Psychol.* **1981**, *17*, 82–86. [CrossRef]

24. Bornstein, M.H.; Krinsky, S.J. Perception of symmetry in infancy—The salience of vertical symmetry and the perception of pattern wholes. *J. Exp. Child Psychol.* **1985**, *39*, 1–19. [CrossRef]

25. Fisher, C.B.; Ferdinandsen, K.; Bornstein, M.H. The role of symmetry in infant form discrimination. *Child Dev.* **1981**, *52*, 457–462. [CrossRef] [PubMed]

26. Humphrey, G.K.; Humphrey, D.E. The role of structure in infant visual pattern perception. *Can. J. Psychol.* **1989**, *43*, 165–182. [CrossRef] [PubMed]

27. Rhodes, G.; Geddes, K.; Jeffery, L.; Dziurawiec, S.; Clark, A. Are average and symmetric faces attractive to infants? Discrimination and looking preferences. *Perception* **2002**, *31*, 315–321. [CrossRef] [PubMed]

28. Balch, W.R. The role of symmetry in the good continuation ratings of two-part tonal melodies. *Percept. Psychophys.* **1981**, *29*, 47–55. [CrossRef] [PubMed]

29. Dowling, W.J. Recognition of interventions of melodies and melodic contours. *Percept. Psychophys.* **1971**, *9*, 348–349. [CrossRef]

30. Dowling, W.J. Recognition of melodic transformations: Inversion, retrograde and retrograde inversion. *Percept. Psychophys.* **1972**, *12*, 417–421. [CrossRef]

31. Krumhansl, C.L.; Sandell, G.J.; Sergeant, D.C. The perception of tone hierarchies and mirror forms in twelve-tone serial music. *Music Percept.* **1987**, *5*, 31–77. [CrossRef]

32. Tovey, D. *The Forms of Music*; Meridian Books: Cleveland, OH, USA, 1956.

33. Dowling, W.J.; Fujitani, D.S. Contour, interval, and pitch recognition in memory for melodies. *Acoust. Soc. Am.* **1971**, *49*, 524–531. [CrossRef]

34. Marks, L. *The Unity of the Senses: Interrelations Among the Modalities*; Academic Press: New York, NY, USA, 1978.

35. Marks, L.E. Cross-modal interactions in speeded classification. In *Handbook of Multisensory Processes*; Calvert, G.A., Spence, C., Stein, B.E., Eds.; MIT Press: Cambridge, MA, USA, 2004; pp. 85–105.

36. Spence, C. Crossmodal correspondences: A tutorial review. *Atten. Percept. Psychophys.* **2011**, *73*, 971–995. [CrossRef] [PubMed]

37. Sperry, R.W. Hemisphere deconnection and unity in conscious awareness. *Am. Psychol.* **1968**, *23*, 723–733. [CrossRef] [PubMed]

38. Köhler, W. *Gestalt Psychology*; Liveright Publication: New York, NY, USA, 1929.

39. Köhler, W. *Gestalt Psychology: An introduction to New Concepts in Modern Psychology*; Liveright Publication: New York, NY, USA, 1947.

40. Bahrick, L.E. Infants' perception of substance and temporal synchrony in multimodal events. *Infant. Behav. Dev.* **1983**, *6*, 429–451. [CrossRef]

41. Bahrick, L.E. Intermodal learning in infancy: Learning on the basis of two kinds of invariant relations in audible and visible events. *Child. Dev.* **1988**, *59*, 197–209. [CrossRef] [PubMed]

42. Lewkowicz, D.J. Infants' response to temporally based intersensory equivalence: The effect of synchronous sounds on visual preferences for moving stimuli. *Infant. Behav. Dev.* **1992**, *15*, 297–323. [CrossRef]

43. Spelke, E.S.; Born, W.S.; Chu, F. Perception of moving, sounding objects by four-month-old infants. *Perception* **1983**, *12*, 719–732. [CrossRef] [PubMed]

44. Barrack, L.E.; Netto, D.; Hernandez-Reif, M. Intermodal perception of adult and child faces and voices by infants. *Child. Dev.* **1998**, *69*, 1263–1275.

45. Walker-Andrews, A.S.; Bahrick, L.E.; Raglioni, S.S.; Diaz, I. Infant's bimodal perception of gender. *Ecol. Psychol.* **1991**, *3*, 55–75. [CrossRef]

46. Allen, T.W.; Walker, K.; Symonds, L.; Marcell, M. Intrasensory and intersensory perception of temporal sequences during infancy. *Dev. Psychol.* **1977**, *3*, 225–229. [CrossRef]

47. Mendelson, M.J.; Ferland, M.B. Auditory-visual transfer in four month old infants. *Child. Dev.* **1982**, *3*, 1022–1027. [CrossRef]

48. Pickens, J.N.; Bahrick, L.E. Do infants perceive invariant tempo and rhythm in auditory-visual events? *Infant. Behav. Dev.* **1997**, *20*, 349–357. [CrossRef]

49. Bahrick, L.E.; Pickens, J.N. Amodal relations: The basis for intermodal perception and learning. In *The Development of Intersensory Perception: Comparative Perspectives*; Lewkowicz, D., Ed.; Erlbaum: Hillsdale, NJ, USA, 1994; pp. 205–233.

50. Stumpf, K. *Tonpsychologie [Psychology of Tones]*; S. Hirzel: Leipzig, Germany, 1883.

51. Pratt, C.C. The spatial character of high and low tones. *J. Exp. Psychol.* **1930**, *13*, 278–285. [CrossRef]

52. Carnevale, M.J.; Harris, L.R. Which direction is up for a high pitch? *Multisens. Res.* **2016**, *29*, 113–132. [CrossRef] [PubMed]

53. White, B.W. Recognition of distorted melodies. *Am. J. Psychol.* **1960**, *73*, 100–107. [CrossRef] [PubMed]

54. Frances, R. *La Perception de la Musique*, 2nd ed.; Librairie Philosophique J. Vrin: Paris, France, 1972. (In French)

55. Pedersen, P. The perception of octave equivalence in twelve-tone rows. *Psychol. Music* **1975**, *3*, 3–8. [CrossRef]

56. Wertheimer, M. Untersuchungen zur Lehre von der Gestalt. II. *Psychol. Forsch.* **1923**, *4*, 301–350. (In German) [CrossRef]

57. Green, D.M.; Swets, J.A. *Signal Detection Theory and Psychophysics*; Wiley: New York, NY, USA, 1966.

58. Stanislaw, H.; Todorov, N. Calculation of signal detection theory measures. *Behav. Res. Methods Instrum. Comput.* **1999**, *31*, 137–149. [CrossRef] [PubMed]

59. Donaldson, W. Measuring recognition memory. *J. Exp. Psychol. Gen.* **1992**, *121*, 275–277. [CrossRef] [PubMed]

60. Nelson, T.O. A comparison of current measures of the accuracy of feeling-of-knowing predictions. *Psychol. Bull.* **1984**, *95*, 109–133. [CrossRef] [PubMed]

61. Smith, W.D. Clarification of sensitivity measure A′. *J. Math. Psychol.* **1995**, *39*, 82–89. [CrossRef]

62. Pollack, I.; Norman, D.A. A nonparametric analysis of recognition experiments. *Psychon. Sci.* **1964**, *1*, 125–126. [CrossRef]

63. Macmillan, N.A.; Creelman, C.D. Triangles in ROC space: History and theory of "nonparametric" measures of sensitivity and bias. *Psychon. Bull. Rev.* **1996**, *3*, 164–170. [CrossRef] [PubMed]

64. Papke, L.E.; Wooldridge, J. Econometric methods for fractional response variables with an application to 401(k) plan participation rates. *J. Appl. Econ.* **1996**, *11*, 619–632. [CrossRef]

65. Baum, C.F. Modeling proportions. *Stata J.* **2008**, *8*, 299–303.

66. Bates, D.; Machler, M.; Bolker, B.M.; Walker, S.C. Fitting linear mixed-effects models using lme4. *arXiv* **2015**, arXiv:1406.5823.

67. Fox, J.; Weisberg, S. *An R Companion to Applied Regression*, 2nd ed.; Sage: Thousand Oaks, CA, USA, 2011.

68. Lenth, R.V. Least-squares means: The R package lsmeans. *J. Stat. Softw.* **2016**, *69*. [CrossRef]

69. Fox, J. Effect Displays in R for Generalised Linear Models. 2003. Available online: http://psfaculty.ucdavis.edu/bsjjones/effectdisplays.pdf (accessed on 7 March 2017).

70. Barr, D.J. Random effects structure for testing interactions in linear mixed-effects models. *Front. Psychol.* **2013**, *4*. [CrossRef] [PubMed]

71. Barr, D.J.; Levy, R.; Scheepers, C.; Tily, H.J. Random effects structure for confirmatory hypothesis testing: Keep it maximal. *J. Mem. Lang.* **2013**, *68*, 255–278. [CrossRef] [PubMed]

72. Bates, D.; Kliegl, R.; Vasishth, S.; Baayen, H. Parsimonious mixed models. *arXiv* **2015**, arXiv:150604967.

73. Singmann, H.; Bolker, B.M.; Westfall, J. AFEX: Analysis of Factorial Experiments. R Package Version 0.16-1. R Foundation for Statistical Computing, Ed.; Vienna. Available online: http://CRAN.R-project.org/package=afex (accessed on 26 January 2017).

74. Von Ehrenfels, C. Über Gestaltqualitäten. *Vierteljahrsschr. Wiss. Philos.* **1890**, *14*, 249–292. (In German)

75. Wagemans, J.; Van Gool, L.; Swinnen, V.; Van Horebeek, J. Higher-order structure in regularity detection. *Vis. Res.* **1993**, *33*, 1067–1088. [CrossRef]

76. Huang, L.; Pashler, H. Symmetry detection and visual attention: A "binary-map" hypothesis. *Vis. Res.* **2002**, *42*, 1421–1430. [CrossRef]

77. Niimi, R.; Watanabe, K.; Yokosawa, K. The dynamic-stimulus advantage of visual symmetry perception. *Psychol. Res.* **2008**, *72*, 567–579. [CrossRef] [PubMed]

78. Baylis, G.C.; Driver, J. Obligatory edge assignment in vision: The role of figure and part segmentation in symmetry detection. *J. Exp. Psychol. Hum. Percept. Perform.* **1995**, *21*, 1323–1342. [CrossRef]

79. Bertamini, M.; Friedenberg, J.D.; Kubovy, M. Detection of symmetry and perceptual organization: The way a lock-and-key process works. *Acta Psychol.* **1997**, *95*, 119–140. [CrossRef]

80. Koning, A.; Wagemans, J. Detection of symmetry and repetition in one and two objects: Structures versus strategies. *Exp. Psychol.* **2009**, *56*, 5–17. [CrossRef] [PubMed]

81. Öğmen, H.; Herzog, M.H. A new conceptualization of human visual sensory-memory. *Front. Psychol.* **2016**, *7*, 830–845. [CrossRef] [PubMed]

82. Winkler, I.; Cowan, N. From sensory to long-term memory: Evidence from auditory memory reactivation studies. *Exp. Psychol.* **2005**, *52*, 3–20. [CrossRef] [PubMed]

83. Bianchi, I.; Savardi, U. *The Perception of Contraries*; Aracne: Roma, Italy, 2008.

84. Bianchi, I.; Savardi, U. The relationship perceived between the real body and the mirror image. *Perception* **2008**, *37*, 666–687. [CrossRef] [PubMed]

85. Diamond, R.; Carey, S. Why faces are and are not special. An effect of expertise. *J. Exp. Psychol. Gen.* **1986**, *115*, 107–117. [CrossRef] [PubMed]

86. Wright, A.A.; Roberts, W.A. Monkey and human face perception: Inversion effects for human faces but not for monkey faces or scenes. *J. Cogn. Neurosci.* **1996**, *8*, 278–290. [CrossRef] [PubMed]

87. Troje, F.N.; Westhoff, C. The inversion effect in biological motion perception: Evidence for a "life detector"? *Curr. Biol.* **2006**, *16*, 821–824. [CrossRef] [PubMed]

88. Dakin, S.C.; Watt, R.J. Detection of bilateral symmetry using spatial filters. *Spat. Vis.* **1994**, *8*, 393–413. [CrossRef] [PubMed]

89. Labonte, F.; Shapira, Y.; Cohen, P.; Faubert, J. A model for global symmetry detection in dense images. *Spat. Vis.* **1995**, *9*, 33–55. [CrossRef] [PubMed]

90. Jenkins, B. Component processes in the perception of bilaterally symmetric dot textures. *Percept. Psychophys.* **1983**, *34*, 433–440. [CrossRef] [PubMed]

91. Ballesteros, S.; Manga, D.; Reales, J.M. Haptic discrimination of bilateral symmetry in 2-dimensional and 3-dimensional unfamiliar displays. *Percept. Psychophys.* **1997**, *59*, 37–50. [CrossRef] [PubMed]

92. Ballesteros, S.; Millar, S.; Reales, J.M. Symmetry in haptic and in visual shape perception. *Percept. Psychophys.* **1998**, *60*, 389–404. [CrossRef] [PubMed]

93. Ballesteros, S.; Reales, J.M. Visual and haptic discrimination of symmetry in unfamiliar displays extended in the *z*-axis. *Perception* **2004**, *33*, 315–327. [CrossRef] [PubMed]

94. Bauer, C.; Yazzolino, L.; Hirsch, G.; Cattaneo, Z.; Vecchi, T.; Merabet, L.B. Neural correlates associated with superior tactile symmetry perception in the early blind. *Cortex* **2015**, *63*, 104–117. [CrossRef] [PubMed]

95. Cattaneo, Z.; Bona, S.; Bauer, C.; Silvanto, J.; Herbert, A.M.; Vecchi, T.; Merabet, L.B. Symmetry detection in visual impairment: Behavioral evidence and neural correlates. *Symmetry* **2014**, *6*, 427–443. [CrossRef]

96. Cattaneo, Z.; Fantino, M.; Silvanto, J.; Tinti, C.; Pascual-Leone, A.; Vecchi, T. Symmetry perception in the blind. *Acta Psychol.* **2010**, *134*, 398–402. [CrossRef] [PubMed]

97. Cattaneo, Z.; Vecchi, T.; Fantino, M.; Herbert, A.M.; Merabet, L.B. The effect of vertical and horizontal symmetry on memory for tactile patterns in late blind individuals. *Atten. Percept. Psychophys.* **2013**, *75*, 375–382. [CrossRef] [PubMed]

98. Driver, J.; Baylis, G.C.; Rafal, R.D. Preserved figure-ground segregation and symmetry perception in visual neglect. *Nature* **1992**, *360*, 73–75. [CrossRef] [PubMed]

99. Verma, A.; Van der Haegen, L.; Brysbaert, M. Symmetry detection in typically and atypically speech lateralized individuals: A visual half-field study. *Neuropsychologia* **2013**, *51*, 2611–2619. [CrossRef] [PubMed]

100. Wagemans, J. Parallel visual processes in symmetry perception: Normality and pathology. *Doc. Ophthalmol.* **1998**, *95*, 359–370. [CrossRef] [PubMed]

101. Bertamini, M.; Makin, A.D.J. Brain activity in response to visual symmetry. *Symmetry* **2014**, *6*, 975–996. [CrossRef]

102. Merabet, L.B.; Thut, G.; Murray, B.; Andrews, J.; Hsiao, S.; Pascual-Leone, A. Feeling by sight or seeing by touch? *Neuron* **2004**, *42*, 173–179. [CrossRef]

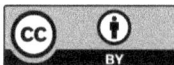

symmetry

MDPI

Article

Anomalous Mirror Symmetry Generated by Optical Illusion

Kokichi Sugihara

Meiji Institute for the Advanced Study of Mathematical Sciences, Meiji University, 4-21-1 Nakano, Nakano-ku, Tokyo 164-8525, Japan; kokichis@meiji.ac.jp; Tel.: +81-3-5343-8366

Academic Editors: Marco Bertamini and Lewis Griffin
Received: 22 January 2016; Accepted: 1 April 2016; Published: 8 April 2016

Abstract: This paper introduces a new concept of mirror symmetry, called "anomalous mirror symmetry", which is physically impossible but can be perceived by human vision systems because of optical illusion. This symmetry is characterized geometrically and a method for creating cylindrical surfaces that create this symmetry is constructed. Examples of solid objects constructed by a 3D printer are also shown.

Keywords: ambiguous cylinder; mirror symmetry; visual illusion; visual perception

1. Introduction

An ordinary planar mirror generates a plane symmetric image of an object, that is, for an arbitrary point of an object and its mirror image, the line segment connecting them crosses the mirror plane at the midpoint in the right angle. Although the concept of the mirror symmetry has been generalized in many directions in mathematics and physics [1,2], the original mirror symmetry with respect to a planar mirror is simple and well understood from a mathematical point of view.

When we see the object and its mirror image, however, what we perceive does not necessarily obey this physical law, because what we perceive is the result of image processing in our brains, and hence optical illusion arises [3,4]. In particular, it was discovered recently that there are cylindrical objects whose mirror images appear to be quite different from what we usually expect [5,6]. Those cylinders seem to defy the law of optical physics. This phenomenon is called ambiguous cylinder illusion.

In this paper, we propose a new concept of symmetry, which we call "anomalous mirror symmetry" ("anomalous symmetry" for short). The anomalous symmetry is a modification of mirror symmetry, but it does not obey the law of optical physics. Hence, it cannot be realized in a purely physical manner. However, we show that anomalous symmetry can be generated if we employ ambiguous cylinder illusion. We characterize the class of cylinders whose mirror images generate anomalous symmetry and moreover the same anomaly is preserved even if the objects are rotated around a vertical axis.

From a mathematical point of view, we solve a problem of finding a pair of mirror symmetric space curves whose projections coincide with a pair of given point symmetric planar curves. The problem of finding symmetric space curves from given planar curves have been studied in many setting. For example, Hong *et al.* [7] showed that both the symmetric space curves and the camera poses can be reconstructed from their perspective images. Sawada *et al.* [8,9] constructed an algorithm for finding a pair of mirror symmetric space curves and the associated mirror from a pair of planar curves. The present problem is similar to them in the sense that we construct symmetric space curves, but simpler because the mirror pose is given.

The paper is organized in the following way. In Section 2, we review the nature of mirror symmetry and introduce a concept of anomalous symmetry. In Section 3, we review a method to generate ambiguous cylinders. In Section 4, we apply this method to design solids that produce the anomalous symmetry. Section 5 gives examples of anomalously symmetric objects and Section 6 gives concluding remarks together with future work.

2. Mirror Symmetry and Anomalous Symmetry

As shown in Figure 1, we consider an (x, y, z) Cartesian coordinate systems, in which the xy plane is horizontal and hence the z axis is vertical.

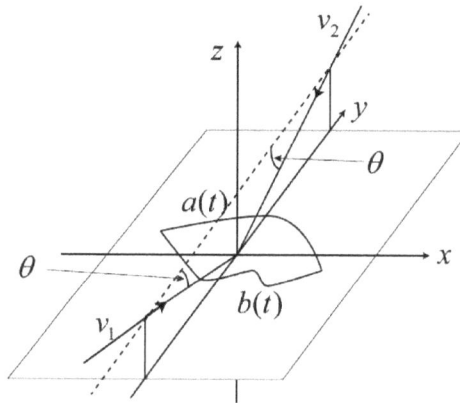

Figure 1. Pair of horizontal curves and a pair of view directions.

Let O be an object and O' be its mirror image with respect to a mirror placed in the xz plane. Then, any point (x, y, z) on O is mapped to the point $(x, -y, z)$. Thus, the y coordinate is reversed while the x and z coordinates are kept unchanged. Hence, we call O' the y-reversal mirror image. We extend the meaning of the term "y-reversal" for any translated version of O'. In other words, we refer to "y-reversal" to represent the posture of O' with respect to O, and do not care about the position of O'. Similarly we name the x-reversal mirror image for the image generated by a mirror in the yz plane, and its translated version.

We are interested in a class of objects whose y-reversal mirror images appear to be x-reversal.

An example is shown in Figure 2. There is a cylinder whose section appears to be an arrow, and a vertical mirror stands behind it. However, the mirror image of the cylinder is anomalous in the sense that the left part and the right part appear to be reversed. Let us consider an (x, y, z) coordinate system such that the mirror is contained in the xz plane. Then, the mirror image of the cylinder should be y-reversal, but the actual mirror image in Figure 2 appears to be x-reversal.

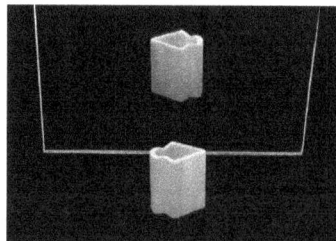

Figure 2. Ambiguous cylinder "Left-Right Reversal Mirror".

If we rotate this cylinder around a vertical axis, the apparent shape of the section changes as shown in Figure 3. Note that in all postures of the cylinder, the corresponding mirror images are *x*-reversal instead of *y*-reversal.

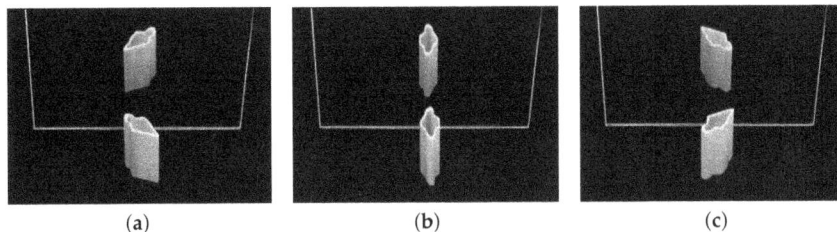

| (a) | (b) | (c) |

Figure 3. Different views of the same cylinder as in Figure 2 rotated around a vertical axis. (**a**) Object and its mirror image after 45 degrees rotation; (**b**) Object and its mirror image after 90 degrees rotation; (**c**) Object and its mirror image after 135 degrees rotation.

Note that the concept of anomalous symmetry is mathematically equivalent to line symmetry with respect to a vertical line. However, we use the term "anomalous mirror" symmetry in order to emphasize that it is physically impossible by a planar mirror.

It might be interesting to note that one of typical errors made by human subjects in predicting motion and orientation in the mirror image is similar to what we call anomalous symmetry. For example, Savardi *et al.* [10] and Bianchi *et al.* [11] made experiments in which they showed motion of an object to subjects and asked them to predict the motion and orientation in its mirror image. They reported that a typical error in estimation is line symmetric with respect to a vertical line instead of mirror symmetric.

The goal of this paper is to characterize the class of cylinders with this anomalous symmetry. For this purpose we review geometric aspects of the class of optical illusion called ambiguous cylinders in the next section.

3. Ambiguous Cylinders

Let $a(t)$ and $b(t)$ be two real-valued continuous functions defined for $-1 \leq t \leq 1$, and let us define three-dimensional vectors,

$$a(t) = (t, a(t), 0), \quad b(t) = (t, b(t), 0)$$

where t is a parameter. The vectors $a(t)$ and $b(t)$ represent planar curves on the xy plane, and they are monotone in the x direction.

As shown in Figure 1, suppose that we see those curves along two view directions $v_1 = (0, \cos\theta, -\sin\theta)$ and $v_2 = (0, -\cos\theta, -\sin\theta)$. They are parallel to the yz plane, and are slanted downward by the same angle θ, $0 < \theta < \pi/2$, with respect to the horizontal plane in mutually opposite directions in the y axis. This means that the two viewpoints are both at infinity. This is a good approximation of actual perspective projection if the viewpoint is sufficiently far from the objects.

We are interested in finding a space curve that coincides with $a(t)$ when it is seen along v_1 and that coincides with $b(t)$ when it is seen along v_2. This space curve can be determined uniquely in the following way. For any $t \in [-1, 1]$, $a(t)$ and $b(t)$ are in the plane $x = t$, which is parallel to the yz plane. Hence the line passing through $a(t)$ and parallel to v_1 and the line passing through $b(t)$ and parallel to v_2 are both in this plane, and consequently they have a point of intersection. Let this point of intersection be denoted by $c(t) = (t, c_1(t), c_2(t))$. As t moves in $-1 \leq t \leq 1$, $c(t)$ traces a space curve. This is the curve that we wanted to get.

The curve $c(t)$ is just a space curve, and it is not necessarily be perceived as the planar curves $a(t)$ and $b(t)$ when it is seen in the corresponding view directions.

However, the human brains prefer right angles in interpreting retinal images as three-dimensional objects; this property is typically observed in Ames's room illusion [3], and is usually understood as a priori constraint for right angles [12–14]. We can use this nature of the brains to guide viewers to perceive the planar curves $a(t)$ and $b(c)$ when they see the space curve $c(t)$ in the following way.

Let l be a vertical line segment, that is, l is parallel to the z axis. Suppose that we move l in a space in such a way that its orientation is fixed and its upper terminal point traces along the curve $c(t)$. Let the surface swept by l be S.

As shown in Figure 4a, the resulting surface S has the same vertical length as the length of l. In this case we are apt to interpret the upper edge $c(t)$ as the intersection of S and a plane perpendicular to l as shown in Figure 4b because of the preference of right angles; we usually do not consider it as the intersection of S and a curved surface as shown in Figure 4c although it is mathematically possible.

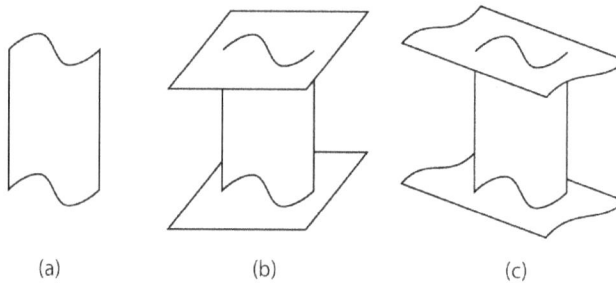

(a)   (b)   (c)

Figure 4. Swept surface and its interpretations: (**a**) Surface swept by a vertical line segment; (**b**) Plane-cut interpretation of the upper edge; (**c**) Another interpretation which is mathematically possible but empirically unnatural.

Therefore, we can expect that when the surface S is seen along the view directions v_1 and v_2, the upper edge $c(t)$ appears to be the planar curves $a(t)$ and $b(t)$, respectively. Moreover, if we place a vertical mirror parallel to the xz plane, the two views of S are obtained simultaneously, the direct view corresponds to v_1 and the mirror image corresponds to v_2. For the solid in Figure 2, we applied the above method twice to the upper curve and the lower curve, resulting in the closed cylinder. This is the mathematical trick to generate ambiguous cylinder illusion.

4. Creation of Anomalous Mirror Symmetry

Our goal is to construct a method for designing the ambiguous cylinders that create anomalous symmetry. For this purpose we replace the pair of x-monotone curves $a(t)$ and $b(t)$ with a pair of closed curves.

Let $a_1(t)$ and $a_2(t)$ be two continuous functions defined in $[-1, 1]$ such that $a_1(-1) = a_2(-1)$ and $a_1(1) = a_2(1)$. Hence $a_1(t) = (t, a_1(t), 0)$ and $a_2(t) = (t, a_2(t), 0)$ altogether form a closed curve on the xy plane. Similarly, let $b_1(t)$ and $b_2(t)$ be two continuous functions defined in $[-1, 1]$ such that $b_1(-1) = b_2(-1)$ and $b_1(1) = b_2(1)$. Hence $b_1(t) = (t, b_1(t), 0)$ and $b_2(t) = (t, b_2(t), 0)$ constitute another closed curve on the xy plane. We want to construct a closed space curve that appears to be the closed curve composed of $a_1(t)$ and $a_2(t)$ when it is seen in the view direction v_1, and that appears to be the closed curve composed of $b_1(t)$ and $b_2(t)$ when it is seen in the view direction v_2, and it generates anomalous symmetry when we place a mirror parallel to the xz plane.

We apply the method for constructing an ambiguous cylinder twice, once to the pair $a_1(t)$ and $b_1(t)$, and once more to the pair $a_2(t)$ and $b_2(t)$. In order to create anomalous symmetry, the curves should satisfy

$$b_1(x) = -a_2(-x) \tag{1}$$
$$b_2(x) = -a_1(-x) \tag{2}$$

This is because, as shown in Figure 5, the two appearances corresponding to the two view directions v_1 and v_2 should be point symmetric with respect to the origin as the center of the symmetry; if they are point symmetric as shown in Figure 5a,b, the mirror parallel to the xz plane will generate a normal image that is y-reversal to Figure 5b, resulting in the curve shown in Figure 5c, which is x-reversal to the curve in Figure 5a, that is, which generates anomalous symmetry.

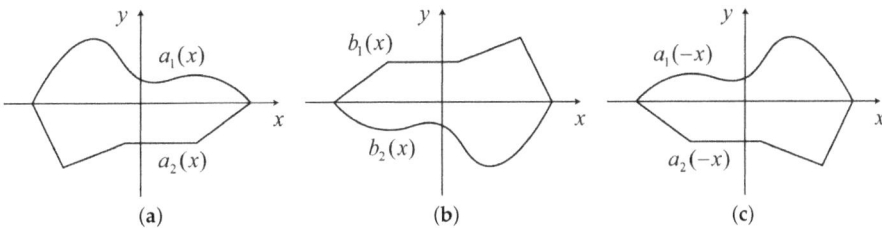

Figure 5. Pair of plane curves that creates anomalous symmetry: (**a**) Arbitrary closed curve compound of upper and lower curves both of which are monotone in the x direction; (**b**) Closed curve that is point symmetric to the curve (a); (**c**) Mirror image of (b) with respect to the mirror parallel to the xz plane.

In Figure 6 we show the intersection of the scene by a plane $x = t$ parallel to the yz plane. As shown in this figure, the space curve $c_1(t)$ that appears $a_1(t)$ when it is seen in the view direction v_1, and that appears $b_1(t)$ when it is seen in the view direction v_2, can be represented as

$$c_1(t) = \left(t, \frac{a_1(t) + b_1(t)}{2}, \alpha \frac{a_1(t) - b_1(t)}{2} \right) \tag{3}$$

where $\alpha = \tan \theta$. Similarly, we get

$$c_2(t) = \left(t, \frac{a_2(t) + b_2(t)}{2}, \alpha \frac{a_2(t) - b_2(t)}{2} \right) \tag{4}$$

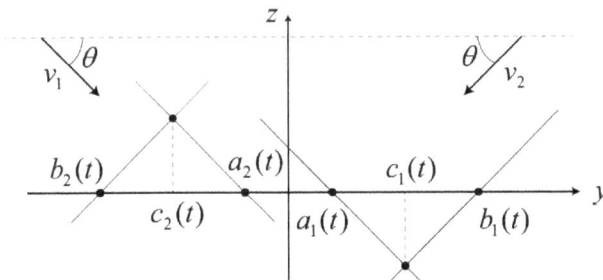

Figure 6. Construction of the space curves from the pair of planar curves on the xy plane.

Substituting Equations (1) and (2), we get the explicit representation of the pair of space curves:

$$c_1(t) = \left(t, \frac{a_1(t) - a_2(-t)}{2}, \alpha \frac{a_1(t) + a_2(-t)}{2} \right) \tag{5}$$

$$c_2(t) = \left(t, \frac{a_2(t) - a_1(-t)}{2}, \alpha \frac{a_2(t) + a_1(-t)}{2} \right) \tag{6}$$

Note that we can choose a pair of functions $a_1(t)$ and $a_2(t)$ arbitrary. Once we choose them, the space curves $c_1(t)$ and $c_2(t)$ are determined by Equations (5) and (6), which create anomalous symmetry.

Next, we consider the conditions such that the anomalous symmetry property is preserved even if the cylinder is rotated around the z axis. Fortunately it turns out that no additional conditions are necessary; the closed curve given by Equations (5) and (6) automatically satisfies the desired property. That is, the next proposition holds.

Proposition.   The closed curve given by Equations (5) and (6) does not destroy the anomalous symmetry property even if it is rotated around the z axis.

Proof.   The rotation around the z axis does not destroy the anomalous symmetry property if the space curve is line symmetric with respect to the z axis. That is,

$$c_1(t)|_y = -c_2(-t)|_y \tag{7}$$

$$c_1(t)|_z = c_2(-t)|_z \tag{8}$$

where $w|_y$ and $w|_z$ represent the y and z coordinates of vector w. Actually the conditions Equations (7) and (8) are satisfied by $c_1(t)$ and $c_2(t)$ defined by Equations (5) and (6). Thus the anomalous symmetry property is preserved when the curve is rotated around the z axis.   (End of proof)

Recall that the object shown in Figure 2 preserves the anomalous symmetry property when it is rotated around a vertical axis, as shown in Figure 3. The above proposition implies that this is not accidental. When we rotate such an object around a vertical axis, we can enjoy an unordinary change of the appearance of the object that always keeps anomalous symmetry. This visual effect might be used as a means for new artistic presentation.

It is interesting to note that a similar non-accidental nature is observed by Sawada *et al.* [8] in the context of reconstructing 3D symmetric curves from 2D projected curves.

5. Examples

We applied our method to various figures whose upper and lower boundaries are both monotone in the x direction. The following are examples.

Figure 7 shows a shape of a fish. Let $a_1(x)$ and $a_2(x)$ be the upper boundary curve and the lower boundary curve, respectively, of this shape. We applied our method to this pair of curves, and constructed a solid object by first making a short cylinder whose edge curve consists of $c_1(t)$ and $c_2(t)$, second making surfaces which cap the top and the bottom of the cylinder, and finally filling material in it.

The resulting object is shown in Figure 8. Figure 8a is a picture of the resulting solid in the original posture and its mirror image. The panels (b), (c) and (d) of this figure show the same object rotated around a vertical axis clockwise step by step in this order.

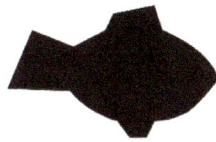

Figure 7. Shape of a fish.

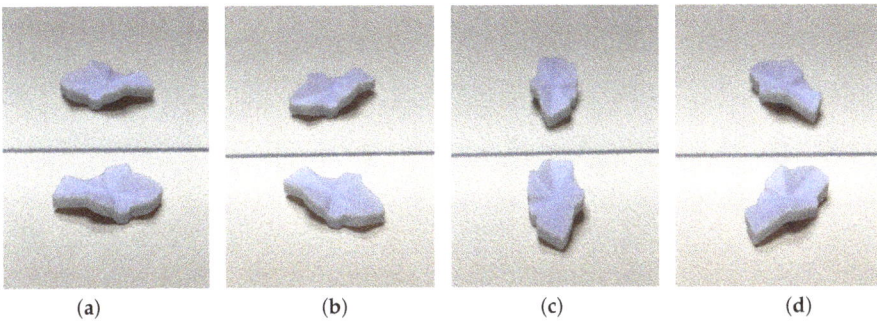

(**a**)	(**b**)	(**c**)	(**d**)

Figure 8. Fish-shape object creating anomalous mirror symmetry. (**a**) Original posture; (**b**) After 30 degrees rotation; (**c**) After 90 degrees rotation; (**d**) After 135 degrees rotation.

Figure 9 is a shape of a car, and Figure 10 shows the object constructed from this shape. Figure 11 is a shape of a ship, and Figure 12 shows the object constructed from this shape. In both Figures 10 and 12, (a) is the original posture, and (b), (c), (d) are the results of rotation.

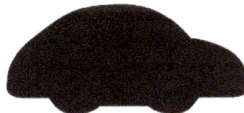

Figure 9. Shape of a car.

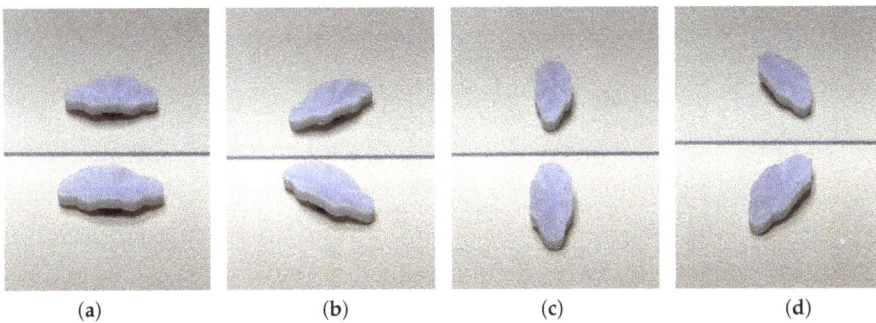

(**a**)	(**b**)	(**c**)	(**d**)

Figure 10. Car-shape object creating anomalous mirror symmetry. (**a**) Original posture; (**b**) After 30 degrees rotation; (**c**) After 90 degrees rotation; (**d**) After 135 degrees rotation.

Figure 11. Shape of a ship.

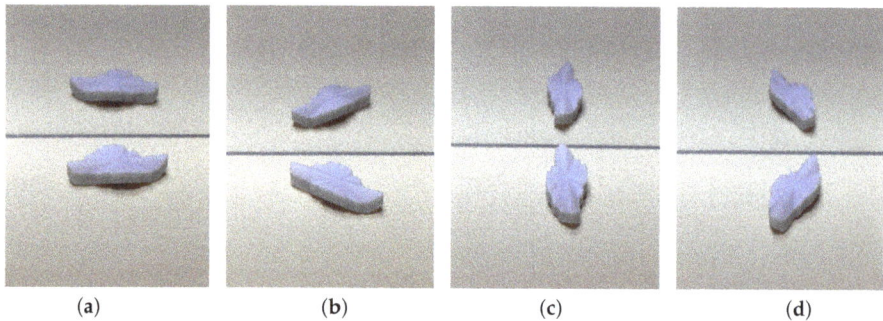

| | | | |
| (a) | (b) | (c) | (d) |

Figure 12. Ship-shape object creating anomalous mirror symmetry. (**a**) Original posture; (**b**) After 30 degrees rotation; (**c**) After 90 degrees rotation; (**d**) After 135 degrees rotation.

From these examples, we can observe that the mirror image of an object appears to be the *x*-reversal mirror image instead of the *y*-reversal, not only in its original posture but also in its rotated versions. Thus, we achieve the anomalous mirror symmetry.

6. Concluding Remarks

We introduced a new concept called "anomalous mirror symmetry", which is not consistent with the law of optical physics, but which can be perceived subjectively because of optical illusion. We characterized this symmetry and constructed a method for designing the class of space curves and the associated cylindrical surfaces that create anomalous symmetry.

The concept of anomalous symmetry we have introduced in this paper might be just one example of many possible new symmetries. The mirror symmetry with respect to a planar mirror is well studied from optical physics point of view. However, if we consider optical illusion, we may be able to extend the concept of mirror symmetry in many directions. The anomalous mirror symmetry introduced in this paper is such that the *y*-reversal image appears to be *x*-reversal. In general, for any pair of mirrors *A* and *B*, we might be able to define anomalous mirror symmetry in such a way that the mirror image with respect to the mirror *A* appears to be a mirror image with respect to the mirror *B*. To study those extensions is one of our future problems.

Acknowledgments: The author expresses his sincere thanks to the anonymous reviewers for their valuable comments, by which the author could improve the manuscript. This work is partly supported by the Grant-in-Aid for Basic Research 24360039 and Challenging Exploratory Research 15K12067 of Ministry of Education, Culture, Sports, Science and Technology of Japan (MEXT).

Conflicts of Interest: The author declares no conflict of interest.

References

1.   Cox, D.A. Mirror symmetry and polar duality of polytopes. *Symmetry* **2015**, *7*, 1633–1645.

Symmetry **2016**, *8*, 21

2. Hori, K.; Katz, S.; Klemm, A.; Pandharipande, R.; Thomas, R.; Vafa, C.; Vakil, R.; Zaslow, E. *Mirror Symmetry*; American Mathematical Society: Providence, RI, USA, 2003.
3. Gregory, R.L. *The Intellignet Eye*; Weidenfeld and Nicolson: London, UK, 1970.
4. Van der Helm, P.A. The influence of perception on the distribution of multiple symmetries in nature and art. *Symmetry* **2011**, *3*, 54–71.
5. Sugihara, K. Design of ambiguous cylinders. In Proceedings of the Asian Forum on Graphic Science, Bangkok, Tailand, 5–9 August 2015; p. 8.
6. Sugihara, K. *Joy of Anomalous Solids: How to Make Anomalous Objects That Change Their Appearances in a Mirror*; Sugi Lab., Inc.: Funabashi, Japan, 2015.
7. Hong, W.; Ma, Y.; Yu, Y. Reconstruction of 3-D deformed symmetric curves from perspective images without discrete features. *Lecture Notes Comput. Sci.* **2004**, *3023*, 533–545.
8. Sawada, T.; Li, Y.; Pizlo, Z. Any pair of 2D curves is consistent with a 3D symmetric interpretation. *Symmetry* **2011**, *3*, 365–388.
9. Sawada, T.; Li, Y.; Pizlo, Z. Detecting 3-D mirror symmetry in a 2-D camera image for 3-D shape recovery. *Proc. IEEE* **2014**, *102*, 1588–1606.
10. Savardi, U.; Bianchi, I.; Bertamini, M. Naive predictions of motion and orientation in mirrors: From what we see to what we expect reflections to do. *Acta Psychol.* **2010**, *134*, 1–15.
11. Bianchi, I.; Bertamini, M.; Savardi, U. Differences between predictions of how a reflection behaves based on the behaviour of an object, and how an object behaves based on the behaviour of its reflection. *Acta Psychol.* **2015**, *161*, 54–63.
12. Perkins, D.N. Visual discrimination between rectangular and nonrectangular parallelopipeds. *Percept. Psychophys.* **1972**, *12*, 293–331.
13. Perkins, D.N. Compensating for distortion in viewing pictures obliquely. *Percept. Psychophys.* **1973**, *14*, 13–18.
14. Perkins, D.N. How good a bet is good form? *Perception* **1976**, *5*, 393–406.

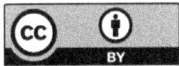

symmetry

MDPI

Review

On the Legibility of Mirror-Reflected and Rotated Text

Gennady Erlikhman *, Lars Strother, Iskra Barzakov and Gideon Paul Caplovitz

Department of Psychology, University of Nevada, Reno, NV 89557, USA; lars@unr.edu (L.S.);
iskrabarzakov@gmail.com (I.B.); gcaplovitz@unr.edu (G.P.C.)
* Correspondence: gerlikhman@unr.edu; Tel.: +1-310-825-4202

Academic Editor: Marco Bertamini
Received: 23 December 2016; Accepted: 17 February 2017; Published: 23 February 2017

Abstract: We happened to observe that text that was reflected about either the horizontal or vertical axis was more difficult to read than text that was reflected about first one and then the other, which amounts to a 180-degree rotation. In this article, we review a number of studies that examine the nature of recognizing reflected and inverted letters, and the frequency of mirror reversal errors (e.g., confusing 'b' for 'd') in children and adults. We explore recent ideas linking the acquisition of literacy with the loss of mirror-invariance, not just for text, but for objects in general. We try to connect these various literatures to examine why certain transformations of text are more difficult to read than others for adults.

Keywords: mirror-reversal; left-right reversal; reading; reversal errors; mirrored text

---

Recently, one of us held up a page of printed text (Figure 1A) to their webcam to take a picture. The camera software by default created a mirror-image snapshot (i.e., the text was reflected or mirrored about the vertical axis, Figure 1B) thereby rendering the text virtually illegible. Correcting or undoing this sort of reflection can be trivially accomplished using any number of image processing software packages that include built-in functions such as 'reflect vertical', 'reflect horizontal', 'rotate left', and 'rotate right'. It was with some surprise that when the wrong function was accidentally applied and instead of reflecting along the vertical axis, the image was reflected along the horizontal axis, the text, although now reflected twice, was now more easily legible (Figure 1D). It is of note that this 'double reflection' is equivalent to a 180° rotation of the text. With only a few mouse clicks, it was clear that when normally-oriented text is mirror reflected about the horizontal axis it again becomes virtually illegible (Figure 1C). This brief series of webcam-picture inspired observations demonstrated a basic property of text perception and reading: the legibility of text is reflection variant and rotation invariant.

Inspired by these observations, we conducted a review of the corresponding work on the intersection of symmetry, reflections, and the legibility of text. We found a large body of literature on mirror-reading and writing; mirror-reversal errors of single letters in reading, copying, and writing; many studies on perception of normal and mirrored single characters; but only a small number of studies on combinations of geometric transformations including both inversion (up-down mirroring) and reflection (left-right mirroring). In this paper, we review the literature on mirror-reversals and inversions of text and synthesize some recent work and ideas on how representational mirror-invariance not only for letters but also for objects may be lost when someone learns how to read.

A OF THE SURFACE OF THINGS

I
In my room, the world is beyond my understanding;
But when I walk I see that it consists of three or four
hills and a cloud.

II
From my balcony, I survey the yellow air,
Reading where I have written,
"The spring is like a belle undressing."

III
The gold tree is blue.
The singer has pulled his cloak over his head.
The moon is in the folds of the cloak.

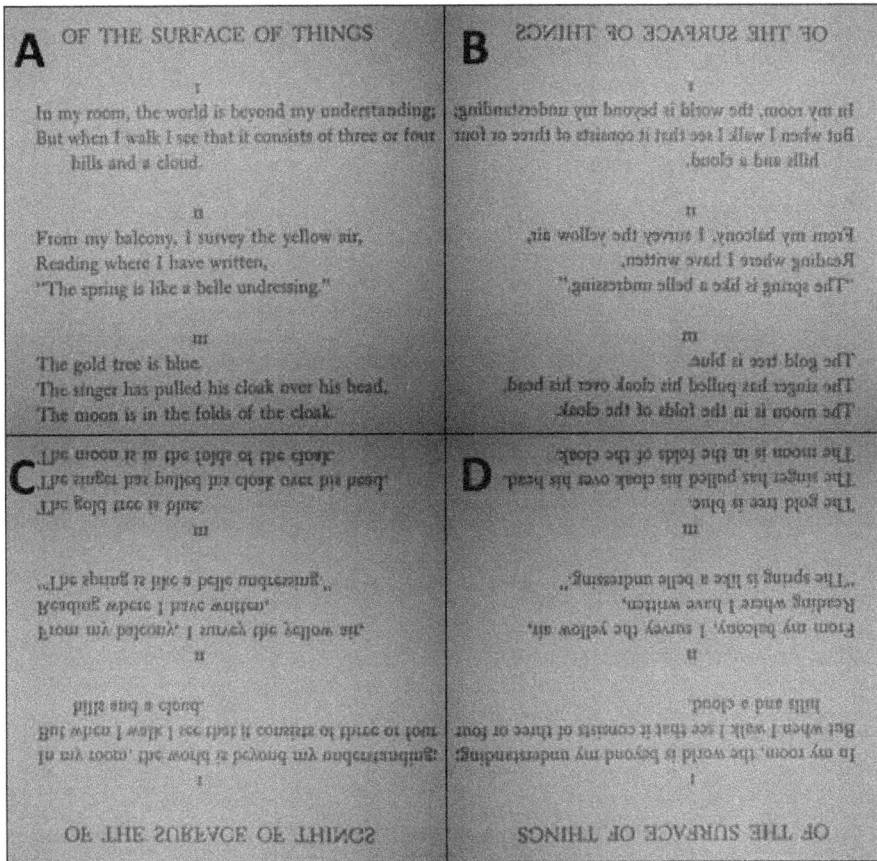

Figure 1. Four examples of the same poem "On the Surface of Things" by Wallace Stevens. (**A**) Normal (upright); (**B**) Reflected about the vertical axis; (**C**) Reflected about the horizontal axis; (**D**) Reflected about the vertical and horizontal axes, which is equivalent to a 180° rotation.

Before proceeding with a survey of the literature, we wish to make several observations about mirrored text as it occurs outside of a laboratory setting. Apart from webcams and mirrors, mirrored text can be seen on the front of ambulances, where the word "AMBULANCE" is mirror-reflected so that it appears correctly in one's rearview mirror (Figure 2A). Mirrored text is also a feature of certain scripts: Boustrophedon, literally meaning "ox-turning", is text that is written left-to-right and right-to-left on alternating lines as one would plow a field, forwards and then backwards. The letters of alternating lines are mirror-reversed (Figure 2B). Some inscriptions in ancient Greek and Latin as well as Luwian (Hittite) hieroglyphics were written in this manner. Tablets found on Easter Island appear to be written in rongorongo (Figure 2C), a script or protoscript that may be in reverse boustrophedon, meaning that alternating lines are flipped about the horizontal axis instead of reflected about the vertical axis. A tablet would be read bottom-to-top, rotating the tablet 180° after every line.

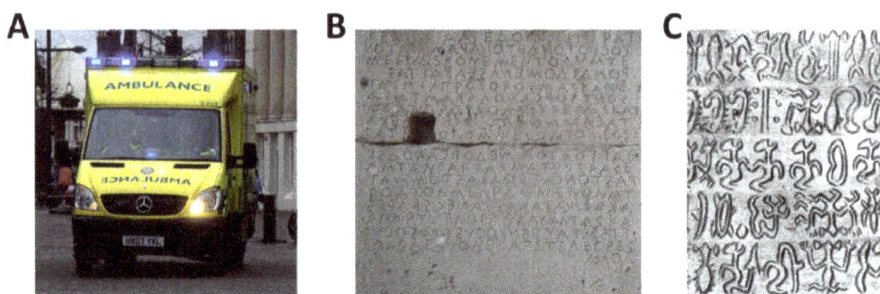

Figure 2. (**A**) An ambulance with mirrored text on the hood so that it appears in the correct orientation in one's rearview mirror. By neiljohnuk from East a bit., ENGLAND! (DSC_0068) CC BY 2.0 via Wikimedia Commons; (**B**) Fragmentary inscription of a code of law from Gortyn (Crete). Written in boustrophedon so that alternating lines are read left-to-right and right-to-left. Each other line is left-right mirror-reversed. By PRA (Own work) CC BY-SA 3.0 via Wikimedia Commons; (**C**) Fragment of rongorongo script.

The fact that the mirror-reversed word "AMBULANCE" can still be read in Figure 2A suggests that the visual system may incorporate some amount of mirror invariance, at least with respect to simple single-letter or single-word representations of text. This notion is bolstered by the fact that young children often make spontaneous mirror-reversals of single letters when learning to read and write [1–4]. Typical errors include reading or writing 'b' for 'd' or transposing the position of letters in a word as in 'was' for 'saw', but also include mirror-reversals of other letters that do not form a new letter upon reversal (e.g., 'a'). Left-right mirror reversal errors are more common than up-down errors [1,5,6]. Confusions between mirror images of letters and letter-like symbols occur when recalling symbols from memory as in writing [7], but also for matching tasks, where a child is asked to pick out a symbol that looks exactly like a target that is continuously visible, even if given explicit instructions and training to not select the mirror image [4]. These results suggest some degree of left-right mirror-invariance in children (see also [8]), which may account for why the left-right mirrored text in Figure 1B may seem easier to read than up-down mirrored text in Figure 1C [9,10].

Initially, however, mirror-reversal errors in children were not thought to be the result of normal developmental or general perceptual process; rather, reading and writing errors were seen as diagnostic of disorders that could persist into adolescence and adulthood. Consistent mirror-reversal errors in identification and reading were called strephosymbolia, meaning "letter turning" [11–15]. Throughout the 20th century, researchers were interested in mirror-reversals in reading and writing as diagnostic features of some disability that predicted good and poor adult readers. Jastak [16] reviewed 170 papers already published by the early 1930s on reading difficulties and their purported causes. We examine several proffered explanations for why mirror-reversals occur any why they may occur more often in poor readers to get a flavor of direction of research at the time and subsequent trends. One theory posited that mirror-reversal errors are perceptual in nature, perhaps having to do with early visual processing of orientation or spatial perception that is underdeveloped or deficient [17–22]. Others suggested possible physiological underpinnings [12,23], differences in memory capacity or ability [24,25], differences in eye movements or oculomotor control [26–28], and differences in mental imagery ability [29]. Attempts had also been made to connect mirror-reversal errors and reading ability more generally to handedness [27,30,31], dyslexia (e.g., that individuals with dyslexia were more fluent at reading and writing inverted and mirrored text than normals, [32–34]), and intelligence [35]. Part of the impetus for considering mirror-reversal errors as symptomatic of disorders were reports of acquired mirror-writing and reading after stroke or injury [36–40] and Gerstmann's syndrome [41,42], of which left-right confusion is a symptom [43,44]. These lines of research emphasized mirror-reversal errors, and therefore mirror-invariance, or an inability to discriminate between left-right mirrored images as an acquired perceptual deficiency.

However, it is ultimately very difficult to conclude anything diagnostic in terms of reading disorders based on reading reversal errors made at a young age [6,45–47]. Nearly all children make reversal errors when learning to read in English [5,48,49]. In addition, mirror reversals of letters are not the most common sort of error in children learning to read [27] (although see [50]), and the amount of reversal errors that children make gradually decreases with age until they almost disappear by age 10 [48,51–53] (although see [54]). Relatively few mirror writing errors occur in children who learn a language in which facing direction does not distinguish between characters, like Japanese [55]. Furthermore, adults also make similar mirror-reversal errors when familiar characters are replaced with reversible, unfamiliar, letter-like symbols [17]. As we will discuss in greater detail later, illiterate adults make the same sorts of mistakes as children [56]. Taken together, these results suggest that there is nothing unusual about mirror-reversal errors in reading and writing, either for children or for adults. One exception may be in the case of dyslexia, where reversal errors may persist for longer [32,57–61].

Towards the latter half of the 20th century, theories for explaining mirror-reversals shifted to attentional and learning-based approaches [48,62]. Some of these ideas had been suggested early on [63,64], but were not popular. According to these perceptual learning accounts, mirror-reversal errors are due to a failure in recognizing facing direction as a relevant stimulus dimension. Gibson, et al. [48] argued that the knowledge of the relevance of this dimension is acquired when learning how to read. That is, learning to read is a perceptual learning problem that requires learning which features are relevant for letter identification, including the facing direction of 2-D symbols [65,66]. This is a matter of feature selection, not feature detection. Mirror images are readily discriminable and look different when presented simultaneously, even for children [67–70] (although see [71]). With age, children learn to discriminate between and remember different types of mirror-symmetric objects [71,72]. Mirror confusions arise because children have not learned that when a letter is reflected or rotated, it is called something else [73]: a 'b' is called "dee" when it is reflected about the vertical axis. This is not true for virtually any other objects, for which infants and adults exhibit some amount of mirror- and rotational-invariance.

In the natural world, there are few objects whose left-right directionality matters for identification—whether you see a tree or car from one side or the other, it is still the same object. Observers have difficulty in distinguishing between previously seen scenes and mirror-reflected images of those scenes in memory tasks [74]. One exception may be the crescent moon, which is illuminated from different sides depending on whether it is new or old, but observers seem not to internalize this difference or remember it in memory tasks [75]. It is with some irony that some of the simple heuristics for determining whether the moon is waxing or waning involve mirror-reflected letters (i.e., in the northern hemisphere, if the moon is shaped like a 'p' it is progressing—waxing, and like a 'q' it is quiescing—waning). Certain man-made artifacts do have distinctive facing directions such as the faces on coins, but these are also notoriously misremembered [76,77]. In fact, Latin letters seem to be one of the few examples where facing direction is a distinguishing feature that we must remember for identification. One exception may be navigation, relative position, and the representation of space (egocentric and allocentric)—it is important to know whether your home is on the left or the right side of the street, whether the train is facing in the correct direction of travel, or which way to turn if you are in a maze [78]. Based on similar observations, Corballis and Beale [79] proposed that mirror discriminability emerges from first acquiring left-right discriminability in the course of learning to distinguish left and right on our own bodies before applying it to the world, objects, and ultimately letters. However, environments are rarely perfectly symmetrical and illiterate adults have no difficulty distinguishing between the sides of their body or navigating in the world, but still make more mirror-reversal errors than literate adults [56,80].

Learning to read calls to attention the fact that facing direction is an important distinguishing feature for a certain class of objects. When one learns to read, one therefore loses mirror-invariance, at least with respect to letters in a reading context. Several studies have indeed found that most mirror-reversal errors occur for children between three and four years of age and the number of errors gradually decreases until about age 10 when performance reaches adult levels [48,62,81]. For age-matched children, weak readers make more errors overall and more of those errors are reversal errors than strong readers [82,83]. Likewise, children for whom learning to read has been deferred by a year make more reversal errors than children of the same age who have started to learn to read [52]. The act of learning to read reduces these errors not solely because they have become more proficient in reading, but because they have improved in discriminating between mirror-symmetric objects.

One of the more compelling tests of this hypothesis has been the investigation of mirror-reversal errors in illiterate and ex-illiterate individuals. Danziger and Pederson [84] tested 10 different language communities for mirror-discriminability of abstract line figures. Literates in almost all tested languages were more sensitive to these differences than illiterates. The one exception were readers of Tamil, a language that has no enantiomorphs (mirror-reversed letters), who were as poor at the task as illiterate individuals. In a follow-up study, it was found that individuals who spoke only Tamil were worse at this task than those who were familiar with both Tamil and a second language that used the Latin alphabet [85]. It was therefore not specific exposure to language in general that led to a loss of mirror-generalization (and therefore a reduction in mirror-reversal errors), but, rather, exposure to a specific stimulus class for which facing direction was a non-accidental, identifying feature. In a more comprehensive study comparing illiterate, ex-illiterate, and literate adults, participants had to sort cards with pictures of circles with a diagonal drawn through them based on either the size of the circle or the orientation of the diagonal [56]. Sometimes, the second feature was uninformative (e.g., small and large circles with vertical lines); sometimes, the second feature was redundant (e.g., all small circles also had left-tilted lines); and sometimes the features were orthogonal to each other such that if the task was to sort based on the orientation of the lines, both small and large circles had left-tilted lines. Illiterates made the most errors in the orthogonal condition, indicating that they were unable to ignore the irrelevant feature of stimulus size, even when told to sort based on the orientation of the diagonal. They had no trouble doing this task if the two dimensions were colors and shapes. This suggests that the effect of literacy is attentional and not perceptual: ex-illiterates and literates were able to perform the task well. It also illustrates that just a small amount of training (ex-illiterates had taken a few courses as adults) could learn that facing direction was a relevant feature rather quickly. Importantly, this effect was observed as a function of reading experience, not instructional manipulation within the experiment. When given more explicit instructions and training trials to point out mirror symmetry and how it can be used to perform the task, illiterates still made errors. In a different study, illiterates, ex-illiterates, and literates performed a same-different matching task with pseudo-words made from letter strings, false fonts (letter-like symbols), and pictures [86]. Illiterates showed no response time difference between normal and mirrored images when the response was "same" for any of the stimulus types. Ex-illiterates and literates, however, were slower at responding "same" to mirror images, with the largest difference being for literates responding to pseudo-words (e.g., "iblo oldi"). This finding is taken to show that, with literacy, the visual system loses some mirror symmetry invariance, especially for letter strings (see also [87]).

Illiteracy and poor reading proficiency not only lead to mirror-reversal errors in identifying and copying letters, but also result in errors for non-letter objects. For example, poor readers tend to make left-right reversals in reassembling matchstick figures from memory [88] and in remembering the facing direction of shapes and asymmetrical figures [89]. The detection of mirror symmetry of figures can also be negatively primed by briefly presented mirror-symmetric letters [90]. This negative priming effect increases with age [91], suggesting that it is the result of inhibition of a mirror generalization process acquired during reading. Recently, Dehaene and colleagues have summarized these results as the "neuronal recycling hypothesis" [92–96]. According to this hypothesis, cultural acquisitions (such as reading) must find a "neuronal niche" in pre-existing, perhaps evolutionarily determined, cortical organization structures. New functions are mapped onto structures that subserved evolutionary older functions, sometimes resulting in small functional losses as those older functions are "overwritten". This may include a repurposing of face-selective neurons for word recognition, resulting in neural competition and left-lateralized word processing (visual word form area, VWFA) and consequently right-lateralized face processing [93,94,97–100]. For a review of the implications and predictions of this idea, see [92,101]. To test this hypothesis, Kolinsky and Fernandes [102] showed illiterates, ex-literates, and literates two sequential pictures of objects and asked them to say whether they were the same or different, ignoring inversions (planar rotations) and mirror reflections (rotations about the vertical axis). Accuracy improved as a function of literacy. Importantly, reaction time for saying "same" for illiterates was no different for identical, rotated, or mirror-reflected objects. However, for ex-literates and literates, reaction times were fastest for second presentations of identical objects, slower for mirror-reflected objects, and slowest for rotated objects. Similar to [86], literacy in adult readers disrupts mirror generalization for objects and abstract geometric shapes, interfering with non-linguistic object recognition. Literacy also has a greater effect on the ability to make mirror-image discriminations than on rotation or orientation-based discriminations [87]. This difference may reflect the special kinds of features that are learned in literacy (i.e., discriminating 'b' from 'd'), although it should be pointed out that 'b' and 'p' are planar rotations that also must be distinguished.

At the same time, adults who are proficient readers often still make reversal errors with novel objects and symbols [17] (although more errors are typically made about an object's axis rather than left-right reflection [103]), suggesting that the unlearning of mirror generalization is somewhat stimulus- or at least domain-specific [33,104,105]. Even for letter stimuli, mirror generalization may be inhibited or unlearned only for certain letters (those that reverse to other letters) and not others [106]. Likewise, training to read mirror-reversed text made up of a specific subset of letters does not transfer to new words composed of unstudied letters [107,108]. It is therefore interesting to examine the extent to which mirror generalization still persists after learning to read.

Acquiring literacy may have a general effect on holistic processing of stimuli. For example, illiterates tend to rely on more holistic processing of faces and show greater influence of irrelevant, aligned facial features on task-specific features [109]. Mirror-reversal errors may arise due to different encoding strategies, in particular, a greater reliance on holistic visual coding of the letters or words than on analytic coding of individual features to allow for greater letter discriminability. For example, poor readers also make more errors in memory for relative spatial positions and orientations of objects [89,110]. Learning to read may therefore engage a more analytic form of processing by which individual letters are identified and special attention is paid to the distinguishing features of, for example, mirror-reversible letters [104,111]. As a result, reading upside-down text (i.e., rotated 180°) may become more difficult with reading experience [112]. Another example of such holistic processing occurs in three- and four-year-old children who were taught to discriminate between differently oriented U-shaped figures [113]. They were readily able to learn the difference between upward and downward facing shapes, but had difficulty with left-right discriminations. Training on this task becomes easier until age 10, when performance stabilizes and resembles that of adults. The largest increase in performance occurs around ages five or six when children learn to read. Similar results obtain for oblique discrimination (/ vs. \), although the results depend on how the stimuli are presented, simultaneously or one at a time, side-by-side, or one above the other [1,67,114–121]. Adults do not show as many errors, but show similar patterns in reaction time, such that same-different judgments on left-right mirror symmetric U-shaped objects are slower than for up-down mirror symmetric objects [122] (see [120] for a review). Children can learn to make left-right mirror discriminations at a young age if given detailed feedback [7,123–125]. However, these results are task dependent, with some tasks in which mirror discriminations must be learned being harder than others [69,115,123]. Overall, children, even before they learn to read, can use orientation and facing direction as a form cue, but it is not the most salient feature, especially when contour and color information can be used instead [126–130]. In all of the above examples, learning to identify and differentiate letters and letter-like forms occurs by focusing attention on specific stimulus features, that is, a transition to a more analytic processing style. These effects, however, appear to be domain- and stimulus-specific as opposed to a broad change in how all objects are represented by the visual system. Furthermore, a general loss of mirror-invariance (or, equivalently, a gain of mirror-discriminability) does not explain why different kinds of transformations of text (left-right mirroring, up-down mirroring, and 180° rotation) result in varying reading difficulty.

We began this article by making the observation that when an entire word or sentence is mirrored first left-right then up-down (or rotated 180°), it is easier to read than when it is mirrored only once. Most of the studies considered thus far have focused on mirror-reversals of single letters, either viewed individually or in the context of a word. There is reason to believe that different processes may be involved in the identification of individual rotated characters or symbols in contrast to reading of rotated or inverted text [131]. For example, in reading passages of text, reading difficulty increases as a function of orientation away from vertical, either upright or upside-down [132–135]. In the following description of results, we will follow Kolers in using "rotation" to refer to rotations in the plane, that is, about the depth axis, "reflection" or "mirroring" to refer to rotations about the vertical axis, and "inversion" to refer to rotations about the horizontal axis.

To our knowledge, Kolers' work in the 1960s is the first systematic investigation of the effect of a large number of geometric transformations on reading speed as a function of practice [136]. In addition to normal text and the three types of transformations mentioned above, reading speed was also examined for text in which each letter was individually reflected about the vertical axis prior to application of the other kinds of transformations. On the first day, it took approximately one minute to read aloud as quickly and accurately as possible 25 lines of the normal (untransformed) text, three minutes to read rotated text and normal text with individual letters left-right reflected, and 4.5–5.5 min to read all other types of transformed text. Participants practiced reading for eight days and on the eighth day showed improvement with all types of transformations. Reading time of normal text with individual letters reversed improved from 3 to 2 minutes, reading time of rotated text improved from 3 to 2.5 min, and all other transformations improved from 4.5–5.5 to 3–3.5 min. Dividing the subjects by familiarity with a language in which text is read right-to-left such as Hebrew or Arabic, it was found that some of those subjects took less time to read left-right mirrored text than inverted (up-down mirrored) text. In a separate study, individuals with familiarity with one of those languages read mirrored text faster than those who only knew English, suggesting that reading direction practice may interact with reading speed in a different language [137]. However, the results were not clear-cut as native speakers of Hebrew who were familiar with English showed a different pattern, with left-right mirrored English text being read the slowest (7 min on the first day and 3.5 min on the eighth), while rotated and inverted text were read faster, but at comparable speeds (5 min on the first day and about 3 min on the last) [136]. Both rotated and mirrored text were read right-to-left so differences in reading time could not solely be explained by reading direction familiarity.

Subsequent work examining training and transfer in English speakers between different types of transformations found that learning to read mirrored text was easiest to do, irrespective of the type of text practiced during training [138]. That is, training on any type of transformed text had almost the same effect on subsequent transfer to mirrored text during testing as initially practicing with mirrored text. Interestingly, when an outlier in transfer from training with normal text with letters left-right reversed to rotated text is excluded, transfer to rotated text is just as good as to mirrored text. The measure used was percentage of transfer from training to test, not reading speed during test. Absolute reading speed was considered a biased measure of trainability because it failed to account for differences in initial difficulty in reading the different transformation types. Therefore, although normal text with letters left-right reversed was fastest to read during test (after normal, un-transformed text) at 3.24 min on average, there was greater transfer (as measured by a difference in reading time before and after training normalized by the difference in reading time between when training and testing with the same transformation type) to mirrored, reversed, and reversed text with individual letters reflected when averaging across training type. That is, learning to read those text transformations was more trainable. When compared to a pre-training baseline, the reading speed of inverted text improved at almost twice the rate of rotated text, but this was likely due to the relatively faster rate at which participants read rotated text before training. There was no correlation, however, between training proficiency and difficulty of the training material. The largest number of geometrical reading errors (e.g., confusing 'b' for 'p') during training occurred not in the inverted, but in the mirrored text condition, while the least number of errors (about half as many) occurred when training with rotated text.

Across these several studies, it is difficult to extract any meaningful patterns. Kolers and Perkins were not able to find a simple set of transformation types whose elements could be combined either additively or multiplicatively in order to predict reading errors, reading time, or trainability [9,136,138]. Combinations of different kinds of rotations did not increase reading difficulty in a linear way, suggesting that readers of geometrically transformed text are not performing sequences of mental rotations or transformations on letters or words in order to read them. Further evidence that readers are not performing rotations of individual letters comes from the fact that when single letters embedded in words are mirror-reversed, reading time is longer than if the entire word is mirror-reversed [9,10,136,139]. Observers are in fact able to identify a rotated letter even before determining whether it is mirror-reflected or not, suggesting that they do not need to perform mental rotation for identification or naming of simple patterns [140–145] and even for novel letter-like shapes [66] (although they can mentally rotate the images if the task demands it [146]). Unlike for objects [147,148], identification time for letters does not depend on letter orientation. It should be noted that while these early studies found no effect of orientation on letter identification reaction time, the data were noisy, sometimes effects were found [141], and single letter identification is not rotation-invariant when accuracy is the dependent measure and presentation times are very brief (<30 ms) [149] or when observers are asked to make same-different judgments of rotated letters [150]. Inverted, reflected, and rotated letter recognition may therefore involve some sort of corrective process such as mental rotation either before or concurrent with identification [135,151–153], but not necessarily performed on a letter-by-letter basis [138]. This may explain why inverted and mirrored texts are more difficult to read than upright and why, when the orientation of a letter is unknown (whether 'p' is upright, rotated, mirrored, or inverted), there is a bias for preferring upright or rotated interpretations [9,10]. Note, however, that only the 180° rotated text can match normal text with a rotation in the plane; left-right and up-down mirrored text must be rotated through the plane in order to return to their normal orientation. There may therefore be something special about the nature of 180° rotated text (Figure 1D) that contributes to its relative readability. Indeed, Kolers suggested that each type of transformation may involve its own decoding mechanism: if correct letter orientation were simply a matter of applying some common mental operation (e.g., mental rotation), then the frequency of errors of mistaking 'u' and 'n' and 'f' and 't', for example, would be the same for all kinds of text transformations, but that is not the case [10].

Another reason why certain transformations are harder to read than others can be explained by familiarity with reading direction. Individuals familiar with Arabic or Hebrew are able to read mirrored text faster than those only familiar with English [136]. There may also be an interaction with writing direction familiarity: letter-facing direction may partially be encoded by pairing motor actions (writing) with orientation direction. When adults learn new characters, they remember their proper facing directions better if they have to write the characters by hand rather than typing them [154]. The production of mirror-reversals during writing, however, is beyond the scope of this review. Mirror-writing involves qualitatively different processes from mirror-reading since, in reading, the letters are continuously visible, but in writing the correct facing direction of letters must be retrieved from memory. For some recent work on mirror-writing see [3,155–161].

Finally, we consider several other factors that may contribute to differential reading times for types of text transformations. One possibility is that difficulty in reading mirrored and inverted text may arise due to temporary lapses of frame of reference—i.e., forgetting which way the entire sentence is oriented [162]. This is particularly problematic if letters face one way and scanning direction is reversed [9]. A letter's facing direction therefore depends on reading direction: the symbol 'b' can be either the letter 'b', 'p', 'q', or 'd' depending on which transformation was applied. When one encounters that symbol, there may be a temporary lapse in the frame of reference rendering the rest of the sentence difficult to read and the reader has to reorient to remember not only which way letters are facing, but also in which direction they should be reading [4,149]. When presented with an inverted word in which several letters are upright, it is difficult to notice that some of the letters are actually upright [163–165]. This has been described as a Thatcher effect for letters [166]. The explanation is that inverted letters become egocentrically upright when we begin to read the word and, in losing the frame of reference, nothing appears out of the ordinary when we encounter an upright letter. When most of the word is upright however, and in the standard egocentric frame, the inverted letters stick out just like inverted parts of a face in the Thatcher illusion.

The idea of a frame of reference can also apply to objects: although it is true that we can recognize a picture of a hammer and a mirror-image of the same hammer equally well, the hammer still has some directionality associated with it [167,168] and a canonical orientation [147,148,169–172]. This notion is supported by the fact that mirror-reversals of letters of children in matching and copying tasks are asymmetric—upright letters are rarely mismatched with their mirror images, but mirror-reversed letters are often copied and matched to normal letters [4]. Young children who have not yet learned to read, make more orientation errors in copying, drawing from memory, and matching shapes with no inherent directionality (e.g., a stretched-out diamond) than with objects, e.g., a spoon, [173].

Under this view, in acquiring literacy, a reader develops templates or schema for letters in canonical orientations [174]. A letter's orientation can be used to determine the frame of reference for an entire word or sentence. For example, an inverted 'A' may provide a cue that the entire text is inverted. Reading of inverted, mirrored, or rotated text involves a detection or an alignment of an appropriate frame of reference [143,167,175–177]. As a result, response time to individual letters at different orientations is predicted by the orientation of the previously seen letter [178]. In the context of an entire word or sentence, therefore, moving from one letter to another could facilitate the maintenance of a consistent frame of reference (as determined by the previous letter) until a reversible letter is encountered, which leads to confusion. When combined with changes in reading direction, this creates additional opportunities for confusion. Although note that the text that 180° rotated text (Figure 1D), which is read right-to-left is easier to read than the up-down mirror reflected text (Figure 1C) which is read left-to-right. Reading direction on its own therefore does not account for the differences in reading difficulty. It is interesting to note that in Kolers' original experiments in which subjects practiced reading aloud geometrically transformed text, the text was transformed one line at a time [136]. For example, 180° rotated text was not read from the bottom of the page to the top, but was still read top-to-bottom because each line was rotated independently. This may have complicated the results by putting into conflict the frame of the text on the whole page with that of a single line. To our knowledge, an experiment that dissociates these confounders has yet to be performed.

The notion of a frame of reference can apply more generally to how individuals understand reflections in mirrors [179,180]. Although we have been describing some text transformations as "left-right mirror reversals", a mirror does not reverse left-right, but through an axis perpendicular to the mirror, i.e., front-to-back [181–187]. When examining their own reflections in mirrors, observers tend describe them as identical instead of reversed or opposite, suggesting an important role for an exocentric (as opposed to egocentric) frame of reference [179]. Familiarity with certain frames of reference over others may account for why the recognition of one's own face is better when it is shown mirrored, while the faces of others are better recognized when shown in the manner in which we are used to seeing them (i.e., not mirrored) [188–192]. In general, however, naïve understanding of how reflections work and appear is quite poor [193–197]. It is possible that given an appropriate frame of reference with many cues to text direction, such as seeing a mirrored image of a person holding a sheet of text, may facilitate the maintenance of a consistent frame of reference during reading. In contrast, in all experiments reviewed here, a reader is presented with mirrored text on a sheet of paper, which, out of context and at odds with the rest of the un-mirrored environment (e.g., their hands holding the paper, the table at which they sit, etc.), may present an especially difficult situation in which the appropriate frame of reference must be maintained for reading. To our knowledge, no experiments have examined the effect of scene and environment context on the reading of transformed text.

We began this article with the observation that certain geometric transformations of text are easier to read than others. We have gone over several lines of research that speak to why mirrored text is more difficult to read: confusions in facing-direction of mirror-symmetric letters like 'b' and 'd', loss of frame of reference, incomplete loss of mirror-invariance (or, conversely, development of mirror-discriminability), etc. Unfortunately, there is not as of yet a conclusive explanation for why text that is reflected twice is easier to read than text that is only reflected once [9]. Part of the effect may be due to reading and writing direction familiarity or the fact that twice-reflected text is equivalent to a 180-degree rotation in the plane and there may be something special about that transformation as opposed to others. What is clear however is that our technological age has taken image transformations out of the reflecting pool and looking glass, and placed them at our fingertips with our webcams, smart-phones, and image processing software packages. This digital proximity reminds us that our curiosity and empirical exploration of symmetries in our environment and in the legibility of text has a long and robust history.

Acknowledgments: This work is supported by the National Eye Institute (1F32EY025520-01A1) to Gennady Erlikhman and the National Science Foundation (NSF 1632738 and NSF 1632849) to Gideon Paul Caplovitz.

Author Contributions: Gennady Erlikhman, Lars Strother, Iskra Barzakov and Gideon Paul Caplovitz wrote the paper.

Conflicts of Interest: The authors declare no conflict of interest.

References

1. Cairns, N.U.; Steward, M.S. Young children's orientation of letters as a function of axis of symmetry and stimulus alignment. *Child Dev.* **1970**, *41*, 993–1002. [CrossRef] [PubMed]
2. Cornell, J.M. Spontaneous mirror-writing in children. *Can. J. Psychol.* **1985**, *39*, 174–179. [CrossRef]
3. Fischer, J.-P.; Koch, A.-M. Mirror writing in typically developing children: A first longitudinal study. *Cogn. Dev.* **2016**, *38*, 114–124. [CrossRef]
4. Frith, U. Why do children reverse letters? *Br. J. Psychol.* **1971**, *62*, 459–468. [CrossRef] [PubMed]
5. Davidson, H.P. A study of the confusing letters b, d, p, and q. *Pedagog. Semin. J. Genet. Psychol.* **1935**, *42*, 458–468. [CrossRef]
6. Liberman, I.Y.; Shankweiler, D.; Orlando, C. Letter confusions and reversals of sequence in the beginning reader: Implications for Orton's theory of developmental dyslexia. *Cortex* **1971**, *7*, 127–142. [CrossRef]
7. Casey, M.B. Individual differences in use of left-right visual cues: A reexamination of mirror-image confusions in preschoolers. *Dev. Psychol.* **1984**, *20*, 551–559. [CrossRef]
8. Bornstein, M.H.; Gross, C.G.; Wolf, J.Z. Perceptual similarity of mirror images in infancy. *Cognition* **1978**, *6*, 89–116. [CrossRef]
9. Kolers, P.A.; Perkins, D.N. Orientation of letters and their speed of recognition. *Percept. Psychophys.* **1969**, *5*, 275–280. [CrossRef]
10. Kolers, P.A.; Perkins, D.N. Orientation of letters and errors in their recognition. *Percept. Psychophys.* **1969**, *5*, 265–269. [CrossRef]
11. Orton, S.T. "Word-blindness" in school children. *Arch. Neurol. Psychiatry* **1925**, *14*, 581–615. [CrossRef]
12. Orton, S.T. Specific reading disability—Strephosimbolia. *J. Am. Med. Assoc.* **1928**, *90*, 1095–1099. [CrossRef]
13. Geschwind, N. Why Orton was right. *Ann. Dyslexia* **1982**, *32*, 13–30. [CrossRef]
14. Orton, S.T. *Reading, Writing and Speech Problems in Children*; William Warder (W. W.) Norton & Company: New York, NY, USA, 1937.
15. Zangwill, O.L. *Cerebral Dominance and Its Relation to Psychological Function*; Oliver & Boyd: Oxford, UK, 1960.
16. Jastak, J. Interferences in reading. *Psychol. Bull.* **1934**, *31*, 244–272. [CrossRef]

17. Krise, M. An experimental investigation of theories of reversals in reading. *J. Educ. Psychol.* **1952**, *43*, 408–422. [CrossRef]
18. Krise, M. Reversals in reading: A problem in space perception? *Elem. Sch. J.* **1949**, *49*, 278–284. [CrossRef]
19. Money, J. *Reading Disability*; Money, J., Ed.; The Johns Hopkins Press: Baltimore, MD, USA, 1962.
20. Fildes, L.G. A psychological inquiry into the nature of the condition known as congenital word-blindness. *Brain* **1921**, *44*, 286–307. [CrossRef]
21. Gates, A.I. A study of reading and spelling with special reference to disability. *J. Educ. Res.* **1922**, *6*, 12–24. [CrossRef]
22. Goins, J.T. *Visual Perceptual Abilities and Early Reading Progress*; The University of Chicago Press: Chicago, IL, USA, 1958.
23. Betts, E.A. Physiological approach to the analysis of reading disabilities. In *Educational Research Bulletin*; Ohio State University: Columbus, OH, USA, 1934; Volume 13.
24. Schubenz, S.; Buchwald, R. Untersuchungen zur Legasthenie. I. Die Beziehung der Legasthenie zur Auftretenshäufigkeit der Buchstaben des Alphabets in der Deutschen Sprache. *Z. Exp. Angew. Psychol.* **1964**, *11*, 155–165.
25. Petty, M.C. An experimental study of certain factors influencing reading readiness. *J. Educ. Psychol.* **1939**, *30*, 215–230. [CrossRef]
26. Rayner, K. The role of eye movements in learning to read and reading disability. *Remedial Spec. Educ.* **1985**, *6*, 53–60. [CrossRef]
27. Monroe, M. *Children Who Cannot Read*; University of Chicago Press: Chicago, IL, USA, 1932.
28. Stein, J.; Talcott, J.; Witton, W. The sensorimotor basis of developmental dyslexia. In *Dyslexia: Theory and Good Practice*; Fawcett, A.J., Ed.; Whurr: London, UK, 2001; pp. 65–88.
29. Silver, A.A.; Hagin, R.A. Visual perception in children with reading disabilities. In *Early Experience and Visual Information Processing in Perceptual and Reading Disorders*; Young, F.A., Ed.; National Academy of Sciences: Washington, DC, USA, 1970; pp. 445–456.
30. Annett, M. Reading upside down and mirror text in groups differing for right minus left hand skill. *Eur. J. Cogn. Psychol.* **1991**, *3*, 363–377. [CrossRef]
31. Woody, C.; Phillips, A.J. The effects of handedness on reversals in reading. *J. Educ. Res.* **1934**, *27*, 651–662. [CrossRef]
32. Lachmann, T.; Geyer, T. Letter reversals in dyslexia: Is the case really closed? A critical review and conclusions. *Psychol. Sci.* **2003**, *45*, 50–72.
33. Lachmann, T.; van Leeuwen, C. Paradoxical enhancement of letter recognition in developmental dyslexia. *Dev. Neuropsychol.* **2007**, *31*, 61–77. [CrossRef]
34. Gross-Glenn, K.; Lewis, D.C.; Smith, S.D.; Lubs, H.A. Phenotype of adult familial dyslexia: Reading of visually transformed texts and nonsense passages. *Int. J. Neurosci.* **1985**, *28*, 49–59. [CrossRef] [PubMed]
35. Gordon, H. Left-handedness and mirror writing, especially among defective children. *Brain* **1921**, *43*, 313–368. [CrossRef]
36. Balfour, S.; Borthwick, S.; Cubelli, R.; Della Sala, S. Mirror writing and reversing single letters in stroke patients and normal elderly. *J. Neurol.* **2007**, *254*, 436–441. [CrossRef] [PubMed]
37. Gottfried, J.A.; Sancar, F.; Chatterjee, A. Acquired mirror writing and reading: Evidence for reflected graphemic representations. *Neuropsychologia* **2003**, *41*, 96–107. [CrossRef]
38. Heilman, K.M.; Howell, G.; Valenstein, E.; Rothi, L. Mirror-reading and writing in association with right-left spatial disorientation. *J. Neurol. Neurosurg. Psychiatry* **1980**, *43*, 774–780. [CrossRef] [PubMed]
39. Paradowski, W.; Ginzburg, M. Mirror writing and hemiplegia. *Percept. Mot. Skills* **1971**, *32*, 617–618. [CrossRef] [PubMed]
40. Turnbull, O.H.; Mccarthy, R.A. Failure to discriminate between mirror-image objects: A case of viewpoint-independent object recognition? *Neurocase* **1996**, *2*, 63–72. [CrossRef]
41. Lebrun, Y. Gerstmann's syndrome. *J. Neurolinguistics* **2005**, *18*, 317–326. [CrossRef]
42. Gerstmann, J. Syndrome of finger agnosia, disorientation from right and left, agraphia and acalculia. *Neurol. Psychiatry* **1940**, *44*, 398–408. [CrossRef]
43. Mayer, E.; Martory, M.D.; Pegna, A.J.; Landis, T.; Delavelle, J.; Annoni, J.M. A pure case of Gerstmann syndrome with a subangular lesion. *Brain* **1999**, *122*, 1107–1120. [CrossRef] [PubMed]
44. Benton, A.L. Gerstmann's syndrome. *Arch. Neurol.* **1992**, *49*, 445–447. [CrossRef] [PubMed]

45. Stanovich, K.E. Explaining the variance in reading ability in terms of psychological processes: What have we learned? *Ann. Dyslexia* **1985**, *35*, 67–96. [CrossRef] [PubMed]
46. Wolff, P.H.; Melngailis, I. Reversing letters and reading transformed text in dyslexia: A reassessment. *Read. Writ.* **1996**, *8*, 341–355. [CrossRef]
47. Vellutino, F. *Dyslexia: Theory and Research*; Massachusetts Institute of Technology (MIT) Press: Cambridge, MD, USA, 1981.
48. Gibson, E.J.; Gibson, J.J.; Pick, A.D.; Osser, H. A developmental study of the discrimination of letter-like forms. *J. Comp. Physiol. Psychol.* **1962**, *55*, 897–906. [CrossRef] [PubMed]
49. Teegarden, L. Tests for the tendency to reversal in reading. *J. Educ. Res.* **1933**, *27*, 81–97. [CrossRef]
50. Ilg, F.; Ames, L.B. Developmental trends in reading behavior. *Pedagog. Semin. J. Genet. Psychol.* **1950**, *76*, 219–312. [CrossRef]
51. Aaron, P.G.; Malatesha, R.N. Discrimination of mirror image stimuli in children. *Neuropsychologia* **1974**, *12*, 549–551. [CrossRef]
52. Hildreth, G. Reversals in reading and writing. *J. Educ. Psychol.* **1934**, *25*, 1–20. [CrossRef]
53. Cole, L. *The Improvement of Reading*; Farrar and Rinehart: New York, NY, USA, 1938.
54. Staller, J.; Sekuler, R.W. Children read normal and reversed letters: A simple test of reading skill. *Q. J. Exp. Psychol.* **1975**, *27*, 539–550. [CrossRef]
55. Makita, K. The rarity of reading disability in Japanese children. *Am. J. Orthopsychiatry* **1968**, *38*, 599–614. [CrossRef] [PubMed]
56. Kolinsky, R.; Verhaeghe, A.; Fernandes, T.; Mengarda, E.J.; Grimm-Cabral, L.; Morais, J. Enantiomorphy through the looking glass: Literacy effects on mirror-image discrimination. *J. Exp. Psychol. Gen.* **2011**, *140*, 210–238. [CrossRef] [PubMed]
57. Badian, N.A. Does a visual-orthographic deficit contribute to reading disability? *Ann. Dyslexia* **2005**, *55*, 28–52. [CrossRef] [PubMed]
58. Willows, D.M.; Terepocki, M. The relation of reversal errors to reading disabilities. In *Visual Processes in Reading and Reading Disabilities*; Willows, D.M., Kruk, R.S., Corcos, E., Eds.; Lawrence Erlbaum Associates: Hillsdale, NJ, USA, 1993; pp. 31–56.
59. Rusiak, P.; Lachmann, T.; Jaskowski, P.; Van Leeuwen, C. Mental rotation of letters and shapes in developmental dyslexia. *Perception* **2007**, *36*, 617–631. [CrossRef] [PubMed]
60. Corballis, M.C.; Macadie, L.; Beale, I.L. Mental rotation and visual laterality in normal and reading disabled children. *Cortex* **1985**, *21*, 225–236. [CrossRef]
61. McMonnies, C.W. Visuo-spatial discrimination and mirror image letter reversals in reading. *J. Am. Optom. Assoc.* **1992**, *63*, 698–704. [PubMed]
62. Gibson, E.J. Learning to read. *Bull. Ort. Soc.* **1965**, *15*, 32–47. [CrossRef]
63. Downey, J. On the reading and writing of mirror-script. *Psychol. Rev.* **1914**, *21*, 408–421. [CrossRef]
64. Stern, W. Uber verlagerte raumformen. *Z. Angew. Psychol.* **1909**, *2*, 498–526.
65. Pick, A. Improvement of visual and tactual form discrimination. *J. Exp. Psychol.* **1965**, *69*, 331–339. [CrossRef] [PubMed]
66. Eley, M.G. Identifying rotated letter-like symbols. *Mem. Cognit.* **1982**, *10*, 25–32. [CrossRef] [PubMed]
67. Bryant, P.E. Perception and memory of the orientation of visually presented lines by children. *Nature* **1969**, *222*, 385–386. [CrossRef]
68. Cronin, V. Mirror-image reversal discrimination in kindergarten and first-grade children. *J. Exp. Child Psychol.* **1967**, *5*, 577–585. [CrossRef]
69. Jeffrey, W.E. Variables in early discrimination learning: I. Motor responses in the training of a left-right discrimination. *Child Dev.* **1958**, *29*, 269–275. [CrossRef] [PubMed]
70. Over, R.; Over, J. Detection and recognition of mirror-image obliques by young children. *J. Comp. Physiol. Psychol.* **1967**, *64*, 467–470. [CrossRef] [PubMed]
71. Bornstein, M.H.; Stiles-Davis, J. Discrimination and memory for symmetry in young children. *Dev. Psychol.* **1984**, *20*, 637–649. [CrossRef]
72. Gregory, E.; Landau, B.; McCloskey, M. Representation of object orientation in children: Evidence from mirror-image confusions. *Vis. Cogn.* **2011**, *19*, 1035–1062. [CrossRef] [PubMed]
73. Bigsby, P. The nature of reversible letter confusions in dyslexic and normal readers: Misperception or mislabelling? *Br. J. Educ. Psychol.* **1985**, *55 Pt 3*, 264–272. [CrossRef] [PubMed]

74. Standing, L.; Conezio, J.; Haber, R.N. Perception and memory for pictures: Single-trial learning of 2500 visual stimuli. *Psychon. Sci.* **1970**, *19*, 73–74. [CrossRef]

75. Martin, M.; Jones, G.V. Memory for orientation in the natural environment. *Appl. Cogn. Psychol.* **1997**, *11*, 279–288. [CrossRef]

76. Nickerson, R.S.; Adams, M.J. Long-term memory for a common. *Cogn. Psychol.* **1979**, *11*, 287–307. [CrossRef]

77. Jones, G.V. Misremembering a common object: When left is not right. *Mem. Cognit.* **1990**, *18*, 174–182. [CrossRef] [PubMed]

78. Spelke, E.; Lee, S.A.; Izard, V. Beyond core knowledge: Natural geometry. *Cogn. Sci.* **2010**, *34*, 863–884. [CrossRef] [PubMed]

79. Corballis, M.C.; Beale, I.L. *The Psychology of Left and Right*; Lawrence Erlbaum Associates, Publishers: Hillsdale, NJ, USA, 1976.

80. Fisher, C.B.; Braine, L.G. Left-right coding in children: implications for adult performance. *Bull. Psychon. Soc.* **1982**, *20*, 305–307. [CrossRef]

81. Davidson, H.P. A study of reversals in young children. *Pedagog. Semin. J. Genet. Psychol.* **1934**, *45*, 452–465. [CrossRef]

82. Cohn, M.; Stricker, G. Reversal errors in strong, average, and weak letter namers. *J. Learn. Disabil.* **1979**, *12*, 533–537. [CrossRef] [PubMed]

83. Terepocki, M.; Kruk, R.S.; Willows, D.M. The incidence and nature of letter orientation errors in reading disability. *J. Learn. Disabil.* **2002**, *35*, 214–233. [CrossRef] [PubMed]

84. Danziger, E.; Pederson, E. Through the looking glass: Literacy, writing systems and mirror image discrimination. *Writ. Lang. Lit.* **1998**, *1*, 153–169. [CrossRef]

85. Pederson, E. Mirror-image discrimination among nonliterate, monoliterate, and biliterate Tamil subjects. *Writ. Lang. Lit.* **2003**, *6*, 71–91. [CrossRef]

86. Pegado, F.; Nakamura, K.; Braga, L.W.; Ventura, P.; Nunes Filho, G.; Pallier, C.; Jobert, A.; Morais, J.; Cohen, L.; Kolinsky, R.; et al. Literacy breaks mirror invariance for visual stimuli: A behavioral study with adult illiterates. *J. Exp. Psychol. Gen.* **2014**, *143*, 887–894. [CrossRef] [PubMed]

87. Fernandes, T.; Kolinsky, R. From hand to eye: The role of literacy, familiarity, graspability, and vision-for-action on enantiomorphy. *Acta Psychol. (Amst.)* **2013**, *142*, 51–61. [CrossRef] [PubMed]

88. Galifret-Granjon, N. Le problème de l'organisation spatiale dans les dyslexies d'évolution. *Enfance* **1951**, *4*, 445–479. [CrossRef] [PubMed]

89. Lyle, J.G.; Goyen, J. Visual recognition, development lag, and strephosymbolia in reading retardation. *J. Abnorm. Psychol.* **1968**, *73*, 25–29. [CrossRef] [PubMed]

90. Borst, J.P.; Nijboer, M.; Taatgen, N.A.; van Rijn, H.; Anderson, J.R. Using data-driven model-brain mappings to constrain formal models of cognition. *PLoS ONE* **2015**, *10*, e0119673. [CrossRef] [PubMed]

91. Ahr, E.; Houdé, O.; Borst, G. Inhibition of the mirror generalization process in reading in school-aged children. *J. Exp. Child Psychol.* **2016**, *145*, 157–165. [CrossRef] [PubMed]

92. Dehaene, S.; Cohen, L. Cultural recycling of cortical maps. *Neuron* **2007**, *56*, 384–398. [CrossRef] [PubMed]

93. Dehaene, S.; Nakamura, K.; Jobert, A.; Kuroki, C.; Ogawa, S.; Cohen, L. Why do children make mirror errors in reading? Neural correlates of mirror invariance in the visual word form area. *Neuroimage* **2010**, *49*, 1837–1848. [CrossRef] [PubMed]

94. Dehaene, S.; Cohen, L.; Morais, J.; Kolinsky, R. Illiterate to literate: Behavioural and cerebral changes induced by reading acquisition. *Nat. Rev. Neurosci.* **2015**, *16*, 234–244. [CrossRef] [PubMed]

95. Dehaene, S. Evolution of human cortical circuits for reading and arithmetic: The "neuronal recycling" hypothesis. In *From Monkey Brain to Human Brain*; Dehaene, S., Duhamel, J.R., Hauser, M., Rizzolatti, G., Eds.; MIT Press: Cambridge, MA, USA, 2005; pp. 133–157.

96. Dehaene, S. *Reading in the Brain: The New Science of How to Read*; Penguin Books: New York, NY, USA, 2010.

97. Cohen, L.; Dehaene, S.; Vinckier, F.; Jobert, A.; Montavont, A. Reading normal and degraded words: Contribution of the dorsal and ventral visual pathways. *Neuroimage* **2008**, *40*, 353–366. [CrossRef] [PubMed]

98. Dehaene, S.; Pegado, F.; Braga, L.W.; Ventura, P.; Nunes Filho, G.; Jobert, A.; Dehaene-Lambertz, G.; Kolinsky, R.; Morais, J.; Cohen, L. How learning to read changes the cortical networks for vision and language. *Science* **2010**, *330*, 1359–1364. [CrossRef] [PubMed]

99. Pegado, F.; Nakamura, K.; Cohen, L.; Dehaene, S. Breaking the symmetry: Mirror discrimination for single letters but not for pictures in the visual word form area. *Neuroimage* **2011**, *55*, 742–749. [CrossRef] [PubMed]

100. Dundas, E.M.; Plaut, D.C.; Behrmann, M. The joint development of hemispheric lateralization for words and faces. *J. Exp. Psychol. Gen.* **2013**, *142*, 348–358. [CrossRef] [PubMed]
101. Behrmann, M.; Plaut, D.C. A vision of graded hemispheric specialization. *Ann. N. Y. Acad. Sci.* **2015**, *1359*, 30–46. [CrossRef] [PubMed]
102. Kolinsky, R.; Fernandes, T. A cultural side effect: Learning to read interferes with identity processing of familiar objects. *Front. Psychol.* **2014**, *5*, 1–11. [CrossRef] [PubMed]
103. Gregory, E.; McCloskey, M. Mirror-image confusions: Implications for representation and processing of object orientation. *Cognition* **2010**, *116*, 110–129. [CrossRef] [PubMed]
104. Lachmann, T.; van Leeuwen, C. Reading as functional coordination: Not recycling but a novel synthesis. *Front. Psychol.* **2014**, *5*, 1–8. [CrossRef] [PubMed]
105. Borst, G.; Ahr, E.; Roell, M.; Houdé, O. The cost of blocking the mirror generalization process in reading: Evidence for the role of inhibitory control in discriminating letters with lateral mirror-image. *Psychon. Bull. Rev.* **2015**, *22*, 228–234. [CrossRef] [PubMed]
106. Perea, M.; Moret-Tatay, C.; Panadero, V. Suppression of mirror generalization for reversible letters: Evidence from masked priming. *J. Mem. Lang.* **2011**, *65*, 237–246. [CrossRef]
107. Masson, M.E. Identification of typographically transformed words: Instance-based skill acquisition. *J. Exp. Psychol. Learn. Mem. Cogn.* **1986**, *12*, 479–488. [CrossRef] [PubMed]
108. Kolers, P.A. Specificity of operations in sentence recognition. *Cogn. Psychol.* **1975**, *7*, 289–306. [CrossRef]
109. Ventura, P.; Fernandes, T.; Cohen, L.; Morais, J.; Kolinsky, R.; Dehaene, S. Literacy acquisition reduces the influence of automatic holistic processing of faces and houses. *Neurosci. Lett.* **2013**, *554*, 105–109. [CrossRef] [PubMed]
110. Kershner, J.R. Rotation of mental images and asymmetries in word recognition in disabled readers. *Can. J. Psychol.* **1979**, *33*, 39–50. [CrossRef] [PubMed]
111. Frith, U. Beneath the surface of developmental dyslexia. *Surface Dyslexia* **1985**, *32*, 301–330.
112. Deich, R.F. Children's perception of differently oriented shapes: Word recognition. *Percept. Mot. Skills* **1971**, *32*, 695–700. [CrossRef] [PubMed]
113. Rudel, R.; Teuber, H.-L. Discrimination of direction of line in children. *J. Comp. Physiol. Psychol.* **1963**, *56*, 892–898. [CrossRef] [PubMed]
114. Barroso, F.; Braine, L.G. "Mirror-image" errors without mirror-image stimuli. *J. Exp. Child Psychol.* **1974**, *18*, 213–225. [CrossRef]
115. Clarke, J.C.; Whitehurst, G.J. Asymmetrical stimulus control and the morror-image problem. *J. Exp. Child Psychol.* **1974**, *17*, 147–166. [CrossRef]
116. Huttenlocher, J. Discrimination of figure orientation: Effects of relative position. *J. Comp. Physiol. Psychol.* **1967**, *63*, 359–361. [CrossRef] [PubMed]
117. Huttenlocher, J. Children's ability to order and orient objects. *Child Dev.* **1967**, *38*, 1169–1176. [CrossRef] [PubMed]
118. Huttenlocher, J. Constructing spatial images: A strategy in reasoning. *Psychol. Rev.* **1968**, *75*, 550–560. [CrossRef]
119. Sekuler, R.W.; Rosenblith, J.F. Discrimination of direction of line and the effect of stimulus alignment. *Psychon. Sci.* **1964**, *1*, 143–144. [CrossRef]
120. Fisher, C.B. The role of stimulus alignment in children's memory for line orientation. *Child Dev.* **1982**, *53*, 1070–1074. [CrossRef] [PubMed]
121. Bornstein, M.H. Perceptual anisotropies in infancy: Ontogenetic origins and implications of inequalities in spatial vision. *Adv. Child Dev. Behav.* **1982**, *16*, 77–123. [PubMed]
122. Sekuler, R.W.; Houlihan, K. Discrimination of mirror-images: Choice time analysis of human adult performance. *Q. J. Exp. Psychol.* **1968**, *20*, 204–207. [CrossRef] [PubMed]
123. Caldwell, E.C.; Hall, V.C. The influence of concept training on letter discrimination. *Child Dev.* **1969**, *40*, 63–71. [CrossRef]
124. Hendrickson, L.N.; Muehl, S. The effect of attention and motor response pretraining on learning to discriminate b and d in kindergarten children. *J. Educ. Psychol.* **1962**, *53*, 236–241. [CrossRef]
125. Koenigsberg, R.S. An evaluation of visual versus sensorimotor methods for improving orientation discrimination of letter reversals by preschool children. *Child Dev.* **1973**, *44*, 764–769. [CrossRef] [PubMed]

126. Owen, D.H. Developmental generality of a form recognition strategy. *J. Exp. Child Psychol.* **1971**, *11*, 194–205. [CrossRef]

127. McGurk, H. The salience of orientation in young children's perception of form. *Child Dev.* **1972**, *43*, 1047–1052. [CrossRef] [PubMed]

128. Watson, J.S. Perception of object orientation in infants. *Merrill-Palmer Q. Behav. Dev.* **1966**, *12*, 73–94.

129. Gellermann, L.W. Form discrimination in chimpanzees and two-year-old children: I. Form (Triangularity) per Se. *J. Genet. Psychol.* **1933**, *42*, 3–27. [CrossRef]

130. Kaufman, N.L. Review of research on reversal errors. *Percept. Mot. Ski.* **1980**, *51*, 55–79. [CrossRef] [PubMed]

131. Koriat, A.; Norman, J. Why is word recognition impaired by disorientation while the identification of single letters is not? *J. Exp. Psychol. Hum. Percept. Perform.* **1989**, *15*, 153–163. [CrossRef] [PubMed]

132. Aulhorn, O. Die Lesegeschwindigkeit als Funktion von Buchstaben und Zeilenlage. *Pflüger's Arch. für die gesamte Physiologie des Menschen und der Tiere* **1948**, *250*, 12–25. [CrossRef]

133. Jordan, K.; Huntsman, L.A. Image rotation of misoriented letter strings: Effects of orientation cuing and repetition. *Percept. Psychophys.* **1990**, *48*, 363–374. [CrossRef] [PubMed]

134. Lavidor, M.; Babkoff, H.; Faust, M. Analysis of standard and non-standard visual word format in the two hemispheres. *Neuropsychologia* **2001**, *39*, 430–439. [CrossRef]

135. Koriat, A.; Norman, J. Reading rotated words. *J. Exp. Psychol. Hum. Percept. Perform.* **1985**, *11*, 490–508. [CrossRef] [PubMed]

136. Kolers, P.A. The recognition of geometrically transformed text. *Percept. Psychophys.* **1968**, *3*, 57–64. [CrossRef]

137. Kolers, P.A. Reading temporally and spatially transformed Text. In *The Psycholinguistic Nature of the Reading Process*; Goodman, K.S., Ed.; Wayne State University Press: Detroit, MI, USA, 1968; pp. 27–40.

138. Kolers, P.A.; Perkins, D.N. Spatial and ordinal components of form perception and literacy. *Cogn. Psychol.* **1975**, *7*, 228–267. [CrossRef]

139. Navon, D. Perception of misoriented words and letter strings. *Can. J. Psychol.* **1978**, *32*, 129–140. [CrossRef] [PubMed]

140. Corballis, M.C.; Nagourney, B.A. Latency to categorize disoriented alphanumeric characters as letters or digits. *J. Psychol.* **1978**, *32*, 186–188. [CrossRef]

141. Corballis, M.C.; Zbrodoff, N.J.; Shetzer, L.I.; Butler, P.B. Decisions about identity and orientation of rotated letters and digits. *Mem. Cognit.* **1978**, *6*, 98–107. [CrossRef] [PubMed]

142. Corballis, M.C.; Macadie, L.; Crotty, A.; Beale, I.L. The naming of disoriented letters by normal and reading-disabled children. *J. Child Psychol. Psychiatry* **1985**, *26*, 929–938. [CrossRef] [PubMed]

143. Simion, F.; Bagnara, S.; Roncato, S.; Umiltá, C. Transformation processes upon the visual code. *Percept. Psychophys.* **1982**, *31*, 13–25. [CrossRef] [PubMed]

144. White, M.J. Naming and categorization of tilted alphanumeric characters do not require mental rotation. *Bull. Psychon. Soc.* **1980**, *15*, 153–156. [CrossRef]

145. Cooper, L.A.; Shepard, R.N. Chronometric studies of the rotation of mental images. In *Visual Information Processing*; Chase, W.G., Ed.; Academic Press: Oxford, UK, 1973; pp. 75–176.

146. Corballis, M.C.; McLaren, R. Winding one's ps and qs: Mental rotation and mirror-image discrimination. *J. Exp. Psychol. Hum. Percept. Perform.* **1984**, *10*, 318–327. [CrossRef] [PubMed]

147. Braine, L.G.; Relyea, L.; Davidman, L. On how adults identify the orientation of a shape. *Percept. Psychophys.* **1981**, *29*, 138–144. [CrossRef] [PubMed]

148. Jolicoeur, P. Time to name disoriented objects. *Mem. Cogn.* **1985**, *13*, 289–303. [CrossRef]

149. Jolicoeur, P.; Landau, M.J. Effects of orientation on the identification of simple visual patterns. *Can. J. Psychol.* **1984**, *38*, 80–93. [CrossRef] [PubMed]

150. Bundesen, C.; Larsen, A.; Farrell, J.E. Mental transformations of size and orientation. *Atten. Perform.* **1981**, *9*, 279–294.

151. Koriat, A.; Norman, J. What is rotated in mental rotation? *J. Exp. Psychol. Learn. Mem. Cogn.* **1984**, *10*, 421–434. [CrossRef] [PubMed]

152. Koriat, A.; Norman, J. Frames and images: Sequential effects in mental rotation. *J. Exp. Psychol. Learn. Mem. Cogn.* **1988**, *14*, 93–111. [CrossRef] [PubMed]

153. Navon, D.; Raveh, O. On the process of recognizing inverted words: Does it rely only on orientation-invariant cues? *Mem. Cognit.* **2004**, *32*, 1103–1117. [CrossRef] [PubMed]

154. Longcamp, M.; Boucard, C.; Gilhodes, J.C.; Velay, J.L. Remembering the orientation of newly learned characters depends on the associated writing knowledge: A comparison between handwriting and typing. *Hum. Mov. Sci.* **2006**, *25*, 646–656. [CrossRef] [PubMed]

155. Sala, S.D.; Cubelli, R. Directional apraxia: A unitary account of mirror writing following brain injury or as found in normal young children. *J. Neuropsychol.* **2007**, *1*, 3–26. [CrossRef] [PubMed]

156. Maass, A.; Suitner, C.; Deconchy, J.-P. *Living in an Asymmetrical World: How Writing Direction Affects thought and Action*; Psychology Press: London, UK; New York, NY, USA, 2014.

157. Fischer, J.P. Character reversal in children: The prominent role of writing direction. *Read. Writ.* **2016**, *30*, 523–542. [CrossRef]

158. Fischer, J.P. Mirror writing of digits and (capital) letters in the typically developing child. *Cortex* **2011**, *47*, 759–762. [CrossRef] [PubMed]

159. Treiman, R.; Gordon, J.; Boada, R.; Peterson, R.L.; Pennington, B.F. statistical learning, letter reversals, and reading. *Sci. Stud. Read.* **2014**, *18*, 383–394. [CrossRef] [PubMed]

160. Treiman, R.; Kessler, B. Similarities among the shapes of writing and their effects on learning. *Writ. Lang. Lit.* **2011**, *14*, 39–57. [PubMed]

161. McIntosh, R.D.; Della Salla, S. Mirror-writing. *Psychologist* **2012**, *25*, 742–746.

162. Kolers, P.A. Three stages of reading. In *Basic Studies on Reading*; Levin, H., Williams, J.P., Eds.; Basic Books, Inc.: New York, NY, USA, 1970; pp. 90–118.

163. Parks, T.E. Misprint. *Perception* **1983**, *12*, 88. [PubMed]

164. Rock, I. On Thompson's inverted-face phenomenon (Research Note). *Perception* **1988**, *17*, 815–817. [CrossRef] [PubMed]

165. Wong, Y.K.; Twedt, E.; Sheinberg, D.; Gauthier, I. Does Thompson's Thatcher effect reflect a face-specific mechanism? *Perception* **2010**, *39*, 1125–1141. [CrossRef] [PubMed]

166. Thompson, P. Margaret thatcher: A new illusion. *Perception* **1980**, *9*, 483–484. [CrossRef] [PubMed]

167. Palmer, S.E. What makes triangles in configurations point: Local and global effects of ambiguous triangles. *Cogn. Psychol.* **1980**, *12*, 285–305. [CrossRef]

168. Nagai, M.; Yagi, A. The pointedness effect on representational momentum. *Mem. Cognit.* **2001**, *29*, 91–99. [CrossRef] [PubMed]

169. McMullen, P.A.; Hamm, J.; Jolicoeur, P. Rotated object identification with and without orientation cues. *Can. J. Exp. Psychol.* **1995**, *49*, 133–149. [CrossRef] [PubMed]

170. McMullen, P.A.; Jolicoeur, P. Reference frame and effects of orientation on finding the tops of rotated objects. *J. Exp. Psychol. Hum. Percept. Perform.* **1992**, *18*, 807–820. [CrossRef] [PubMed]

171. Jolicoeur, P.; Milliken, B. Identification of disoriented objects: Effects of context of prior presentation. *J. Exp. Psychol. Learn. Mem. Cogn.* **1989**, *15*, 200–210. [CrossRef] [PubMed]

172. McMullen, P.A.; Jolicoeur, P. The spatial frame of reference in object naming and discrimination of left-right reflections. *Mem. Cognit.* **1990**, *18*, 99–115. [CrossRef] [PubMed]

173. Rice, C. The orientation of plane figures as a factor in their perception by children. *Child Dev.* **1930**, *1*, 111–143. [CrossRef]

174. Frith, U. Internal schemata for letters in good and bad readers. *Br. J. Psychol.* **1974**, *65*, 233–241.

175. Humphreys, G.W. Reference frames and shape perception. *Cogn. Psychol.* **1983**, *15*, 151–196. [CrossRef]

176. Attneave, F.; Reid, K.W. Voluntary control of frame of reference and slope equivalence under head rotation. *J. Exp. Psychol.* **1968**, *78*, 153–159. [CrossRef] [PubMed]

177. Corballis, M.C. Recognition of disoriented shapes. *Psychol. Rev.* **1988**, *95*, 115–123. [CrossRef] [PubMed]

178. Robertson, L.C.; Palmer, S.E.; Gomez, L.M. Reference frames in mental rotation. *J. Exp. Psychol. Learn. Mem. Cogn.* **1987**, *13*, 368–379. [CrossRef] [PubMed]

179. Bianchi, I.; Savardi, U. The relationship perceived between the real body and the mirror image. *Perception* **2008**, *37*, 666–688. [CrossRef] [PubMed]

180. Ittelson, W.H.; Mowafy, L.; Magid, D. The perception of mirror-reflected objects. *Perception* **1991**, *20*, 567–584. [CrossRef] [PubMed]

181. Morris, R.C. Mirror image reversal: Is what we see what we present? *Perception* **1993**, *22*, 869–876. [CrossRef] [PubMed]

182. Ittelson, W.H. Mirror reversals: Real and perceived. *Perception* **1993**, *22*, 855–861. [CrossRef] [PubMed]

183. Corballis, M.C. Much ado about mirrors. *Psychon. Bull. Rev.* **2000**, *7*, 163–169. [CrossRef] [PubMed]

184. Haig, N.D. Reflections on inversion and reversion. *Perception* **1993**, *22*, 863–868. [CrossRef] [PubMed]
185. Gregory, R.L. Mirror reversal. In *The Oxford Companion to the Mind*; Gregory, R.L., Ed.; Oxford University Press: Oxford, UK, 1987.
186. Gardner, M. *The Ambidextrous Universe*; Basic Books: New York, NY, USA, 1964.
187. Block, N.J. Why do mirrors reverse right/left but not up/down. *J. Philos.* **1974**, *9*, 259–277. [CrossRef]
188. Bredart, S. Recognising the usual orientation of one's own face: The role of asymmetrically located details. *Perception* **2003**, *32*, 805–812. [CrossRef] [PubMed]
189. Rhodes, G. Memory for lateral asymmetries in well-known faces: Evidence for configural information in memory representations of faces. *Mem. Cognit.* **1986**, *14*, 209–219. [CrossRef] [PubMed]
190. Mita, T.H.; Dermer, M.; Knight, J. Reversed facial images and the mere-exposure hypothesis. *J. Pers. Soc. Psychol.* **1977**, *35*, 597–601. [CrossRef]
191. Brady, N.; Campbell, M.; Flaherty, M. Perceptual asymmetries are preserved in memory for highly familiar faces of self and friend. *Brain Cogn.* **2005**, *58*, 334–342. [CrossRef] [PubMed]
192. Smith, E.L.; Grabowecky, M.; Suzuki, S. Self-awareness affects vision. *Curr. Biol.* **2008**, *18*, 414–415. [CrossRef] [PubMed]
193. Bertamini, M.; Parks, T.E. On what people know about images on mirrors. *Cognition* **2005**, *98*, 85–104. [CrossRef] [PubMed]
194. Dieguez, S.; Scherer, J.; Blanke, O. My face through the looking-glass: The effect of mirror reversal on reflection size estimation. *Conscious. Cogn.* **2011**, *20*, 1452–1459. [CrossRef] [PubMed]
195. Savardi, U.; Bianchi, I.; Bertamini, M. Naïve predictions of motion and orientation in mirrors: From what we see to what we expect reflections to do. *Acta Psychol. (Amst.)* **2010**, *134*, 1–15. [CrossRef] [PubMed]
196. Bertamini, M.; Spooner, A.; Hecht, H. Naive optics: Predicting and perceiving reflections in mirrors. *J. Exp. Psychol. Hum. Percept. Perform.* **2003**, *29*, 982–1002. [CrossRef] [PubMed]
197. Croucher, C.J.; Bertamini, M.; Hecht, H. Naive optics: Understanding the geometry of mirror reflections. *J. Exp. Psychol. Hum. Percept. Perform.* **2002**, *28*, 546–562. [CrossRef] [PubMed]

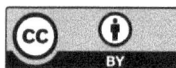

![symmetry logo] *symmetry*

MDPI

Article

Affine Geometry, Visual Sensation, and Preference for Symmetry of Things in a Thing

Birgitta Dresp-Langley

ICube Laboratory UMR 7357 CNRS, University of Strasbourg, Strasbourg 67000, France;
birgitta.dresp@unistra.fr

Academic Editor: Marco Bertamini
Received: 4 August 2016; Accepted: 9 November 2016; Published: 14 November 2016

Abstract: Evolution and geometry generate complexity in similar ways. Evolution drives natural selection while geometry may capture the logic of this selection and express it visually, in terms of specific generic properties representing some kind of advantage. Geometry is ideally suited for expressing the logic of evolutionary selection for symmetry, which is found in the shape curves of vein systems and other natural objects such as leaves, cell membranes, or tunnel systems built by ants. The topology and geometry of symmetry is controlled by numerical parameters, which act in analogy with a biological organism's DNA. The introductory part of this paper reviews findings from experiments illustrating the critical role of two-dimensional (2D) design parameters, affine geometry and shape symmetry for visual or tactile shape sensation and perception-based decision making in populations of experts and non-experts. It will be shown that 2D fractal symmetry, referred to herein as the "symmetry of things in a thing", results from principles very similar to those of affine projection. Results from experiments on aesthetic and visual preference judgments in response to 2D fractal trees with varying degrees of asymmetry are presented. In a first experiment (psychophysical scaling procedure), non-expert observers had to rate (on a scale from 0 to 10) the perceived beauty of a random series of 2D fractal trees with varying degrees of fractal symmetry. In a second experiment (two-alternative forced choice procedure), they had to express their preference for one of two shapes from the series. The shape pairs were presented successively in random order. Results show that the smallest possible fractal deviation from "symmetry of things in a thing" significantly reduces the perceived attractiveness of such shapes. The potential of future studies where different levels of complexity of fractal patterns are weighed against different degrees of symmetry is pointed out in the conclusion.

Keywords: visual symmetry; affine projection; fractals; visual sensation; aesthetics; preference

1. Introduction

Brain evolution has produced highly specialized processes which enable us to effectively exploit the geometry of visual perceptual space. Some data suggest that the human brain is equipped with an in-built sense of geometry [1,2] which provides a key to recognizing specific object properties, associations between two-dimensional projections, and their correlated three-dimensional structures in the real world [3–6]. These associations favour structural regularities and, very often, symmetry [6,7], while asymmetry plays a critical role in processes of perceptual discrimination, as discussed recently regarding music and sounds [8]. In the domain of visual objects, symmetry plays an important role in conceptual processes for structural design, and is abundantly exploited by engineers and architects. The following paragraphs will expand on the importance of affine geometry, the symmetry of curves, which may be perceived as single things or as multiples of one and the same thing in a complex shape or object [9,10], and visual sensation. Thereafter, two-dimensional fractal trees based on geometrical principles which produce symmetry of things in a thing will be discussed and made use of psychophysically. The symmetrical structure of these fractal trees results, like 2D curve symmetry, from principles of affine projection, as will become clear in light of further discussions here below.

The use of symmetrical curves dates back to the dawn of building shelter and vernacular architecture, which relies, given the nature of the materials and construction techniques used, almost entirely on symmetry (Figure 1, left). In the Middle Ages, descriptive geometry was used for the planning and execution of building projects for which symmetric curves were the reference model, as in the design of arched hallways and corridors (Figure 1, middle). In the last century, the Spanish designer and architect Antoni Gaudi used the same kind of geometry for the design of the *Sagrada Familia* in Barcelona (Figure 1, right) and many of his other fabulous structures, which can be appreciated by taking a walk through the Park Guëll, or by visiting the Guëll museum in Barcelona. In Antoni Gaudi's three-dimensional design of arches, for churches or natural environments, there is a clear distinction between physical (objective) and subjective (perceived) symmetry. Physical symmetry takes into account the principles of gravity. As a consequence, a resulting real-world structure may not necessarily be perceived as perfectly symmetrical (cf. Figure 1, image on right).

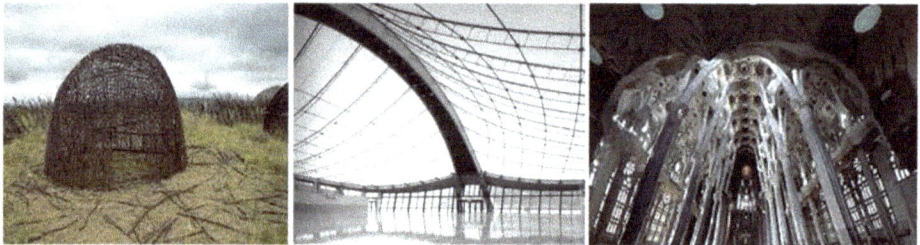

Figure 1. The importance of curve symmetry for human endeavour dates back to the dawn of building shelter and to vernacular architecture (**left**). Similar geometry is currently used in contemporary free-form architecture (**middle**), which has been much inspired by the Spanish architect Gaudi, who largely exploited symmetry for the design of the hall and archways of the *Sagrada Familia* in Barcelona (**right**).

Antoni Gaudi's structures were inspired by nature, which abounds with curved shapes and features, and our perception uses these features as cues to shape or object recognition, and for image interpretation [9–16]. In biology, curvature guides physical, chemical, and biological processes, such as protein folding, membrane binding, and other biophysical transformations [17]. The representation and cognition of curvature ranges from the biochemical level of living organisms capable of sensing this property in their near or distant physical environments [18] to perceptual properties extracted from physical stimuli by the human brain, the ultimate product of evolution. In terms of a mathematical property of the physical world, curve symmetry is directly linked to affine geometry [19].

1.1. Affine Geometry and Visual Sensation

In affine geometry, curves derived from circles and ellipses share certain properties, the circle being a particular case of the ellipse. Projective geometry permits generating symmetric curves from ellipses by affinity with concentric circles (Figure 2). Their perception is grounded in biology in the sense that most natural objects can be represented in 2D as symmetrically curved shapes with Euclidean properties of ellipses. Studies comparing between visually perceived curvature by experts in geometry (architects and design engineers) and non-experts [12] by using symmetric curves derived from concentric circles by affine projection have shown that their perceived magnitude is determined by a single geometric parameter, the curves' aspect ratio. The perceptual responses to such curves are independent of both expertise and sensory modality, given that tactile sensing by sighted blindfolded and congenitally blind observers produces the same results [14]. The symmetry of the curves, however, is a critical factor to these geometry-based perceptual responses [15]. The aspect ratio relates the height (*sagitta*) to the width of a curve, and in symmetric curves of variable size but constant aspect ratio directly taken from concentric circles (no projection by affinity), perceived curvature is also constant, in both vision and touch. This observation is directly linked to the phenomenon of scale-invariance in visual curvature discrimination [20] and the detection and recognition of shapes in general.

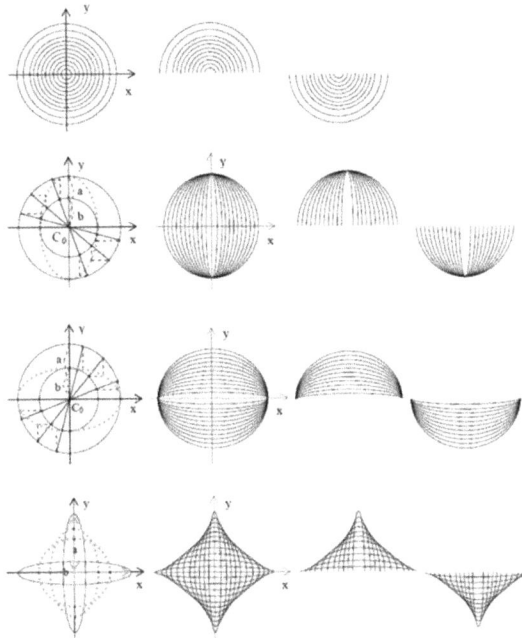

Figure 2. Projective geometry permits generating symmetric curves from ellipses by affinity with concentric circles. Each such curve may be perceived as a single thing or as a multiple of one and the same thing in a complex shape or object, as shown here. This perception is grounded in biology in the sense that most natural objects can be represented as images of symmetrically curved shapes with the Euclidean properties of ellipses. Symmetric curves yield visual and tactile sensations of curvature which increase exponentially with the *aspect ratio* of the curves.

1.2. Reflection and Rotational Shape Symmetry

The role of reflection symmetry in visual perception was pointed out by Gestalt psychologists at the beginning of the 20th century [21] as a major factor in shape perception. It refers to specific transformations by transition of points in Euclidean space resulting in mirrored representations. Axial symmetry e.g., which results from point-by-point mirroring across an axis (f $(x, y, z) =$ f $(-x, y, z)$), is an important factor in visual recognition [22–24]. Reflection or mirror symmetry is detected quickly [25,26] in foveal and in peripheral vision [27]. Vertical mirror symmetry facilitates face recognition by human [28] and non-human primates [29], and is used by the human visual system as a second-order cue to perceptual grouping [30].

Rotational symmetry of shape plays an important role in architecture and design. The design of complex modern spatial structures is a domain of contemporary relevance. Visual-spatial experiments on expert architects as well as novices have shown that perceiving the rotational symmetry of partial shapes, which constitute the simplest possible tensegrity (tensile integrity) structure, is an important part of our understanding how they are put together. Only once this symmetry is perceived by the expert or novice, will he/she be able to draw the structure from memory into axonometric or topological reference frames provided to that effect [31]. Tensegrity structures have inspired current biological models [32], from the level of single cells to that of the whole human body. They possess what Mandelbrot [33] called "fractal consistency across spatial scales", or "fractal iterations", like those seen in large trees that appear to be composed of many smaller trees of the same structure.

1.3. Nature-Inspired Design and the Symmetry of "Things in a Thing"

Fractal geometry is also inspired by nature and its many symmetric visual structures like those found in cells, trees, butterflies and flowers. The term "fractal" was first introduced by Mandelbrot [33] based on the meaning "broken" or "fractured" (*fractus*). A fractal may be defined as a complex whole (object or pattern) that has the same structural characteristics as its constituent parts. The structural symmetry that results from fractal iterations may be described as the "symmetry of things in a thing". The radial symmetry of a sunflower is a choice example of fractal symmetry as it exists in nature. Behavioural studies have shown that various animal species are naturally attracted to two-dimensional representations of objects exhibiting flower-like radial symmetry [34,35]. In complex 3D fractal trees, single fractals ("things") have a symmetrical counterpart within the whole structure ("the thing"), which may possess radial symmetry, reflection symmetry and manifold rotational symmetries, like many objects in nature (plants, snowflakes, etc.) are bound by both reflection and rotational symmetry, and exhibit multiples of one and the same shape (things) repeated in all directions.

Nature-inspired design occupies an important place in contemporary graphic art, and symmetry has been identified as a major defining feature of visual beauty, compositional order, and harmony. Symmetry directly determines aesthetic preferences and the subjectively perceived beauty of two-dimensional visual images and patterns [36–41], and symmetrical visual patterns are also more easily remembered and recognized [42–44] compared with asymmetrical ones. Sabatelli et al. [8] suggested that natural and artistic creative processes rely on common, possibly fractal transformations. Fractal transformations may describe iterative transitions from simplicity and order (symmetry) to complexity and chaos (asymmetry). Again, fractal trees seem to be a pertinent example here, where simple 2D mirror trees (Figure 3) with reflection and/or radial symmetry open an almost infinite number of possibilities for adding complexity through further transformations leading to complex projections of 3D structures with multiple rotational symmetries (not shown here).

Whether nature-inspired fractal design appeals to our senses in the same way as the real objects found in nature was studied by [45], who found that human observers produce highly consistent aesthetic preference judgments across fractal images produced by nature, algorithm, or by the human hand. Hagerhall, Purcell, and Taylor [46] found that fractal characteristics of landscape silhouette outlines reliably predict landscape preferences. Fractal characteristics provide a consistent measure of complexity, and were shown to account for judgments of perceived beauty in visual art [47]. Here, we make the prediction that the "symmetry of things in a thing" in 2D fractal objects plays a decisive role in our perception of their aesthetic content and thereby influences visual preference judgments. Given the multiple levels of complexity of fractal objects, trying to address this question requires starting with simple examples. For this pilot study here, we created a series of basic fractal mirror trees based on geometric transformations as shown in Figures 2 and 3. In two psychophysical experiments, one using an aesthetic rating procedure, the other a preference judgment design, we tested whether the subjective attractiveness of such trees is affected by different degrees of violation of symmetry, from an almost imperceptible lack of mirror detail to massive asymmetry.

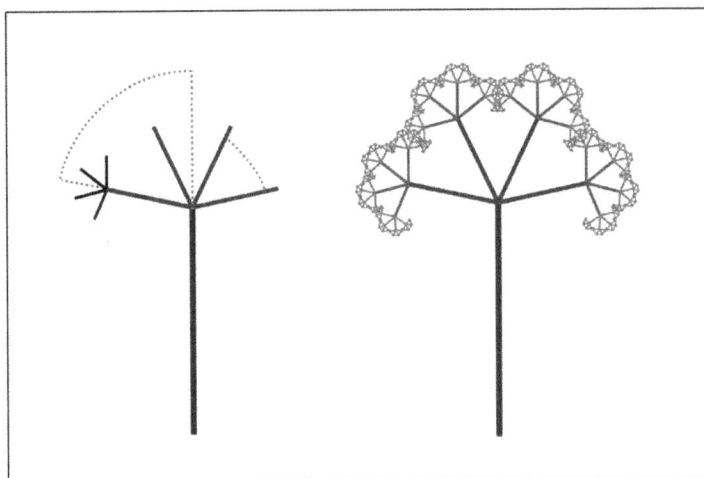

Figure 3. Fractal geometry and affine geometry share principles of projection in Euclidean space, as illustrated in this example here. Fractal trees, inspired by nature, may be defined as complex wholes where every part repeats itself across multiple fractal iterations, producing "symmetry of things in a thing". In the 2D fractal mirror-tree shown here, concentric circles and affine projection are the mathematical basis for describing structural regularities with vertical reflection (mirror) symmetry, which has been identified as a major determinant of the visual attractiveness of image configurations.

2. Materials and Methods

The experiments were conducted in accordance with the Declaration of Helsinki (1964) and with the full approval of the corresponding author's institutional (CNRS) ethics committee. Informed written consent was obtained from each of the participants. Experimental sessions were organized following conditions of randomized, trial-by-trial free image viewing using Python for Windows 7 and a computer with a keyboard and a high resolution monitor. 15 mirror tree images were generated using a comprehensive vector graphics environment (Adobe Illustrator CC) and computer shape library.

2.1. Subjects

30 observers, ranging in age between 25 and 70 and unaware of the hypotheses of the study, participated in the experiments. All subjects had normal or corrected-to-normal visual acuity.

2.2. Stimuli

The stimuli for the two experiments were generated on the basis of 15 images of fractal trees drawn in a vector graphics environment (Adobe illustrator CC) using simple principles of 2D geometry, as shown here above. Five of these images (Figure 4, top row) were mirror trees with vertical reflection symmetry and perfect symmetry of things in a thing. Five of them (Figure 4, middle row) were imperfect mirror trees in the sense that their vertical reflection symmetry excluded one of the elementary parts, which was not mirrored on the right side of the tree. In the asymmetrical images (Figure 4, bottom row), elementary shapes "growing" on the branches of the left side of the trees were not mirrored on the right side. The luminance contrast between figures and backgrounds was constant in the 15 images (same RGB (200, 200, 200) for all figures, same RGB (20, 20, 20) for all backgrounds). The approximate angular height of a fractal tree was 2.25° (vertical mid-axis), the angular width 1.64° (horizontal mid-axis). A trial-loop algorithm written in Python for Windows 7 selected the images or image pairs in random order, and recorded the individual key board responses from the experimental trials.

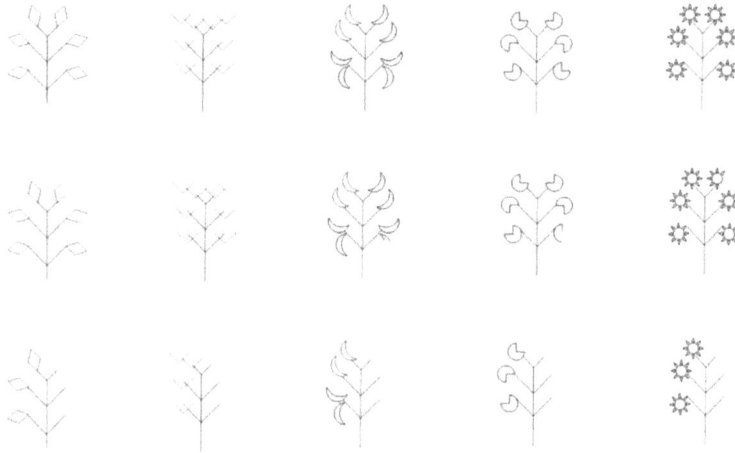

Figure 4. Fifteen images of fractal mirror trees were designed using some of the principles of transformation shown in Figures 2 and 3. The first five trees (**top**) possess perfect "symmetry of things in a thing" across the vertical axis. In the next set of five (**middle**), the smallest of fractal details is missing on the right. The remaining five trees (**bottom**) are asymmetrical. It is noted that in these tree structures here, only the symmetrical ones (**top**) appear perceptually complete.

2.3. Task Instructions

In the aesthetic rating experiment, subjects were instructed to type a number on the keyboard rating the beauty of each of the fifteen individual images on a subjective psychophysical scale from 0 (zero) for "very ugly" to ten (10) for "very beautiful". In the preference judgment experiment, subjects were instructed to indicate whether they spontaneously preferred the left (hit "1") or the right (hit "2") of an image pair. Hitting the response key initiated the next image pair. Half of the subjects started with the rating experiment, the other half with the preference judgment experiment.

2.4. Procedure

Subjects were seated at a distance of about 90 cm from the screen and looked at the center. The images were displayed centrally and presented in random order. In the aesthetic rating experiment, each of the 15 images was presented once to each of the 30 subjects. In the preference judgment experiment, each image from a group of five was paired with its counterpart from the two other groups, and spatial position in a pair (left/right) was counterbalanced (Figure 5). This produced 30 image pairs with 20 presentations for each figure type (10 times on the left, and 10 times on the right). The image pairs were displayed in random order and each pair was displayed twice in an individual session, yielding 60 preference judgments from each of the 30 subjects.

The intervals between stimulus presentations were under the control of the observer, who initiated the next image presentation by striking a given response key ("1" for "left", "2" for "right") on the computer keyboard. The individual keyboard responses were coded and automatically written into text files. These were then imported into *SYSTAT 11* software for processing and statistical analysis.

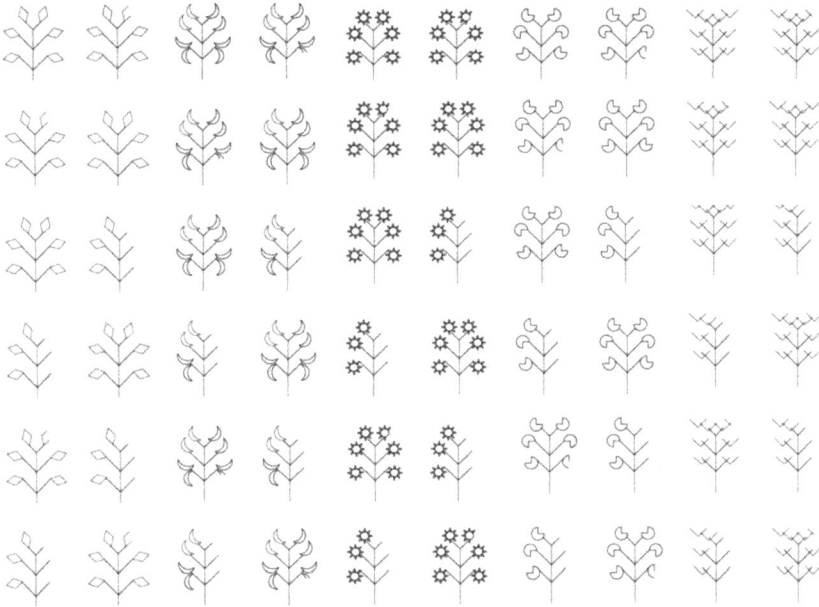

Figure 5. 30 image pairs with 20 presentations for figures of a given type (10 times on the left, and 10 times on the right). The image pairs were displayed in random order, and each pair was displayed twice in an individual session, yielding 60 preference judgments from each of the 30 subjects.

3. Results

The raw data were analyzed using *Systat/Sigmaplot 11* (Systat Software Inc., 2010, San Jose, CA, USA). One-way analysis of variance (ANOVA) for repeated measures was performed to assess the statistical significance of differences in means across subjects and figure types: 'symmetrical', 'detail missing' and 'asymmetrical'. In the data from the preference judgment experiment with figure pairs, a first check of the means showed no effect of secondary variables such as the spatial position (left vs. right) of figures of a type in a pair (M_{left} = 4.92 vs. M_{right} = 5.07), or the order (first vs. second) in which a judgment was formed in response to a figure pair (M_{first} = 5.02 vs. M_{second} = 4.95).

3.1. Aesthetic Ratings

The results of the ANOVA on average aesthetic ratings for each individual as a function of the three figure types are given in Table 1. The table summarizes, for each figure type, the sample size (N), the mean (M), the standard error (SEM), and the F value and its probability limits (*p*). Effect sizes in terms of differences between the means (*dM*), and the corresponding *t* values and probability limits for each paired comparison are given. From the results in Table 1 we conclude that symmetrical figures received a significantly higher average aesthetic rating compared with figures where a small detail was missing, which received a significantly higher average aesthetic rating than the asymmetrical figures. A graphic representation of these effects is shown below in Figure 6.

Table 1. Results from the one-way repeated measures ANOVA on aesthetic ratings for each of the three figure types: Number of observations (N) per figure type, means (M) and standard errors (SEM), and the *F* value with probability limits (*p*) are given. Effect sizes, *t* values and the corresponding probability limits are given at the bottom.

One Way Repeated Measures Analysis of Variance AESTHETIC RATINGS			
Treatment	N	M	SEM
Symmetrical	30	6.347	0.222
Detail missing	30	4.487	0.258
Asymmetrical	30	3.053	0.308
Source of Variation	**DF**	*F*	*p*
Between Subjects	29	-	-
Between Treatments	2	64.323	<0.001
Residual	58	-	-
Total	89	-	-
Comparison	*d*M	*t*	*p*
Symmetrical vs. Asymmetrical	3.293	11.311	<0.001
Symmetrical vs. Detail missing	1.860	6.388	<0.001
Detail missing vs. Asymmetrical	1.433	4.923	<0.001

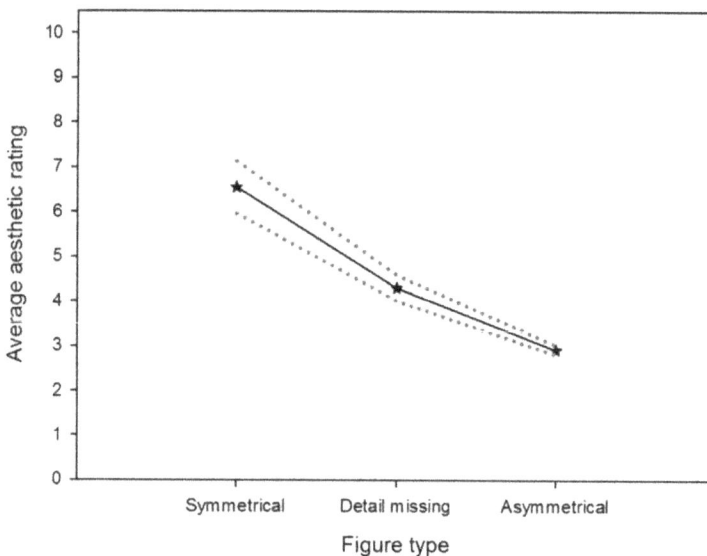

Figure 6. Average aesthetic ratings on a scale between zero and ten are shown as a function of the figure type.

3.2. Preference Judgments

The *SYSTAT* results of the ANOVA on average preference judgments of each individual as a function of the three figure types are summarized in Table 2. The table shows, for each figure type, the sample size (N), the mean (M), the standard error (SEM), and the *F* value and probability limits (*p*). Effect sizes in terms of differences between the means (*d*M), and the corresponding *t* values and probability limits for each paired comparison are given.

Table 2. Results from the one-way ANOVA for repeated measures of preference judgments for each of the three figure types.

One Way Repeated Measures Analysis of Variance PREFERENCES			
Treatment	N	M	SEM
Symmetrical	30	8.942	0.163
Detail missing	30	4.542	0.094
Asymmetrical	30	1.517	0.145
Source of Variation	**DF**	***F***	***p***
Between Subjects	29	-	-
Between Treatments	2	195.399	<0.001
Residual	58	-	-
Total	89	-	-
Comparison	***d*M**	***t***	***p***
Symmetrical vs. Asymmetrical	7.425	31.299	<0.001
Symmetrical vs. Detail missing	4.400	18.547	<0.001
Detail missing vs. Asymmetrical	3.025	12.751	<0.001

From the results in Table 2 we conclude that symmetrical figures were significantly more often preferred than figures with a detail missing, which were significantly more often preferred than asymmetrical figures. These observations are fully consistent with the effects on aesthetic ratings shown in Figure 6.

4. Discussion

As illustrated by examples from the introduction here above, shape sensation and perception can be related to affine design geometry [15,19,21,22,48,49]. The topology and geometry of fractal objects is controlled in similar ways, as shown in the fractal mirror trees used as stimuli here. The findings show that the smallest "fractal" deviation from perfect "symmetry of things in a thing" in basic mirror trees (any computer shape library can generate them) with vertical reflection symmetry when no fractals are removed, significantly diminishes subjectively perceived beauty and visual preference. These results confirm previous observations from aesthetic perception studies using different two-dimensional configurations [36–41]. Perfectly symmetrical trees also produced the strongest consensual results, for both subjective aesthetic ratings and visual preferences, while the ones with a small detail missing and the asymmetrical trees produced more disparate data, indicating higher uncertainty (i.e., less confidence) in the subjects' perceptual responses.

In the experiments here, subjects could look at the figures or pairs for as long as they wanted to make a perceptual decision and no instruction to respond as swiftly as possible were given, as is often the case in reaction time studies. Reaction times were not measured here. It is to be noted that aesthetic ratings and preference judgments may be driven by low-level heuristics or by higher order cognitive processes [50,51]. Measuring reaction times in future studies will be useful to shed light on how one or the other type of processing may have influenced response strategies. Whenever a figure was symmetrical here, it was also perceptually complete; whenever it was not, it was perceptually incomplete. Using simple response heuristics based on this kind of local detail analysis instead of forming an overall global aesthetic appreciation, for example, would certainly yield faster responses. A way of disentangling perceptual completeness and symmetry in the stimuli is to include a group of perceptually incomplete but symmetrical figures, like fractal trees with a local detail missing on both sides.

In nature, it is difficult to find complete things which do not have at least one axis of mirror or reflection symmetry. On the other hand, things which are incomplete and at the same time symmetrical are very hard to find. Our aesthetic preferences are well-primed for symmetrical objects [41], yet results from earlier studies [52] suggest that things may not be that simple when complexity and symmetry are weighed against each other, and when socio-cultural factors are brought into the equation. Personality and creativity [30,53,54] have been identified as two such variables. Highly creative individuals may have a stronger tendency to prefer asymmetrical objects, especially when these exhibit high levels of complexity, as in the case of fractal objects with multiple rotational symmetries, for example.

Recent work has highlighted that our aesthetic appreciation is essentially dynamic [55,56], and involves reflexive processes which drive cultural evolution and changes in the *Zeitgeist*, or what the French call *l'esprit du temps*. The human mind has the ability to master perceptual input which challenges current preferences (otherwise, creative fashion designers would go out of business). By way of cognitive processes these preferences may be overruled and replaced by new ones. Recent studies [51] have identified double mechanisms of preference formation. One is reflected by an immediate and basically conservative perceptual response to what is familiar [57], or deemed the current aesthetic norm, the other by a slowly strengthening disposition to adopt what is new, unusual, or challenging. As pointed out earlier [8], symmetry stands for order, asymmetry for disorder. Their dual subjective appreciation is likely to influence preferences.

Fractal objects offer new perspectives for research on complementary aspects of symmetry and asymmetry in processes of increasing complexity, including processes of visual perception. Fractals are different from other geometric figures because of the way in which they scale across multiple iterations, yielding increasingly complex repetitive structures which are symmetrical by nature. Fractal symmetry is also referred to as "expanding symmetry" or "evolving symmetry," especially if replication is exactly the same at every scale, as in a detailed pattern that repeats itself across multiple fractal iterations. For the visual scientist, this opens many perspectives as it permits the finely controlled manipulation of each and every shape detail in a given configuration and thereby allows creating visual stimuli where variations in complexity and symmetry can be effectively weighed against each other in further studies.

5. Conclusions

The visual attractiveness of 2D fractal design shapes greatly depends on the "symmetry of things in a thing" in configurations with simple geometry, as shown in this pilot study here on the example of a few very basic fractal mirror-trees. In simple displays, which are often surprisingly well suited for probing the most complex perceptual mechanisms [58], the smallest fractal deviation from a perfect "symmetry of things in a thing" is shown here to have significantly negative effects on subjectively perceived beauty and preference judgments. These findings are to encourage further studies with more sophisticated fractal design objects, and an increasingly large number of fractal iterations, producing more and more complex 2D mirror designs, and shapes with increasing levels of rotational symmetry in 3D. Such design objects are ideally suited for a numerically controlled manipulation of the "symmetry of things in a thing", and can be tailored for investigating complex interactions between symmetry and complexity in their effects on visual sensation and aesthetic perception.

Conflicts of Interest: The author declares no conflict of interest.

References

1. Amir, O.; Biederman, I.; Hayworth, K.J. Sensitivity to non-accidental properties across various shape dimensions. *Vis. Res.* **2012**, *62*, 35–43. [CrossRef] [PubMed]
2. Amir, O.; Biederman, I.; Herald, S.B.; Shah, M.P.; Mintz, T.H. Greater sensitivity to non-accidental than metric shape properties in preschool children. *Vis. Res.* **2014**, *97*, 83–88. [CrossRef] [PubMed]
3. Biederman, I. Recognition-by-components: A theory of human image understanding. *Psychol. Rev.* **1987**, *94*, 115–117. [CrossRef] [PubMed]
4. Wilson, H.R.; Wilkinson, F. Symmetry perception: A novel approach for biological shapes. *Vis. Res.* **2002**, *42*, 589–597. [CrossRef]
5. Pizlo, Z.; Sawada, T.; Li, Y.; Kropatsch, W.G.; Steinman, R.M. New approach to the perception of 3D shape based on veridicality, complexity, symmetry and volume: A mini-review. *Vis. Res.* **2010**, *50*, 1–11. [CrossRef] [PubMed]

6.   Li, Y.; Pizlo, Z.; Steinman, R.M. A computational model that recovers the 3D shape of an object from a single 2D retinal representation. *Vis. Res.* **2009**, *49*, 979–991. [CrossRef] [PubMed]

7.   Li, Y.; Sawada, T.; Shi, Y.; Steinman, R.M.; Pizlo, Z. Symmetry is the *sine qua non* of shape. In *Shape Perception in Human and Computer Vision*; Dickinson, S., Pizlo, Z., Eds.; Springer: London, UK, 2013; pp. 21–40.

8.   Sabatelli, H.; Lawandow, A.; Kopra, A.R. Asymmetry, symmetry and beauty. *Symmetry* **2010**, *2*, 1591–1624. [CrossRef]

9.   Stevens, K.A. The visual interpretation of surface contours. *Artif. Intell.* **1981**, *17*, 47–73. [CrossRef]

10.   Stevens, K.A. The information content of texture gradients. *Biol. Cybern.* **1981**, *42*, 95–105. [CrossRef] [PubMed]

11.   Foley, J.M.; Ribeiro-Filho, N.P.; Da Silva, J.A. Visual perception of extent and the geometry of visual space. *Vis. Res.* **2004**, *44*, 147–156. [CrossRef] [PubMed]

12.   Dresp, B.; Silvestri, C.; Motro, R. Which geometric model for the perceived curvature of 2-D shape contours? *Spat. Vis.* **2007**, *20*, 219–264. [CrossRef] [PubMed]

13.   Dresp-Langley, B. Why the brain knows more than we do: Non-conscious representations and their role in the construction of conscious experience. *Brain Sci.* **2012**, *2*, 1–21. [CrossRef] [PubMed]

14.   Dresp-Langley, B. Generic properties of curvature sensing by vision and touch. *Comput. Math. Methods Med.* **2013**, *2013*, 634168. [CrossRef] [PubMed]

15.   Dresp-Langley, B. 2D geometry predicts perceived visual curvature in context-free viewing. *Comput. Intell. Neurosci.* **2015**, *9*. [CrossRef] [PubMed]

16.   Strother, L.; Killebrew, K.W.; Caplovitz, G.P. The lemon illusion: Seeing curvature where there is none. *Front. Hum. Neurosci.* **2015**, *9*, 95. [CrossRef] [PubMed]

17.   Groves, J.T. The physical chemistry of membrane curvature. *Nat. Chem. Biol.* **2009**, *5*, 783–784. [CrossRef] [PubMed]

18.   Hatzakis, N.S.; Bhatia, V.K.; Larsen, J.; Madsen, K.L.; Bolinger, P.Y.; Kunding, A.H.; Castillo, J.; Gether, U.; Hedegård, P.; Stamou, D. How curved membranes recruit amphipathic helices and protein anchoring motifs. *Nat. Chem. Biol.* **2009**, *5*, 835–841. [CrossRef] [PubMed]

19.   Gerbino, W.; Zhang, L. Visual orientation and symmetry detection under affine transformations. *Bull. Psychon. Soc.* **1991**, *29*, 480.

20.   Whitaker, D.; McGraw, P.W. Geometric representation of the mechanisms underlying human curvature detection. *Vis. Res.* **1998**, *38*, 3843–3848. [CrossRef]

21.   Bahnsen, P. Eine Untersuchung über Symmetrie und Asymmetrie bei visuellen Wahrnehmungen. *Z. Psychol.* **1928**, *108*, 129–154.

22.   Braitenberg, V. Reading the structure of brains. *Network* **1990**, *1*, 1–11. [CrossRef]

23.   Beck, D.M.; Pinsk, M.A.; Kastner, S. Symmetry perception in humans and macaques. *Trends Cogn. Sci.* **2005**, *9*, 405–406. [CrossRef] [PubMed]

24.   Tjan, B.S.; Liu, Z. Symmetry impedes symmetry discrimination. *J. Vis.* **2005**, *5*, 88–900. [CrossRef] [PubMed]

25.   Barlow, H.B.; Reeves, B.C. The versatility and absolute efficiency of detecting mirror symmetry in random dot displays. *Vis. Res.* **1979**, *19*, 783–793. [CrossRef]

26.   Wagemans, J.; Van Gool, L.; D'Ydewalle, G. Detection of symmetry in tachistoscopically presented dot patterns: Effects of multiple axes and skewing. *Percept. Psychophys.* **1991**, *50*, 413–427. [CrossRef] [PubMed]

27.   Barrett, B.T.; Whitaker, D.; McGraw, P.V.; Herbert, A.M. Discriminating mirror symmetry in foveal and extra-foveal vision. *Vis. Res.* **1999**, *39*, 3737–3744. [CrossRef]

28.   Thornhill, R.; Gangestad, S.W. Facial attractiveness. *Trends Cognit. Sci.* **1999**, *3*, 452–460. [CrossRef]

29.   Anderson, J.R.; Kuwahata, H.; Kuroshima, F.; Leighty, K.A.; Fujita, K. Are monkeys aesthetists? Rensch (1957) revisited. *J. Exp. Psychol.* **2005**, *31*, 71–78. [CrossRef] [PubMed]

30.   Machilsen, B.; Pauwels, M.; Wagemans, J. The role of vertical mirror symmetry in visual shape perception. *J. Vis.* **2009**, *9*. [CrossRef] [PubMed]

31.   Silvestri, C.; Motro, R.; Maurin, B.; Dresp-Langley, B. Visual spatial learning of complex object morphologies through the interaction with virtual and real-world data. *Des. Stud.* **2010**, *31*, 363–381. [CrossRef]

32.   Levin, S.M. Biotensegrity: The tensegrity truss as a model for spine mechanics. *J. Mech. Med. Biol.* **2002**, *3–4*, 375–388. [CrossRef]

33.   Mandelbrot, B. *The Fractal Geometry of Nature*; Freeman & Co.: San Francisco, CA, USA, 1982.

34. Lehrer, M.; Horridge, G.A.; Zhang, S.W.; Gadagkar, R. Shape vision in bees: Innate preference for flower-like patterns. *Philos. Trans. R. Soc. Lond. B* **1995**, *347*, 123–137. [CrossRef]

35. Giurfa, M.; Eichmann, B.; Menzl, R. Symmetry perception in an insect. *Nature* **1996**, *382*, 458–461. [CrossRef] [PubMed]

36. Eisenman, R. Complexity–simplicity: I. Preference for symmetry and rejection of complexity. *Psychon. Sci.* **1967**, *8*, 169–170. [CrossRef]

37. Berlyne, D.E. *Aesthetics and Psychobiology*; Appleton: New York, NY, USA, 1971.

38. Jacobsen, T.; Hofel, L. Aesthetics judgments of novel graphic patterns: Analyses of individual judgments. *Percept. Motor Skills* **2002**, *95*, 755–766. [CrossRef] [PubMed]

39. Jacobsen, T.; Hofel, L. Descriptive and evaluative judgment processes: Behavioral and electrophysiological indices of processing symmetry and aesthetics. *Cognit. Affect. Behav. Neurosci.* **2003**, *3*, 289–299. [CrossRef] [PubMed]

40. Jacobsen, T.; Schubotz, R.I.; Hofel, L.; van Cramon, D.Y. Brain correlates of aesthetic judgment of beauty. *NeuroImage* **2006**, *29*, 276–285. [CrossRef] [PubMed]

41. Tinio, P.P.L.; Leder, H. Just how stable are stable aesthetic features? Symmetry, complexity, and the jaws of massive familiarization. *Acta Psychol.* **2009**, *130*, 241–150. [CrossRef] [PubMed]

42. Deregowski, J.B. Symmetry, Gestalt and information theory. *Q. J. Exp. Psychol.* **1971**, *23*, 381–385. [CrossRef] [PubMed]

43. Deregowski, J.B. The role of symmetry in pattern reproduction by Zambian children. *J. Cross-Cult. Psychol.* **1972**, *3*, 303–307. [CrossRef]

44. Kayaert, G.; Wagemans, J. Delayed shape matching benefits from simplicity and symmetry. *Vis. Res.* **2009**, *49*, 708–717. [CrossRef] [PubMed]

45. Spehar, B.; Clifford, C.W.G.; Newell, B.; Taylor, R.P. Universal aesthetics of fractals. *Comput. Graph.* **2003**, *27*, 813–820. [CrossRef]

46. Hagerhall, C.M.; Purcell, T.; Taylor, R. Fractal dimension of landscape silhouette outlines as a predictor of landscape preference. *J. Environ. Psychol.* **2004**, *24*, 247–255. [CrossRef]

47. Forsythe, A.; Nadal, M.; Sheehy, N.; Cela-Conde, C.J.; Sawey, M. Predicting beauty: Fractal dimension and visual complexity in art. *Br. J. Psychol.* **2011**, *102*, 49–70. [CrossRef] [PubMed]

48. Dresp-Langley, B. Principles of perceptual grouping: implications for image-guided surgery. *Front. Psychol.* **2015**, *6*, 1565. [CrossRef] [PubMed]

49. Dresp, B. On illusory contours and their functional significance. *Curr. Psychol. Cognit.* **1997**, *16*, 489–518.

50. Samuel, F.; Kerzel, D. Judging whether it is aesthetic: Does equilibrium compensate for lack of symmetry? *I-Perception* **2013**, *4*, 57–77. [CrossRef] [PubMed]

51. Belke, B.; Leder, H.; Carbon, C.C. When challenging art gets liked: Evidences for a dual preference formation process for fluent and non-fluent portraits. *PLoS ONE* **2015**, *10*, e0131796.

52. Eisenman, R.; Rappaport, J. Complexity preference and semantic differential ratings of complexity-simplicity and symmetry-asymmetry. *Psychon. Sci.* **1967**, *7*, 147–148. [CrossRef]

53. Eisenman, R.; Gellens, H.K. Preference for complexity—Simplicity and symmetry-asymmetry. *Percept. Motor Skills* **1968**, *26*, 888–890. [CrossRef] [PubMed]

54. Cook, R.; Furnham, A. Aesthetic preferences for architectural styles vary as a function of personality. *Imagin. Cognit. Personal.* **2012**, *32*, 103–114. [CrossRef]

55. Carbon, C.C. The cycle of preference: Long-term dynamics of aesthetic appreciation. *Acta Psychol.* **2010**, *134*, 233–244. [CrossRef] [PubMed]

56. Carbon, C.C. Cognitive mechanisms for explaining dynamics of aesthetic appreciation. *I-Perception* **2011**, *2*, 708–719. [CrossRef] [PubMed]

57. Grammer, K.; Thornhill, R. Human (Homo sapiens) facial attractiveness and sexual selection: The role of symmetry and averageness. *J. Comp. Psychol.* **1994**, *108*, 233–242. [CrossRef] [PubMed]

58. Dresp-Langley, B.; Grossberg, S. Neural computation of surface border ownership and relative surface depth from ambiguous contrast inputs. *Front. Psychol.* **2016**, *7*, 1102. [CrossRef] [PubMed]

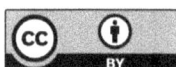

symmetry

MDPI

Article

Opposition and Identicalness: Two Basic Components of Adults' Perception and Mental Representation of Symmetry

Ivana Bianchi [1,*], Marco Bertamini [2], Roberto Burro[3] and Ugo Savardi [3]

[1]   Department of Humanities, University of Macerata, 62100 Macerata, Italy
[2]   Department of Psychological Sciences, University of Liverpool, Liverpool L69 7ZA, UK;
       M.Bertamini@liverpool.ac.uk
[3]   Department of Human Sciences, University of Verona, 37129 Verona, Italy; roberto.burro@univr.it (R.B.);
       ugo.savardi@univr.it (U.S.)
*   Correspondence: ivana.bianchi@unimc.it; Tel.: +39-0733-258-4320

Academic Editors: Sergei D. Odintsov and Christopher W. Tyler
Received: 25 June 2017; Accepted: 21 July 2017; Published: 25 July 2017

Abstract: Symmetry is a salient aspect of biological and man-made objects, and has a central role in perceptual organization. Two studies investigate the role of opposition and identicalness in shaping adults' naïve idea of "symmetry". In study 1, both verbal descriptions of symmetry (either provided by the participants or selected from among alternatives presented by the experimenter) and configurations drawn as exemplars of symmetry were studied. In study 2, a pair comparison task was used. Both studies focus on configurations formed by two symmetrical shapes (i.e., between-objects symmetry). Three main results emerged. The explicit description of symmetry provided by participants generally referred to features relating to the relationship perceived between the two shapes and not to geometrical point-by-point transformations. Despite the fact that people tended to avoid references to opposition in their verbal definition of symmetry in study 1, the drawings that they did to represent their prototypical idea of symmetry manifested opposition as a basic component. This latter result was confirmed when the participants were asked to select the definition (in study 1) or the configuration (in study 2) that best fitted with their idea of symmetry. In conclusion, identicalness is an important component in people's naïve idea of symmetry, but it does not suffice: opposition complements it.

Keywords: visual symmetry; bilateral symmetry; identicalness; opposition; between-objects symmetry; mirror-reflected pairs; mirrors

1. Introduction

The perception of symmetry has always been an intriguing subject for psychologists (for a review, see [1,2]). It has also been studied in relation to aesthetics (e.g., [3–9]) and, in recent times, to neuroscience [10,11].

Various studies have consistently demonstrated higher sensitivity (from the age of about four months) for bilateral symmetry around a vertical axis even at very short exposure times [12–15] and in various sense modalities [16,17]. Some studies have shown that the ability to detect mirror symmetry around a particular axis depends on the frequencies of various different orientations within a block of trials (e.g., [14,18]). This implies that the effect of orientation on the detection of symmetry is not completely determined by a fixed neural architecture in the visual system but can be modulated by scanning or attentional strategies. These findings do not negate the aforementioned preference for bilateral symmetry around a vertical axis, they indicate that it may be necessary to adjust the hypotheses regarding the causes of the phenomena. Since the structure of the ecological world and of artifacts is predominantly bilateral around a vertical axis, the preference for this type of symmetry might depend on exposure.

As noted by Wagemans ([19], p. 346), much of what is known about the effects of several factors on human detection of symmetry (thanks to decades of experimental work) has been inspired by phenomenological observation. Regularity, for example, defined as the salience or perceptual strength of a given pattern, is a classic phenomenological notion (or Gestalt notion) which has inspired a large number of studies on symmetry (e.g., [20–33]). The study described in this paper starts from a similar basis with the aim of analyzing whether and to what extent two phenomenological relationships, namely opposition and identicalness, are salient components of adults' naïve idea of symmetry.

Identicalness, opposition, similarity and diversity are directly perceived relationships, which are basic to human perception and categorization [34–42]. Every time we make a comparison between two stimuli these relationships inevitably emerge. Therefore, a reasonable question for a psychologist to ask concerns the relationship which is perceived between two shapes recognized as being "symmetrical" (e.g., Figure 1). This has been referred to as "between-object" symmetry to distinguish it from "within-object" symmetry, i.e., when a single figure is involved and symmetry exists between its individual parts [43,44].

Independently of whether we are talking of a within-object symmetry or between-object symmetry, in geometrical terms symmetry is an isometry, that is, it is a transformation that maps elements to the same or another metric space such that the distance between the elements in the new metric space is equal to the distance between the elements in the original metric space (usually assumed to be bijective). There are four plane isometries: reflection, rotation, translation and glide reflection. Here we focus on reflection and we will reserve the word symmetry for reflectional symmetry. According to a standard definition (see Figure 1): "a spatial configuration is symmetrical with respect to a given plane *E* if it is carried into itself by reflection in *E*. Take any line *l* perpendicular to *E* and any point *p* on *l*: there exists one and only one point *p′* on *l* which has the same distance from *E* but lies on the other side. The point *p′* coincides with *p* only if *p* is on *E*. Reflection in *E* is that mapping of space upon itself, $S: p \rightarrow p'$, that carries the arbitrary point *p* into its mirror image *p′* with respect to *E*" ([45], pp. 4–5).

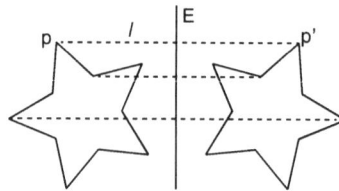

Figure 1. The point by point transformation underlying the geometry of mirror symmetry (around a vertical axis). "Take any line *l* perpendicular to *E* and any point *p* on *l* (...). Reflection in *E* is that mapping of space upon itself, $S: p \rightarrow p'$, that carries the arbitrary point *p* into its mirror image *p′* with respect to *E*" ([45], pp. 4–5).

Is this what people have in mind when they think of "symmetry"? In Euclidean geometry and its applications, any reference to qualitative features which reveal experiential spatial constructs are eliminated and replaced by abstract entities, definitions and terms. Conversely, the objective of Experimental Phenomenology (e.g., [46–49]) is to identify, describe and define the properties and relationships that are salient from the point of view of human direct experiences. The constructs of "symmetry", "identicalness" and "opposition" which are used in this paper, as well as those of "regularity" or "goodness" which have been used in relation to symmetry, are all connected with this theoretical perspective. In particular, we hypothesize that since bilateral symmetry is modelled on a mirror reflection and since identicalness and opposition are salient features (as reviewed in Section 2), opposition and identicalness should emerge as a salient integral part of people's perception and mental representation of "symmetry". The two studies presented in this paper test this hypothesis.

From Mirrors to Mirror Symmetry

Studies in the field of naïve optics [50] have revealed that when people are asked to determine the reflected world from the "real world" they do not rely on the optical-geometrical point-by-point rule (shown in Figure 1) even though they have explicit knowledge of this [50,51]. This is the same as the evidence found in studies on naïve or intuitive Physics concerning movement. It was discovered that when adults are asked to make predictions about simple physical phenomena—for example the case of free falling objects [52–55], the trajectory of objects which have been thrown [56,57] or the orientation of the surface of liquids in variously inclined containers [58,59]—many observers forget about what they have learnt in school. Instead they base their responses on prototypical models that they have in mind [60].

Among the proposals put forward to explain the systematic mistakes that adults make when asked to predict the behavior of reflections (e.g., [61–64]) one concerns the hypothesis that people think of reflections in terms of Identity and/or Opposition [65–67]. Most of the errors made [67–69] are compatible with a generalization of the rule which states that "the reflection does the same" (see Figure 2c) and/or "the reflection does the opposite" (see Figure 2b), which forms the basis of the macroscopic geometry of the relationship seen between a "real object" and its reflection ([67] (studies 4–5), [70]).

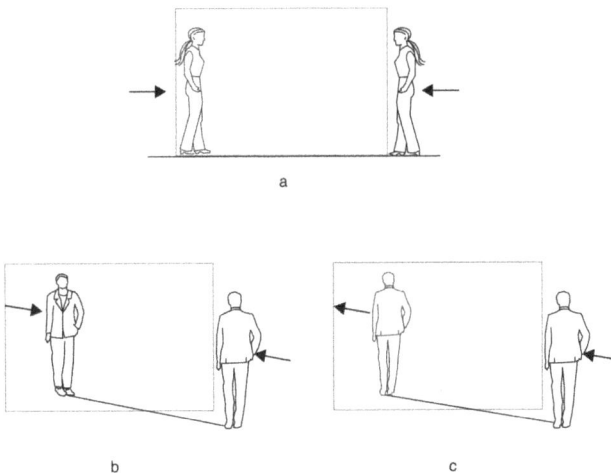

Figure 2. Some errors emerged in tasks which required participants to predict the location and direction of motion in a reflection: (**a**) when the "real" person moved parallel to a vertical mirror on a wall, many people expected her reflection to appear at the farther edge of the mirror walking towards the "real person"; (**b,c**) when the "real person" moved at an angle towards a mirror, some people expected the reflection to move along the same trajectory with an opposite orientation (**b**) or along the same trajectory but with an identical orientation (**c**).

When people observe simple objects positioned in front of a vertical plane mirror or in motion at various angles of incidence towards or away from the mirror, descriptions such as "the reflection has an identical orientation/direction of motion" or "the reflection has an opposites orientation/direction of motion as compared to that of the real object" are judged to be accurate (see [67] studies 4–5). Similarly, when naïve observers see their own image in a plane mirror (or another person's image), they report that they perceive the orientation of the reflection to be opposite with respect to the real body [70]. The fact that our left arm in the reflection is our right arm is a visual characteristic which we notice, especially when we are encouraged to focus on the lateralization of our body. However, we also immediately notice that we are facing in one direction (e.g., north) while the reflection is facing the opposite direction (i.e., south) and when we walk towards the mirror, the person in the reflection moves in the opposite direction (i.e., representing opposition on the sagittal axis). When the mirror is on the wall to the side of an observer, the reflection has an identical sagittal and gravitational orientation with respect to the real person but is opposite in terms of the coronal axis; if the person then moves laterally to his/her right (e.g., eastwards), the reflection moves in the opposite direction (i.e., to the left and westwards). If the observer then positions him/herself on top of a mirror lying on the floor, he/she again perceives the reflection as having an opposite orientation along the gravitational axes (as the reflection is upside-down). In all of these conditions, the *orientation* of the reflection is consistently described as "opposite" (rather than "identical", "similar", or "different") in a percentage of cases ranging between 80% and 100% of the participants, depending on the position of the mirror (see [70], Figure 3). This concurs with the fact that participants in mirror tasks describe their *reflection* as "identical" to themselves when looking at their reflection in a mirror set vertically in front of them or to their side, or as "opposite" or "similar" to themselves when looking at their reflection in a mirror set horizontally under their feet [70]. These findings are in agreement with studies carried out with various types of visual stimuli which show that transforming the orientation of something into its opposite orientation guarantees an overall perception of clear contrast and clear invariance at the same time, and these seem to be the two conditions which are necessary for the relationship between two things or events to be specifically recognized as contrary/opposite, rather than generically different [34,35,71].

In this study, we posed the question of whether the fact that reflections are phenomenally associated with the recognition of identity and opposition (as mentioned above) can be generalized to the naïve idea of symmetry, which adults have in mind. If so, the configurations that people consider to be good examples of a "symmetrical configuration" should reveal not only identity but also opposition. In other words, they should look more like those shown on the right side in Figure 3 than those shown on the left.

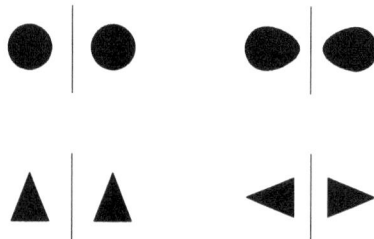

Figure 3. Mirror symmetry applied to configurations that have different symmetrical structures. On the left: shapes which are symmetrical along the axis parallel to the mirror minimize the perception of contrariety (which remains relative only to the *position* of the shapes, i.e., one to the left and the other to the right of the mirror axis) and maximize perception of identicalness. On the right: shapes which are symmetrical only with respect to the axis which is orthogonal to the mirror axis but which are asymmetrical with respect to the axis parallel to the mirror axis make the opposite orientation easier to see (for farther explanations, see text).

The configurations displayed in Figure 3 are, from a geometrical point of view, equally valid examples of reflections around a vertical axis. However, the configurations on the left look identical and the only recognizable element of opposition concerns the localization of the two shapes with respect to the mirror axis. Conversely, the configurations on the right show opposition as they show shapes which are oppositely oriented. If visible opposition, in addition to visible identity, is an important component of people's naïve idea of symmetry, then these configurations would not be equally good and we should expect those on the right to be better examples.

2. Study 1

The aim of this study was to ascertain how important the role of identicalness and opposition is in the explicit idea (i.e., verbal description) and implicit idea (i.e., mental representation or "prototypical mental image" in Yates et al.'s terms [60]) that naïve subjects have of symmetry. The former was assessed by asking participants to verbally describe the features characterizing two symmetrical shapes (the 1st question in the experiment) and at the end of the session, requesting them to choose which description out of three fit in best with their idea of symmetry (the 4th question). The implicit idea of symmetry was tested by assessing the drawings done by the participants as examples of their idea of symmetry (the 2nd and 3rd questions).

Since we were interested in understanding the relational aspects which characterize two symmetrical figures and to prevent the participants from simply drawing stereotypical images of symmetry such as a butterfly or a human face, we asked them to draw configurations consisting of two shapes which were symmetrical to each other.

We expected explicit and implicit descriptions to be related, but not necessarily to coincide. For example, participants might omit explicit references to opposition in their verbal description in response to question 1, but then draw configurations that manifest the opposite orientation of two figures (as those represented on the right in Figure 3) or, conversely, give verbal descriptions referring to the opposition component and then draw configurations that do not display opposition (such as the configurations on the left in Figure 3). Since we hypothesize that opposition is a structural implicit component of symmetry, we anticipated that the former expectation would be more likely to occur.

The drawings were analyzed according to a series of features of interest for the purposes of this study. These concerned, first of all, the *shape* of the figures forming the configuration (i.e., were they symmetrical or asymmetrical?) and the *orientation* of the two shapes with respect to the mirror axis. The reason why these features are important will become evident in Figure 4. The Figure represents various examples of symmetrical configurations around a vertical mirror axis, black circles in the first row, isosceles triangles in the second row and isosceles triangles with a piece missing in the third row. The difference between these concerns: (i) the structure of the *shapes* forming the configuration in terms of whether they are symmetrical or asymmetrical and the *orientation* of the shapes with respect to the mirror axis ($0°$, $20°$, or $90°$). The structure of the shapes (symmetry or lack of symmetry) is defined by two internal axes which are orthogonal to each other, represented by dashed lines in Figure 4. The orientation of the shapes with respect to the mirror axis is determined by three different angles: in the first column ($0°$), the shapes are positioned so that one of the internal axes is parallel and the other is orthogonal to the mirror axis; in the second column, the shapes have been rotated by $20°$ with respect to the original position and in the third column, they have been rotated by $90°$ with respect to the original position.

If the shapes forming the configuration are symmetrical with respect to both of their internal axes (Sym in Figure 4), it is impossible for the two shapes to be oppositely oriented, whatever their position with respect to the mirror axis is. Conversely, if the shapes are symmetrical with respect to one axis but asymmetrical with respect to the other axis (Asym 1 in Figure 4), it is only when the shapes are positioned so that their internal axis of symmetry is parallel to the mirror axis (i.e., Asym 1 at $0°$ in Figure 4) that the two shapes look identical to each other. In all other positions, the two shapes display an opposite orientation and this becomes particularly salient when the internal axis of symmetry is orthogonal to the mirror axis (i.e., Asym 1 at $90°$ in Figure 4). If the shapes are asymmetrical with respect to both of their internal axes (Asym 2 in Figure 4), it is impossible for them to be organized in such a way that they look identical and do not display an opposite orientation.

In order to determine whether opposition was visually evident or masked in the participants' drawings, it was therefore critical to analyze the shapes in terms of whether they were Sym, Asym

1 or Asym 2 and, in the case of shapes with one internal axis of symmetry (i.e., Asym 1), to analyze how the participants positioned them with respect to the mirror axis, i.e., whether the internal axis of symmetry was parallel to the mirror axis, as in the 0° column in Figure 4, or orthogonal to the mirror axis, as in the 90° column in Figure 4.

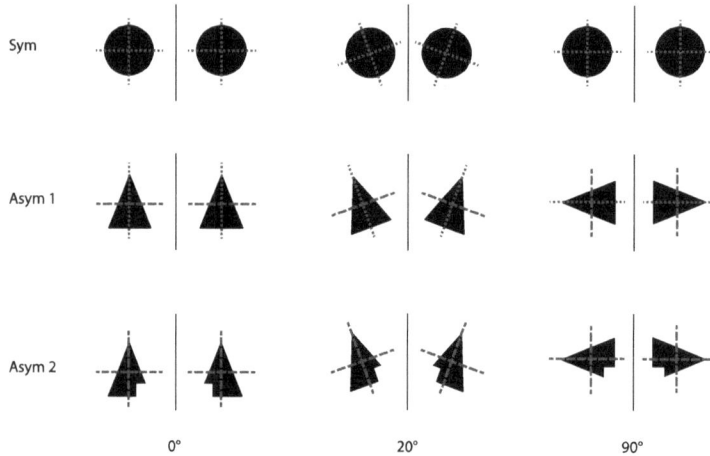

Figure 4. The differences in perceptual impact of rotating the black shapes (original position: 0°) by, respectively, 20° and 90° angles with respect to the "mirror axis" (the solid vertical line). The dashed lines indicate the two internal orthogonal symmetry axes. The shapes in the first row (**Sym**) are symmetrical with respect to both their internal axes (indicated by small dashes); the shapes in the second row (**Asym 1**) are symmetrical with respect to one axis (small dashes) and asymmetrical with respect to the other axis (large dashes) and the shapes in the third row (**Asym 2**) are asymmetrical with respect to both internal axes (large dashes). For a further explanation, see the text.

We also took into consideration, in the case of shapes that clearly pointed in a particular direction, whether there was a preference for divergent or convergent patterns. Furthermore, we explored whether the mirror axis of the prototypical configurations that the participants had in mind was more frequently oriented vertically. If so, we further investigated how robust this aspect was in terms of whether it was invariant in both drawings.

2.1. Materials and Method

2.1.1. Participants

109 undergraduate students of Psychology and Education at the University of Verona, Italy (mean age 21.2; 74 females; 35 males). The study was approved by the Ethics Committee of the University of Verona as the local ethics committee responsible and was conducted in accordance with the Declaration of Helsinki (revised 2008). All participants gave their written informed consent in accordance with the local ethics committee requirements.

2.1.2. Materials

A 5 page booklet with each page containing a different request:

(1) *How would you define the relationship between two symmetrical shapes?*
(2) *Draw a clear example of your idea of two symmetrical shapes.*
(3) *Draw another clear example (radically different from the first two) of your idea of two symmetrical shapes.*
(4) *Which of the following three definitions best describes your idea of symmetry?*

(a)   *Two identical shapes*

(b)   *Two opposite shapes*

(c)   *Two identical and opposite shapes*

The order of the four questions was the same for all participants; the order of the three definitions in question four was randomized between participants.

2.1.3. Procedure

The experiment was conducted at the beginning of a class on a topic which was totally unrelated to the issue. Participants were seated 6 seats apart in order to prevent them from influencing each other. Each participant received a booklet. They were told to start from the first page and move to the next one only after having completed the previous page. There were no time limits. All of the participants took less than 10 min to complete the task.

2.1.4. Statistical Analysis

Responses were analyzed using Generalized Mixed effect Models (GLMM) [72]. All of the variables analyzed in Study 1 are categorical variables. Responses were coded binomially (i.e., in terms of use or non-use of each level of the categorical variable), and binomial family GLMMs (with logit link function) were then conducted on the frequency of use of each level of the categorical variable (i.e., proportion of use over non-use). Mixed effect models allowed us to deal with the variability between participants as a Random effect. In cases involving significant main effects or interactions, post-hoc tests using the Bonferroni correction were conducted and estimates were made of both the non-standardized size of the effect (i.e., EST, which indicates the log odd ratio) and the standardized size of the effect (i.e., Cohen's index d; see [73–75]).

All analyses were carried out using the statistical software program R 3.3.1, with the "lme4", "car", "lsmeans", and "effects" packages. We performed Mixed Model ANOVA Tables (Type 3 tests) via likelihood ratio tests implemented in the "afex" package.

2.1.5. Results

In this section, we will focus first on the verbal descriptions of symmetry given by the participants in answer to question 1 and chosen in question 4; then we will analyze the drawings showing examples of the idea of symmetry (questions 2 and 3). Lastly, we will assess any association between the verbal descriptions in questions 1 and 4 and the drawings.

(I)   *Verbal descriptions of symmetry*

The definitions produced by the participants in response to question 1 were classified into different categories based on their content. The categories were defined by the experimenters after an initial inspection of the responses. The classification was then conducted by two independent judges based on these categories (with almost perfect agreement, Cohen's κ index = 0.92). Four responses were excluded from the analyses since they were either missing or tautological. The categories are listed in Table 1, together with some examples of descriptions and the frequency of each category. Less than 3% of the descriptions given by the participants referred to a point-by-point transformation such that shown in Figure 1 (see category a in Table 1). All the other responses referred to features relating to the relationship perceived between the two shapes.

A GLMM (binomial family) tested whether some types of description were more frequently given and this turned out to be the case ($\chi^2_{(7, 105)} = 77.189$, $p < 0.0001$, see top graph in Figure 5). As post-hoc tests revealed, responses referring exclusively to the sameness of the two symmetrical shapes (either in general, or specifying that they were the same in terms of shape and/or size—see examples of the descriptions under the category b in Table 1) were significantly more frequent than all of the other response categories except for those responses which made exclusive and explicit reference to a specular configuration (i.e., category c in Table 1; EST = 9.074, SE = 0.309, z-ratio = 2.934, p = 0.093). The findings were as follows:

(a) Exclusive references to Sameness were significantly more frequent than references to both Sameness and Opposition (categories b versus f in Table 1: EST = 1.292, SE = 0.334, z-ratio = 3.863, p = 0.003, d = 0.376);

(b) The two most frequent types of description (i.e., categories b and c in Table 1), which together amount to 61% of the total number of responses, do not explicitly refer to opposition;

(c) Only one response (i.e., less than 1%) mentioned the opposition component exclusively (category e in Table 1: "Two symmetrical shapes are two opposite shapes");

(d) Overall Opposition, in one way or another (i.e., categories e, f, and g in Table 1) was mentioned in only 20 out of the 105 descriptions collected (i.e., 19.04%).

These results suggest that the perception of opposition was not prominent in the verbal definitions.

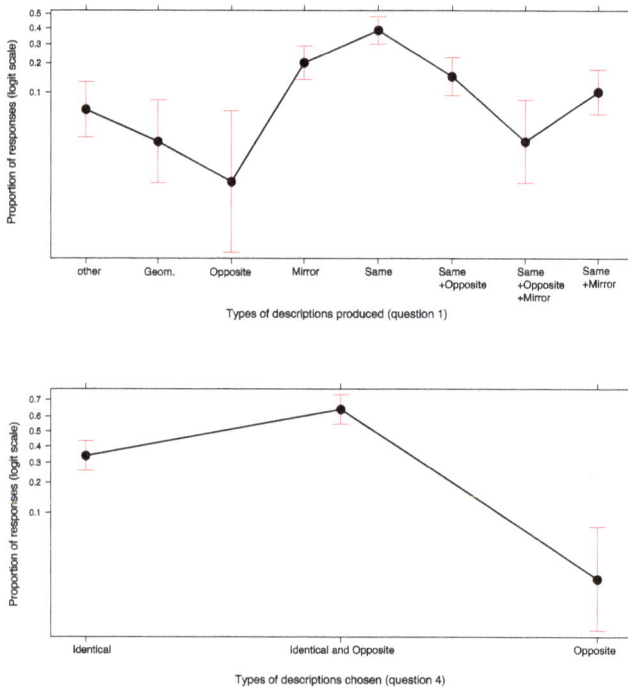

Figure 5. Effect plot of the proportional use of each of the various response categories for question 1 (**top graph**) or chosen from among the three alternatives in question 4 (**bottom graph**). Proportions are reported on a logit link scale (as computed by the GLMMs described in the main text). Error bars represent a 95% confidence interval.

A different picture emerged in the case of responses to question 4, for which participants were asked to choose which out of the three descriptions ("Two identical shapes", "Two opposite shapes" and "Two identical and opposite shapes") best fitted their idea of symmetry ($\chi^2_{(2, 109)}$ = 48.769, p < 0.0001; see bottom graph in Figure 5). "Identical and Opposite" was more frequently chosen as compared to exclusive references to Opposition (EST = 4.564, SE = 0.741, z-ratio = 6.159, p < 0.0001, d = 0.601) but "Identical and Opposite" was also more frequently chosen as compared to exclusive references to Identicalness (EST = 1.250, SE = 0.284, z-ratio = 4.398, p < 0.001, d = 0.429).

Table 1. The categories used to classify the definitions of symmetry produced by the participants in study 1 (in response to question 1). Examples of each type of description and the frequency of each category are presented.

Types of Descriptions	Examples	Counts (and %)
a. Geometrical	[Shapes with corresponding points at the same distance from the axis of symmetry]	3 (2.9%)
b. Same	[Identical shapes] [Perfectly overlapping shapes] [Identical, coincident shapes] [shapes of the same form] [Shapes of the same form and size]	42 (40.0%)
c. Mirror	[Specular shapes] [Reflected shapes]	22 (21.0%)
d. Same + Mirror	[Shapes with same form and size, specular to each other] [Similar shapes, as if reflected in a mirror] [Specular/shapes with the same characteristics]	11 (10.5%)
e. Opposite	[Two opposite shapes]	1 (1.0%)
f. Same + Opposite	[Identical shapes, but with one reversed with respect to the other] [Same but contrary shapes] [Same and opposite shapes] [Shapes with the same features but which are inverted left to right]	16 (15.2%)
g. Same + Opposite + Mirror	[Reflected shapes: identical but reversed] [Specular shapes: identical but inverted] [Equal and opposite shapes, as if reflected in a mirror]	3 (2.9%)
h. Other	[Two shapes, one near the other] [Shapes which are parallel to each other]	7 (6.7%)
Total		105
Missing	(missing responses or tautological responses)	4

(II) *Prototypical representations*

The following analyses was conducted on 76 of the first drawings and 75 of the second drawings (some of them are shown in Figure 6). The other drawings were not considered either because they showed only one shape and not two as requested or because they were incorrect (i.e., they did not display symmetry). The latter was the case for 6 (i.e., 5.5%) of the drawings done as a first representation and 8 (i.e., 7%) of the drawings done as a second representation.

For all the variables considered in the following analyses, the assessment of the drawings was conducted by two independent judges, with inter-rater agreement ranging from very good (Cohen's κ = 0.84) to excellent (Cohen's κ = 0.94).

Figure 6. Some of the drawings done by the participants as examples of their idea of symmetry (in response to questions 2 or 3).

Mirror axis: vertical, horizontal or oblique? A GLMM was performed to analyze the orientation of the mirror axis in relation to the two drawings (first and second). A main effect of Orientation of the mirror axis emerged ($\chi^2_{(2, 86)}$ = 123.448, $p < 0.0001$). As shown in Figure 7 (top graph), participants more frequently drew configurations displaying a Vertical mirror axis than a Horizontal mirror axis (EST = −3.855, SE = 0.392; z-ratio = −9.843, $p < 0.0001$, $d = -1.061$), which in turn was more frequently used than an Oblique mirror axis (EST = 1.835, SE = 0.685, z-ratio = 2.678, $p = 0.022$, $d = 0.288$). As shown in the central graph in Figure 7 (which shows the interaction between Drawing and Orientation: $\chi^2_{(2, 87)} = 14.677$, $p = 0.0006$), this distribution held for both the first and the second drawings. However, configurations displaying a horizontal mirror axis tended to be drawn more frequently in the second drawing as compared to the first (EST = −1.666, SE = 0.592; z-ratio = −2.816, $p = 0.07$, $d = 0.274$).

A combined analysis of the two drawings done by each participant was performed to determine whether the participants had used vertical axes in both drawings, horizontal axes in both drawings or had opted for a mixed solution. This allowed us to assess how robust the idea of a specific orientation of the mirror axis was in the participants' minds. A combined GLMM was conducted on the mirror axes in Drawings 1 and 2 and the results are represented in the bottom graph in Figure 7 ($\chi^2_{(4, 56)} = 57.357$, $p < 0.0001$). As confirmed by the post-hoc tests, the most frequent orientation was vertical in both the first and second drawings (EST = 3.152, SE = 0.58, z-ratio = 5.352, $p < 0.0001$, $d = 0.715$) despite the fact that participants had been explicitly told in the instructions that the second drawing should present a radically different example of symmetry to the first drawing.

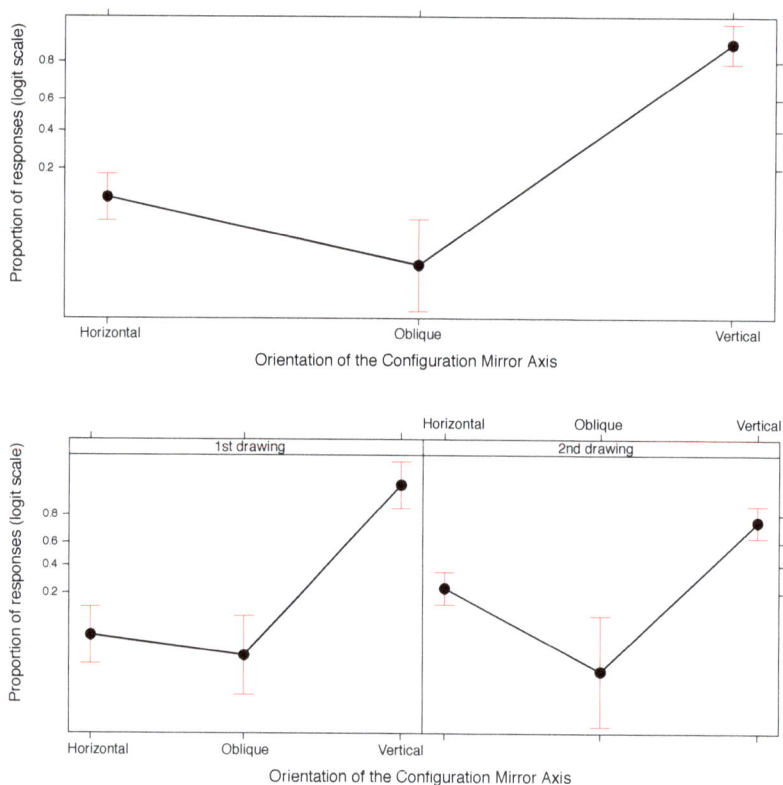

Figure 7. *Cont.*

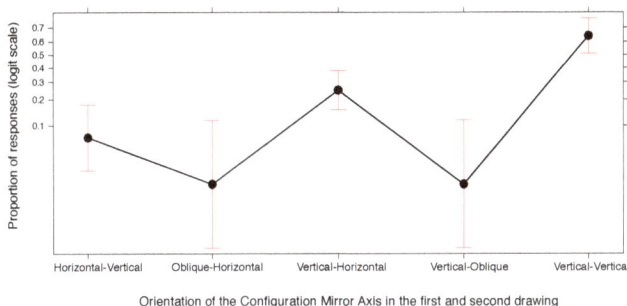

Figure 7. Effect plots of the Orientation of the mirror axis in the configurations drawn by participants. Top graph: Main effect of mirror axis Orientation. Central graph: interaction between mirror axis Orientation and Drawing. Bottom graph: Main effect of a combined analysis of the two drawings done by each participant. In all plots, error bars represent a 95% confidence interval.

Symmetrical or asymmetrical shapes? The shapes in the drawings were classified according to whether they were symmetrical around both their vertical and horizontal axes (see the configurations in the top row in Figures 4 and 6), asymmetrical with respect to both the vertical and horizontal axes (see the configurations in the third row in Figure 4 and in the third and fourth rows in Figure 6) or symmetrical around one axis and asymmetrical with respect to the other (see the configurations in the second row in Figures 4 and 6). As explained in the introduction of the study, when commenting on Figure 4, the symmetry/asymmetry of the shape is relevant since opposition emerges only with shapes which are asymmetrical with respect to at least one axis.

A GLMM was conducted to analyze the shapes in the two drawings according to the level of Symmetry/Asymmetry they displayed. The main effect of Symmetry/Asymmetry was confirmed ($\chi^2_{(2, 86)} = 17.758$, $p < 0.0001$), with no interaction with Drawing ($\chi^2_{(2, 86)} = 2.412$, $p = 0.299$). As shown in Figure 8, the drawings were based on asymmetrical shapes in the majority of cases: asymmetrical shapes (either Asym 1 or Asym 2) constituted around 75% of the total, including both the first and second exemplars. Perfectly symmetrical shapes, i.e., shapes that minimized the opposition component, accounted for less than 25% of the configurations.

Post hoc tests revealed that participants had a preference for shapes which were symmetrical around one axis and asymmetrical around the other axis (i.e., Asym 1 in Figures 4 and 8). This was more frequent than either perfectly symmetrical figures (EST = 1.113, SE = 0.264, z-ratio = 4.208, $p < 0.0001$, $d = 0.453$) or figures which were asymmetrical with respect to both the horizontal and vertical axes (EST = 0.600, SE = 0.248, z-ratio = 2.414, $p < 0.05$, $d = 0.260$).

How were the shapes which were symmetrical around one axis (i.e., Asym 1) *oriented with respect to the mirror axis?* We analyzed the positioning of the shapes when they were symmetrical with respect to one axis and asymmetrical with respect to the other axis (i.e., Asym 1, see the configurations in the second row in Figures 4 and 6). We studied whether the opposite orientation of the shapes was manifested (i.e., with the symmetrical axis orthogonal to the mirror axis) or absent (i.e., with the symmetrical axis parallel to the mirror).

We performed another GLMM on the Orientation of the shapes (both the first and second Drawing) with respect to the Mirror axis (Parallel or Orthogonal). A main effect of Orientation emerged ($\chi^2_{(1, 57)} = 38.572$, $p < 0.0001$). As shown in Figure 9, participants more frequently positioned the shapes with their internal axis of symmetry orthogonal with respect to the mirror axis rather than parallel to it (EST = 3.434, SE = 0.516, z-ratio = 6.657, $p < 0.0001$, $d = 0.882$). This means that they chose a configuration that made the opposite orientation of the two shapes evident.

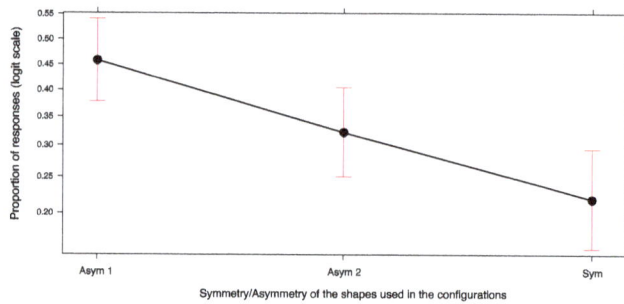

Figure 8. Effect plot of the use of symmetrical and asymmetrical shapes in the drawings done by the participants to exemplify their idea of a "symmetrical configuration" (Asym 2 = asymmetrical with respect to both the vertical and horizontal axes; Asym 1 = symmetrical around one axis and asymmetrical with respect to the other; Sym = symmetrical with respect to both the vertical and horizontal axes). Error bars represent a 95% confidence interval.

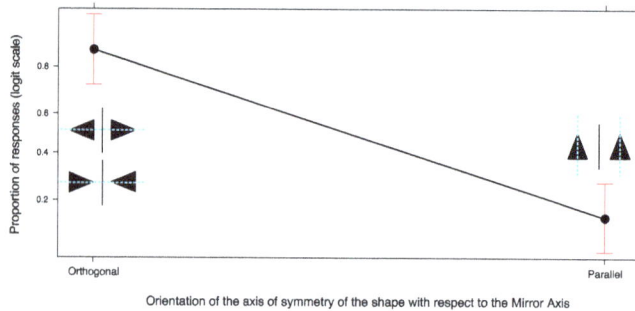

Figure 9. Effect plot of the Orientation (Orthogonal or Parallel) of the internal axis of symmetry of the shapes drawn by participants with respect to the mirror axis. Two examples of orthogonal configurations are shown on the left and one example of parallel configuration is shown on the right. Error bars represent a 95% confidence interval.

A further GLMM was conducted to ascertain whether, in cases in which the two shapes pointed in a direction which was orthogonal to the mirror, the participants more frequently drew two shapes pointing away from the mirror axis (i.e., a divergent configuration) or two shapes pointing towards the mirror axis (i.e., a convergent configuration). No significant effect of Convergent/Divergent Orientation emerged, either as a main effect ($\chi^2_{(1, 43)} = 1.490$, $p < 0.222$), or interacting with Drawing, ($\chi^2_{(1, 43)} = 0.043$, $p = 0.835$).

(III)   *Associations between verbal and iconic descriptions*

We wondered whether there was an association between the descriptions given in answer to question 1 or selected from among alternatives in question 4 and the drawings. In particular, we wished to determine whether definitions which made reference exclusively to identicalness were associated with drawings showing shapes that maximized identicalness and minimized opposition (i.e., perfectly symmetrical shapes, i.e., Sym) and, conversely, definitions that mentioned an opposition component were associated with drawings showing asymmetrical shapes (i.e., Asym 1 and Asym 2).

We created a new three level variable labelled Iconic Pair to further classify the shapes in the drawings: (1) both shapes symmetrical (i.e., Sym); (2) both shapes asymmetrical (i.e., Asym 1 or Asym 2) and (3) mixed, i.e., one symmetrical (i.e., Sym) and the other asymmetrical (i.e., Asym 1 or Asym 2).

A first GLMM was carried out to determine whether there was any association between Iconic Pair levels and the responses to question 1 which had been re-coded according to three Categories: responses referring exclusively to identicalness (i.e., category b in Table 1); responses referring explicitly to Opposition (i.e., categories e + f + g in Table 1) and responses generically referring to a specular configuration, without mentioning opposition (categories c and d in Table 1). The interaction between the response categories in question 1 and the three Iconic Pair levels turned out to be significant ($\chi^2_{(4, 57)} = 9.353$, $p = 0.05$). A second GLMM was then carried out to assess any association between the Iconic Pair levels and the responses to question 4 (Identical; Identical and Opposite; Opposite). In this case, too, the interaction between the responses to question 4 and the Iconic Pair levels turned out to be significant ($\chi^2_{(4, 57)} = 27.312$, $p < 0.0001$).

We used mosaic plots to represent the association between the two variables [76–78]. A mosaic plot represents the observed frequencies of a contingency table by means of the size of the tiles; the interaction between variables by means of the asymmetrical non-alignment of the tiles and the significance of the difference between observed and expected frequencies according to a specific model (in our case a log-linear model of independence between variables) by means of the color of the tiles. The color of the tiles corresponds to Pearson residuals and the bars to the right of each mosaic show which color corresponds to residuals greater than the cut-off points |2| (corresponding to $\alpha = 0.05$).

As shown in Figure 10, in the mosaic plot on the left, the responses to question 1 that mentioned only identicalness were more frequently associated with iconic representations that used symmetrical shapes (either in both the 1st and the 2nd drawings or in one of the two). Similarly, as shown in the mosaic plot on the right, those responses to question 4 that mentioned only identicalness were less frequently associated with iconic representations that used asymmetrical shapes in both the 1st and the 2nd drawings. Conversely an association emerged between using asymmetrical shapes in both the first and second drawings and selecting Identical and Opposite as the most fitting description in question 4.

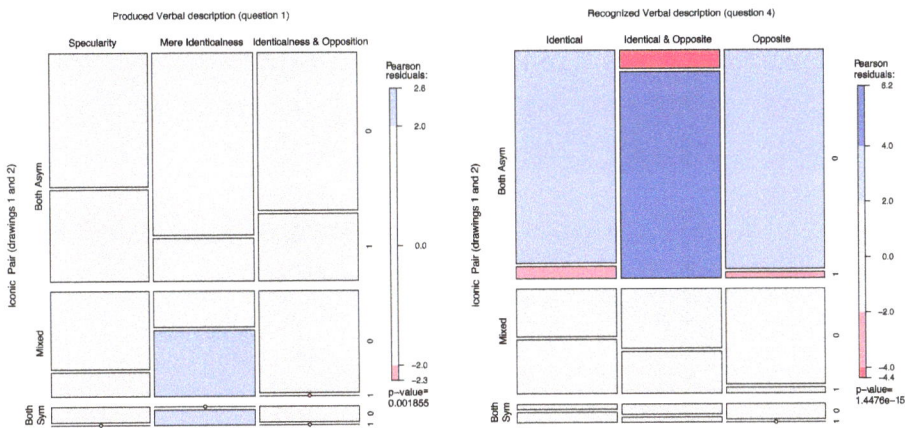

Figure 10. Mosaic plot showing the association between the three Iconic Pair levels relating to the shapes drawn by participants as exemplar configurations (in terms of symmetry/asymmetry) and the responses to question 1 (mosaic on the left) and question 4 (mosaic on the right).

3. Study 2

Study 2 was designed to further test (by means of a comparison task) the hypothesis that the phenomenal evidence of symmetry is more aligned with a perception of opposition in addition to identicalness, as compared to identicalness alone. Participants were asked to choose which of the two matched configurations better represented their idea of symmetry.

Various types of configurations and pair comparisons were presented in order to prevent participants from responding strategically (demand characteristics). In some cases, there were two configurations, both of which only showed evidence of identicalness; in other cases there were configurations that both showed evidence of identicalness and opposition and in another case the match was between a configuration which only showed identicalness and a configuration which showed both identicalness and opposition. The latter case was critical as it enabled us to test our hypothesis. If identicalness and opposition are the two salient components underlying the perception of symmetry, then the pairs showing opposition should be chosen over those showing only identicalness.

3.1. Materials and Method

3.1.1. Participants

70 undergraduate students of Psychology and Education at the University of Verona, Italy (mean age 23.8; 45 females; 25 males).

3.1.2. Materials

A 36-page booklet with each page containing two different configurations each consisting of a pair of shapes (the order of the pairs was randomized between participants and the order of the two configurations forming each pair was counterbalanced). Eight of the 36 pairs presented were catch trials and these consisted of a symmetrical configuration and a non-symmetrical configuration. They were introduced to check participants' understanding of the task, but were then excluded from data analysis. The other pairs are shown in Figure 11.

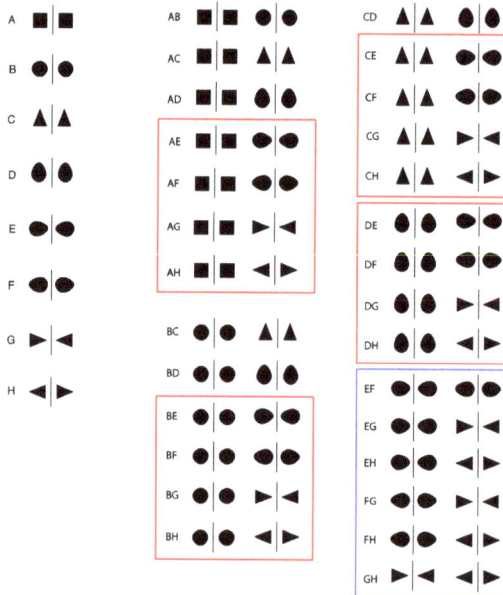

Figure 11. The configurations used in the pair comparison task in study 2. The pairs inside the red borders are those instantiating a match between a configuration which shows only identicalness and another which shows both identicalness and opposition. The pairs inside the blue border are formed of two configurations both of which show identicalness and opposition. The configurations which are not inside a border are the pairs which are formed of two configurations, both of which only show identicalness.

3.1.3. Procedure

The experiment was conducted at the beginning of a class on a topic which was totally unrelated to the issue. Participants were seated 6 seats apart to prevent them from influencing each other. Each participant received a booklet. They were asked to choose which of two matched configurations they considered the best fit to their idea of a "symmetrical configuration". They were told to start from the first page and move to the next one only after having completed the previous page. There were no time limits. All of the participants took less than 10 min to complete the task.

3.1.4. Statistical Analysis

The responses were analyzed using the Thurston Case V scaling (package "psych" [79]) and Generalized Mixed effect Models (GLMM).

3.1.5. Results

Figure 12 shows the scaling of the configurations based on a paired comparison model (goodness of fit of the model = 0.98). The results of the scaling are in clear agreement with the hypothesis; the configurations showing identicalness and opposition were generally preferred as representatives of symmetry as compared to configurations showing only identicalness.

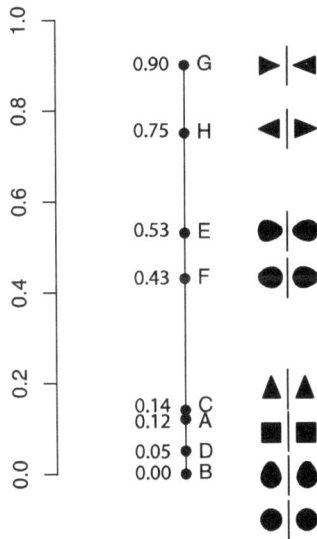

Figure 12. Scaling of the configurations used in the pair comparison task (based on the Thurston Case V scaling).

Two further analyses were conducted on two subsets of the original data in order to analyze whether the perception of symmetry was preferentially associated with divergent configurations or convergent configurations or whether there was no difference between the two. A first GLMM (binomial family, with Participants and Stimulus pair as Random effects) was performed on the subset of stimuli with red borders in Figure 10 which consist of a configuration showing identicalness and another showing identicalness and opposition in a convergent pattern (i.e., AE, AG, BE, BG, CE, CG, DE, DG in Figure 10) as compared to a configuration showing identicalness and another showing identicalness and opposition in a divergent pattern (i.e., AF, AH, BF, BH, CF, CH, DF, DH in Figure 10). No significant difference emerged ($\chi^2_{(1, 70)} = 1.861$, $p = 0.172$). It should be noted that participants were not directly asked to choose between a convergent configuration versus a divergent configuration but between a pattern showing identicalness and a pattern showing opposition (either divergent or convergent).

Conversely, when the participants were presented with the subset of stimuli in the blue border in Figure 10 (i.e., EF, EH, FG, GH) they were asked to make a forced choice between a divergent configuration and a convergent configuration. The GLMM performed on the responses to this set of stimuli revealed a significant effect of Orientation ($\chi^2_{(1, 70)} = 7.422$, $p = 0.006$). Convergent patterns were selected more frequently than divergent patterns (EST = 0.536; SE = 0.197; z-ratio = 2.724; $p = 0.006$; $d = 0.326$).

4. Discussion

The study aimed to investigate adults' naïve implicit and explicit idea of symmetry by means of various tasks. We started by studying the verbal definitions of "symmetrical configuration" provided by the participants. They rarely (3%) referred to the type of transformation that is usually presented as an example of symmetry in geometry textbooks, i.e., a point-by-point correspondence (see Figure 1) or a rotation around an axis of symmetry. It should be noted that demonstrating that two symmetrical objects correspond by rotating one object on a 3D dimension around the axis of symmetry in order to make it match the other, is a shortcut that works specifically for geometry on a plane. We cannot exclude the possibility that the participants ($n = 12/105$) who explicitly mentioned a coincidence between the two figures in response to question 1 were thinking in terms of this type of rotational transformation. However, since they did not explicitly state this, it cannot be taken for granted that this was the case.

The participants usually described symmetry in terms of an overall relationship of identicalness (cited in around 68% of the responses, see Table 1, b + d + f + g) or a mirror reflection (cited in around 35% of the total number of responses, see Table 1, c + d + g). Opposition was mentioned in less than 20% of the total number of responses (see Table 1, e + f + g). These findings indicate that the relationship which is perceptually evident between two shapes is a salient aspect of adults' idea of symmetry (and that people refer to this rather than to geometry), but opposition seems not to be a salient aspect *per se*. One could argue that the participants in our study who mentioned the mirror structure in response to question 1 might have been thinking precisely of the oppositional component which characterizes mirror reflections. Again, this is not something that we can take for granted. What is clear is that, when in question 4, Study 1, the participants were asked to select which of three definitions represented the best description of symmetry, only 1/3 of them chose the reference to mere identicalness. The majority (2/3) preferred "identical and opposite" as the most fitting definition. This last finding is also in line with the results of the analyses of the drawings done by the participants which in the majority of cases (around 80%) used asymmetrical shapes rather than perfectly symmetrical shapes, i.e., their drawings clearly showed a reversed orientation of the two shapes around a mirror axis rather than configurations that masked this oppositional component. When the shapes had one internal axis of symmetry, the opposition element was evident, i.e., the participants had positioned the "Asym 1" shapes so that their internal axis of symmetry was orthogonal to the mirror axis, rather than parallel to the mirror axis which would have made their identicalness more evident. There was also a strong preference for symmetry around a vertical axis. This result confirms a finding which has been discussed at length in previous literature (see the introduction) and provides evidence that this preference can be extended not only to the visual detection of symmetry or to aesthetic preferences but also to the prototypical representation of symmetry that people have in mind.

In study 2, participants were presented with images and were asked to select the one which fit in better with their idea of symmetry. Again, a strong preference for configurations showing opposition emerged. However, it is not clear whether the participants' perception of symmetry tended more towards convergent or divergent patterns, as defined by the orientation of the shapes, i.e., whether they pointed towards or away from the mirror axis. There were no indications of this in the configurations drawn in study 1 and only a partial preference for convergent configurations emerged in study 2 from an analysis of the pair comparisons which showed a direct match between convergent and divergent patterns.

In conclusion, the studies presented in this paper support the conclusion that identicalness is an important component in people's naïve idea of symmetry, but it does not suffice: opposition complements it.

Potential Impact and Limitations of the Study

Both of the studies presented in this paper focus on configurations formed of two shapes with symmetry defining the relationship between them, rather than on configurations formed of one shape in which the symmetry is determined by the relationship between individual parts of the shape. We know from previous literature that symmetry is not detected in exactly the same way when it is a "within-object" relationship as compared to a "between-objects" relationship [43,44,80]. We also know that this distinction is not simply related to whether one shape/object or more shapes/objects are involved since, for instance, in band patterns, grouping establishes phenomenal motifs that parse the band in sub-unities thus transforming what, locally defined, are between-objects relationships into within-object relationships [81]. Our decision to concentrate on a specific type of configuration (formed of two shapes) was motivated by our interest in exploring symmetry as a specific visual relationship between two objects. This was the specific aim of the research and the generalizability of the results discussed here are of course limited to this area.

Despite this, the results of this research provide new evidence regarding the existence of a qualitative aspect which is inherent to the structure of what people think of as "symmetrical" and that it makes sense, therefore, to consider the issue of how well a configuration represents "symmetry". This is not related to its geometrical definition or to aesthetic considerations but rather regards structural aspects related to the perceived relationship between two shapes. From a geometrical point of view, there are various different types of symmetry (e.g., central, bilateral etc.) and there may be various symmetrical axes but this does not make the property of "being symmetrical" qualitatively gradable. On the other hand, studies on aesthetic judgments of symmetry can assess and measure to what extent people appreciate a particular shape or configuration (e.g., [82–85]) and this goes to show that symmetrical patterns can be graded from a qualitative point of view based on the observer's assessment of pleasantness. The studies presented in this paper, however, take a different approach. They show that a configuration may be perceived as being a better or worse exemplar of symmetry on the basis of some relational features which are evident, namely, opposition and identicalness. Our findings add to previous results which have shown, for instance, that the perception of symmetry is sensitive to aspects such as changes in the spatial arrangement of motifs, even when these alterations do not modify their formal classification [86].

One might raise the issue of whether the participants in study 2 chose images that made both identicalness and opposition evident since they were more salient (i.e., less redundant) and therefore attracted their attention. This would be interesting to investigate in the future. Since salience is closely linked to perceptual organization (e.g., [48]) and salient stimuli tend to be associated with beauty (e.g., [87]), one might also raise the question of whether the participants selected configurations which showed both identicalness and opposition because those were more aesthetically pleasing. However, we have no reason to believe that they had understood that the task involved indicating a preference. In effect, this issue is more promising when considered in the light of whether these "prototypical features" influence judgments of beauty and pleasantness. For example, it might be interesting to test whether judgments of beauty are associated with a specific balance between opposition and identicalness or with extreme evidence of one of these two elements or whether they are totally independent from these relational aspects.

Lastly, another issue concerns the potential influence of literacy. It has been shown that the spontaneous inclination to identify an image as the same, regardless of its left-right orientation (a phenomenon known as "mirror invariance" or "mirror generalization"), is inhibited by literacy. While mirror generalization is spontaneously found in infants (for a review, see [88]), in a same-different task involving mirror-reflected pairs, literate adults familiar with the Latin alphabet found it difficult to answer "same" to mirror-reversed stimuli than illiterate adults [89–91]. This has been explained in terms of the acquisition of a written system that incorporates mirrored letters (e.g., b and d), in the sense that this enhances sensitivity in the discrimination of lateral mirror-images (see also [92]). The participants in our study were all adults familiar with the Latin alphabet. A cross-cultural study in order to verify whether the sensitivity to contrasts in orientation which is a characteristic of the idea of symmetry according to our study is related to literacy or is a more general phenomenon may be worthwhile.

Acknowledgments: We thank Paola Boccacci for help in data collection (study 1).

Author Contributions: Ivana Bianchi, Marco Bertamini and Ugo Savardi conceived and designed the experiments; Ivana Bianchi and Ugo Savardi performed the experiments; Ivana Bianchi and Roberto Burro analyzed the data; Ivana Bianchi, Marco Bertamini, Roberto Burro and Ugo Savardi wrote the paper.

Conflicts of Interest: The authors declare no conflict of interest.

References

1. Wagemans, J. Detection of visual symmetries. *Spat. Vis.* **1995**, *9*, 9–32. [CrossRef] [PubMed]
2. Treder, M.S. Behind the looking-glass: A review on human symmetry perception. *Symmetry* **2010**, *2*, 1510–1543. [CrossRef]
3. Eisenman, R. Preference for symmetry and the rejection of complexity. *Psychon. Sci.* **1967**, *8*, 169–170. [CrossRef]
4. Enquist, M.; Arak, A. Symmetry, beauty and evolution. *Nature* **1994**, *372*, 169–172. [CrossRef] [PubMed]
5. Enquist, M.; Johnstone, R.A. Generalization and the evolution of symmetry preferences. *Proc. R. Soc. B Biol. Sci.* **1997**, *264*, 1345–1348. [CrossRef]
6. Jacobsen, T.; Hofel, L. Descriptive and evaluative judgment processes: Behavioral and electrophysiological indices of processing symmetry and aesthetics. *Cognit. Affect. Behav. Neurosci.* **2003**, *3*, 289–299. [CrossRef]
7. Chen, C.C.; Wu, J.H.; Wu, C.C. Reduction of image complexity explains aesthetic preference for symmetry. *Symmetry* **2011**, *3*, 443–456. [CrossRef]
8. Makin, A.D.J.; Bertamini, M.; Jones, A.; Holmes, T.; Zanker, J.M. A gaze-driven evolutionary algorithm to study aesthetic evaluation of visual symmetry. *i-Perception* **2016**, *7*. [CrossRef] [PubMed]
9. Pecchinenda, A.; Bertamini, M.; Makin, A.D.J.; Ruta, N. The pleasantness of visual symmetry: Always, never or sometimes. *PLoS ONE* **2014**, *9*, e92685. [CrossRef] [PubMed]
10. Bertamini, M.; Makin, A. Brain activity in response to visual symmetry. *Symmetry* **2014**, *6*, 975–996. [CrossRef]
11. Cattaneo, Z. The neural basis of mirror symmetry detection: A review. *J. Cognit. Psychol.* **2017**, *29*, 259–268. [CrossRef]
12. Pornstein, M.H.; Krinsky, S.J. Perception of symmetry in infancy—The salience of vertical symmetry and the perception of pattern wholes. *J. Exp. Child Psychol.* **1985**, *39*, 1–19. [CrossRef]
13. Tyler, C.W.; Hardage, L.; Miller, R.T. Multiple mechanisms for the detection of mirror symmetry. *Spat. Vis.* **1995**, *9*, 79–100. [CrossRef] [PubMed]
14. Wenderoth, P. The salience of vertical symmetry. *Perception* **1994**, *23*, 221–236. [CrossRef] [PubMed]
15. Wenderoth, P. The effects of dot pattern parameters and constraints on the relative salience of vertical bilateral symmetry. *Vis. Res* **1996**, *36*, 2311–2320. [CrossRef]
16. Bianchi, I.; Burro, R.; Pezzola, R.; Savardi, U. Matching visual and acoustic mirror forms. *Symmetry* **2017**, *9*, 39. [CrossRef]
17. Cattaneo, Z.; Vecchi, T.; Fantino, M.; Herbert, A.M.; Merabet, L.B. The effect of vertical and horizontal symmetry on memory for tactile patterns in late blind individuals. *Atten. Percept. Psychophys.* **2013**, *75*, 375–382. [CrossRef] [PubMed]
18. Wagemans, J.; Vangool, L.; Dydewalle, G. Detection of symmetry in tachistoscopically presented dot patterns—Effects of multiple axes and skewing. *Atten. Percept. Psychophys.* **1991**, *50*, 413–427. [CrossRef]

19. Wagemans, J. Characteristics and models of human symmetry detection. *Trends Cognit. Sci.* **1997**, *1*, 346–352. [CrossRef]
20. Csatho, A.; van der Vloed, G.; van der Helm, P.A. Blobs strengthen repetition but weaken symmetry. *Vis. Res.* **2003**, *43*, 993–1007. [CrossRef]
21. Csatho, A.; van der Vloed, G.; van der Helm, P.A. The force of symmetry revisited: Symmetry-to-noise ratios regulate (a) symmetry effects. *Acta Psychol.* **2004**, *117*, 233–250. [CrossRef] [PubMed]
22. Dastani, M.; Scha, R. Languages for gestalts of line patterns. *J. Math. Psychol.* **2003**, *47*, 429–449. [CrossRef]
23. Nucci, M.; Wagemans, J. Goodness of regularity in dot patterns: Global symmetry, local symmetry, and their interactions. *Perception* **2007**, *36*, 1305–1319. [CrossRef] [PubMed]
24. Olivers, C.N.L.; Chater, N.; Watson, G.D. Holography does not account for goodness: A critique of van der Helm and Leeuwenberg (1996). *Psychol. Rev.* **2004**, *11*, 242–260. [CrossRef] [PubMed]
25. Palmer, S.E. Symmetry, transformation, and the structure of perceptual systems. In *Organization and Representation in Perception*; Beck, J., Ed.; Lawrence Erlbaum Associates: Hillsdale, NJ, USA, 1982; pp. 95–144.
26. Palmer, S.E. The psychology of perceptual organization: A transformational approach. In *Human and Machine Vision*; Beck, J., Hope, B., Rosenfeld, A., Eds.; Academic Press: New York, NY, USA, 1983; Volume 1, pp. 269–339.
27. Vanderhelm, P.A.; Leeuwenberg, E.L.J. Accessibility—A criterion for regularity and hierarchy in visual-pattern codes. *J. Math. Psychol.* **1991**, *35*, 151–213. [CrossRef]
28. VanderHelm, P.A.; Leeuwenberg, E.L.J. Goodness of visual regularities: A nontransformational approach. *Psychol. Rev.* **1996**, *103*, 429–456. [CrossRef]
29. VanderHelm, P.A.; Leeuwenberg, E.L.J. A Better Approach to Goodness: Reply to Wagemans. *Psychol. Rev.* **1999**, *106*, 622–630. [CrossRef]
30. VanderHelm, P.A.; Leeuwenberg, E.L.J. Holographic Goodness Is Not That Bad: Reply to Olivers, Chater, and Watson. *Psychol. Rev.* **2004**, *111*, 261–273. [CrossRef]
31. Wagemans, J.; Van Gool, L.; Swinnen, V.; Van Horebeek, J. Higher-order structure in regularity detection. *Vis. Res.* **1993**, *33*, 1067–1088. [CrossRef]
32. Wagemans, J. Toward a better approach to goodness: Comments on van der helm and leeuwenberg (1996). *Psychol. Rev.* **1999**, *106*, 610–621. [CrossRef]
33. Makin, A.D.; Wright, D.; Rampone, G.; Palumbo, L.; Guest, M.; Sheehan, R.; Cleaver, H.; Bertamini, M. An electrophysiological index of perceptual goodness. *Cereb. Cortex* **2016**, *26*, 4416–4434. [CrossRef] [PubMed]
34. Bianchi, I.; Savardi, U. The opposite of a figure. *Gestalt Theory* **2006**, *4*, 354–374.
35. Bianchi, I.; Savardi, U. *The Perception of Contraries*; Aracne: Roma, Italy, 2008.
36. Gati, I.; Tversky, A. Weighting Common and Distinctive Features in Perceptual and Conceptual Judgments. *Cognit. Psychol.* **1984**, *16*, 341–370. [CrossRef]
37. Gati, I.; Tversky, A. Recall of common and distinctive features of verbal and pictorial stimuli. *Mem. Cognit.* **1987**, *15*, 97–100. [CrossRef] [PubMed]
38. Goldmeier, E. Similarity in visually perceived forms. *Psychol. Issues* **1972**, *29*, 1–131.
39. Medin, D.L.; Goldston, R.L.; Gentner, D. Similarity involving attributes and relations: Judgments of similarity and difference are not inverses. *Psychol. Sci.* **1990**, *1*, 64–69. [CrossRef]
40. Rock, I. *Orientation and Form*; Academic Press: New York, NY, USA, 1973.
41. Sattath, S.; Tversky, A. On the Relation between Common and Distinctive features Models. *Psychol. Rev.* **1987**, *94*, 16–22. [CrossRef]
42. Tversky, A. Features of similarity. *Psychol. Rev.* **1977**, *84*, 327–352. [CrossRef]
43. Baylis, G.C.; Driver, J. Obligatory edge assignment in vision: The role of figure and part segmentation in symmetry detection. *J. Exp. Psychol. Hum. Percept. Perform.* **1995**, *21*, 1323–1342. [CrossRef]
44. Koning, A.; Wagemans, J. Detection of symmetry and repetition in one and two objects: Structures versus strategies. *Exp. Psychol* **2009**, *56*, 5–17. [CrossRef] [PubMed]
45. Weyl, H. *Symmetry*; Princeton University Press: Princeton, NJ, USA, 2016.
46. Kubovy, M. Phenomenology, psychological. In *Encyclopedia of Cognitive Science*; Nadel, L., Ed.; Macmillan: Hampshire, UK, 2002; pp. 579–586.
47. Thinés, G.; Costall, A.; Butterworth, G. *Michotte's Experimental Phenomenology of Perception*, 2nd ed.; Routledge: Oxford, UK, 2015.

48. Wagemans, J.; Elder, J.H.; Kubovy, M.; Palmer, S.E.; Peterson, M.A.; Singh, M. A Century of Gestalt Psychology in Visual Perception I. Perceptual Grouping and Figure-Ground Organization. *Psychol. Bull.* **2012**, *138*, 1172–1217. [PubMed]

49. Wagemans, J.; Feldman, J.; Gepshtein, S.; Kimchi, R.; Pomerantz, J.R.; van der Helm, P.A.; van Leeuwen, C. A century of Gestalt psychology in visual perception: II. Conceptual and theoretical foundations. *Psychol. Bull.* **2012**, *138*, 1218–1252. [CrossRef] [PubMed]

50. Croucher, C.J.; Bertamini, M.; Hecht, H. Naïve optics: Understanding the geometry of mirror reflections. *J. Exp. Psychol. Hum.* **2002**, *28*, 546–562. [CrossRef]

51. Bianchi, I.; Savardi, U. What fits into a mirror: Naïve beliefs about the field of view. *J. Exp. Psychol. Hum. Percept. Perform.* **2012**, *38*, 1144–1158. [CrossRef] [PubMed]

52. Kaiser, M.K.; Proffitt, D.R.; McCloskey, M. The development of beliefs about falling objects. *Percept. Psychophys.* **1985**, *38*, 533–539. [CrossRef] [PubMed]

53. Huber, S.; Krist, H. When is the ball going to hit the ground? Duration estimates, eye movements, and mental imagery of object motion. *J. Exp. Psychol. Hum. Percept. Perform.* **2004**, *30*, 431–444. [CrossRef] [PubMed]

54. McCloskey, M.; Washburn, A.; Felch, L. Intuitive physics: The straight-down belief and its origin. *J. Exp. Psychol. Learn. Mem. Cognit.* **1983**, *9*, 636–649. [CrossRef]

55. Shanon, B. Aristotelianism, newtonianism and the physics of the layman. *Perception* **1976**, *5*, 241–243. [CrossRef] [PubMed]

56. Hecht, H.; Bertamini, M. Understanding projectile acceleration. *J. Exp. Psychol. Hum. Percept. Perform.* **2000**, *26*, 730–746. [CrossRef] [PubMed]

57. McCloskey, M.; Caramazza, A.; Green, B. Curvilinear motion in the absence of external forces: Naïve beliefs about the motion of objects. *Science* **1980**, *210*, 1139–1141. [CrossRef] [PubMed]

58. McAfee, E.A.; Proffitt, D.R. Understanding the surface orientation of liquids. *Cognit. Psychol.* **1991**, *23*, 483–514. [CrossRef]

59. Sholl, M.J.; Liben, L.S. Illusory tilt and Euclidean schemes as factors in performance on the water-level task. *J. Exp. Psychol. Learn. Mem. Cognit.* **1995**, *21*, 1624–1638. [CrossRef]

60. Yates, J.; Bessman, M.; Dunne, M.; Jertson, D.; Sly, K.; Wendelboe, B. Are conceptions of motion based on a naïve theory or on prototypes? *Cognition* **1988**, *29*, 251–275. [CrossRef]

61. Gregory, R.L. *Mirrors in Mind*; Freeman Spektrum: New York, NY, USA, 1966.

62. Gregory, R.L. Mirror reversals. In *The Oxford Companion to the Mind*; Gregory, R.L., Ed.; Oxford University Press: Oxford, UK, 1987; pp. 491–493.

63. Hecht, H.; Bertamini, M.; Gamer, M. Naïve optics: Acting on mirror reflections. *J. Exp. Psychol. Hum. Percept. Perform.* **2005**, *31*, 1023–1038. [CrossRef] [PubMed]

64. Muelenz, C.; Hecht, H.; Gamer, M. Testing the egocentric mirror-rotation hypothesis. *Seeing Perceiving* **2010**, *23*, 373–383. [CrossRef] [PubMed]

65. Bianchi, I.; Savardi, U. Contrariety in plane mirror reflections. In *The Perception and Cognition of Contraries*; Savardi, U., Ed.; Mc-Graw Hill: Milan, Italy, 2009; pp. 113–128.

66. Bianchi, I.; Savardi, U. Grounding naïve physics and optics in perception. *Balt. Int. Yearb. Cognit. Log. Commun.* **2014**, *6*. [CrossRef]

67. Savardi, U.; Bianchi, I.; Bertamini, M. Naïve predictions of motion and orientation in mirrors: From what we see to what we expect reflections to do. *Acta Psychol.* **2010**, *134*, 1–15. [CrossRef] [PubMed]

68. Bertamini, M.; Spooner, A.; Hecht, H. Naïve optics: Predicting and perceiving reflections in mirrors. *J. Exp. Psychol. Hum. Percept. Perform.* **2003**, *29*, 982–1002. [CrossRef] [PubMed]

69. Bianchi, I.; Bertamini, M.; Savardi, U. Differences between predictions of how a reflection behaves based on the behaviour of an object, and how an object behaves based on the behaviour of its reflection. *Acta Psychol.* **2015**, *161*, 54–63. [CrossRef] [PubMed]

70. Bianchi, I.; Savardi, U. The relationship perceived between the real body and the mirror image. *Perception* **2008**, *37*, 666–687. [CrossRef] [PubMed]

71. Bianchi, I.; Savardi, U.; Burro, R.; Martelli, M.F. Doing the opposite to what another person is doing. *Acta Psychol.* **2014**, *151*, 117–133. [CrossRef] [PubMed]

72. Bates, D.; Machler, M.; Bolker, B.M.; Walker, S.C. Fitting linear mixed-effects models using lme4. *arXiv* **2015**, arXiv:1406.5823.

73. Lenth, R.V. Least-squares means: The R package lsmeans. *J. Stat. Softw.* **2016**, *69*, 1–33. [CrossRef]

74. Kuznetsova, A.; Bruun, B.P.; Haubo, B.C.R. lmerTest: Tests in Linear Mixed Effects Models. R Package Version 2.0-33. 2016. Available online: https://CRAN.R-project.org/package=lmerTest (accessed on 3 December 2016).

75. Cohen, J. *Statistical Power Analysis for the Behavioral Sciences*, 2nd ed.; Academic Press: New York, NY, USA, 1988.

76. Friendly, M. Mosaic displays for multi-way contingency tables. *J. Am. Stat. Assoc.* **1994**, *89*, 190–200. [CrossRef]

77. Friendly, M. Visualizing Categorical Data. SAS Institute: Cary, NC, USA, 2000. Available online: http://www.math.yorku.ca/SCS/vcd/ (accessed on 25 December 2000).

78. Meyer, D.; Zeileis, A.; Hornik, K. The Strucplot framework: Visualizing multi-way contingency tables with vcd. *J. Stat. Softw.* **2006**, *17*, 1–48. [CrossRef]

79. Ravelle, W. *psych: Procedures for Personality and Psychological Research*; Northwestern University: Evanston, IL, USA, 2017.

80. Bertamini, M.; Friedenberg, J.D.; Kubovy, M. Detection of symmetry and perceptual organization: The way a lock-and-key process works. *Acta Psychol.* **1997**, *95*, 119–140. [CrossRef]

81. Strother, L.; Kubovy, M. Perceived complexity and the grouping effect in band patterns. *Acta Psychol.* **2003**, *114*, 229–244. [CrossRef]

82. Bertamini, M.; Makin, A.D.J.; Rampone, G. Implicit association of symmetry with positive valence, high arousal and simplicity. *i-Perception* **2013**, *4*, 317–327. [CrossRef]

83. Cardenas, R.A.; Harris, L.J. Symmetrical decorations enhance the attractiveness of faces and abstract designs. *Evol. Hum. Behav.* **2006**, *27*, 1–18. [CrossRef]

84. Eysenck, H.J.; Castle, M. Training in art as a factor in the determination of preference judgements for polygons. *Br. J. Psychol.* **1970**, *61*, 65–81. [CrossRef] [PubMed]

85. Jacobsen, T.; Hofel, L. Aesthetic judgments of novel graphic patterns: Analyses of individual judgments. *Percept. Mot. Skills* **2002**, *95*, 755–766. [CrossRef] [PubMed]

86. Kubovy, M.; Strother, L. The perception of band patterns: Going beyond geometry. In *Embedded Symmetries, Natural and Cultural*; Washburn, D., Ed.; Amerind Foundation and University of New Mexico Press: Albuquerque, NM, USA, 2004; pp. 19–26.

87. Makin, A.D.J.; Pecchinenda, A.; Bertamini, M. Implicit affective evaluation of visual symmetry. *Emotion* **2012**, *12*, 1021–1030. [CrossRef] [PubMed]

88. Erlikhman, G.; Strother, L.; Barzakov, I.; Caplovitz, G.P. On the Legibility of Mirror-Reflected and Rotated Text. *Symmetry* **2017**, *9*, 28. [CrossRef]

89. Danziger, E.; Pederson, E. Through the looking glass: Literacy, writing systems and mirror image discrimination. *Writ. Lang. Lit.* **1998**, *1*, 153–169. [CrossRef]

90. Kolinsky, R.; Verhaeghe, A.; Fernandes, T.; Mengarda, E.J.; Grimm-Cabral, L.; Morais, J. Enantiomorphy through the looking glass: Literacy effects on mirror-image discrimination. *J. Exp. Psychol. Gen.* **2011**, *140*, 210–238. [CrossRef] [PubMed]

91. Pegado, F.; Nakamura, K.; Braga, L.W.; Ventura, P.; Nunes Filho, G.; Pallier, C.; Jobert, A.; Morais, J.; Cohen, L.; Kolinsky, R.; et al. Literacy breaks mirror invariance for visual stimuli: A behavioral study with adult illiterates. *J. Exp. Psychol. Gen.* **2014**, *143*, 887–894. [CrossRef] [PubMed]

92. Borst, G.; Ahr, E.; Roell, M.; Houdé, O. The cost of blocking the mirror generalization process in reading: Evidence for the role of inhibitory control in discriminating letters with lateral mirror-image counterparts. *Pysychon. Bull. Rev.* **2015**, *22*, 228–234. [CrossRef] [PubMed]

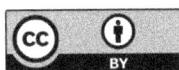

MDPI AG

St. Alban-Anlage 66

4052 Basel, Switzerland

Tel. +41 61 683 77 34

Fax +41 61 302 89 18

http://www.mdpi.com

Symmetry Editorial Office

E-mail: symmetry@mdpi.com

http://www.mdpi.com/journal/symmetry

www.ingramcontent.com/pod-product-compliance
Lightning Source LLC
Chambersburg PA
CBHW051314020426
42333CB00028B/3334